AF701652

Nursing, Policy and Politics in Twentieth-century Chile

"A much-needed study that reveals the fundamental significance of the nursing profession in the history of public health and that traces the important contributions nurses made to the creation of a functioning healthcare system. It explores vital questions of gender, medical practice, and power – all placed in the context of the dramatic political transitions of twentieth-century Chilean history."

—Jadwiga E. Pieper Mooney, *Executive Council of Latin American Studies, University of Arizona*

"Among other things, a piece of research that has tackled in great detail the influence of the US on nursing systems in Latin America."

—SusaneKreutzer, *Münster University of Applied Sciences*

"The authors convincingly demonstrate the links between nurses, past and present. This is an essential read for both studying processes of yesteryear and reviewing health policy of today."

—Karina Ramacciotti, *National University of Quilmes*

"It was about time that nurses in Latin America had their proper share in historiography. This book sits at the intersection of social history, history of welfare and women's history. Thulin and Ayala have produced fineresearch which sheds a different light on the development of professional women in the health sector."

—Barbara Potthast, *University of Cologne*

"The book offers an extraordinarily well documented narrative on Chilean nursing. The political economic and historical analysis allows to profile the social history of Chilean nursing policymaking within the political process. A book that will be a reference book in its genre."

—Jaime Llambias-Wolff, *York University, Canada*

"A thoroughly researched and engaging social history of healthcare policy in Chile in the twentieth century. Thulin and Ayala have contributed an important work of critical scholarship on nursing agency in both shaping and mobilizing health policy to the benefit of society and the profession itself. This book is an essential read for students and teachers of social and healthcare policy, labour history, nursing history and women's history. It addresses the ways that women navigated power, patriarchy, and class structures."

—Gerard Fealy, *University College Dublin*

Markus Thulin • Ricardo A. Ayala

Nursing, Policy and Politics in Twentieth-century Chile

Reforming Health, 1920s–1990s

palgrave
macmillan

Markus Thulin
Inst of Iberian & Latin
American History
University of Cologne
Cologne, Germany

Brauweiler Memorial Site
Rhineland Regional Council (LVR)
Pulheim, Germany

Ricardo A. Ayala
Faculty of Health & Social Sciences
University of the Americas
Santiago, Chile

Department of Sociology
Ghent University
Belgium

ISBN 978-3-030-90834-8 ISBN 978-3-030-90835-5 (eBook)
https://doi.org/10.1007/978-3-030-90835-5

© The Editor(s) (if applicable) and The Author(s), under exclusive licence to Springer Nature Switzerland AG 2023
This work is subject to copyright. All rights are solely and exclusively licensed by the Publisher, whether the whole or part of the material is concerned, specifically the rights of reprinting, reuse of illustrations, recitation, broadcasting, reproduction on microfilms or in any other physical way, and transmission or information storage and retrieval, electronic adaptation, computer software, or by similar or dissimilar methodology now known or hereafter developed.
The use of general descriptive names, registered names, trademarks, service marks, etc. in this publication does not imply, even in the absence of a specific statement, that such names are exempt from the relevant protective laws and regulations and therefore free for general use.
The publisher, the authors, and the editors are safe to assume that the advice and information in this book are believed to be true and accurate at the date of publication. Neither the publisher nor the authors or the editors give a warranty, expressed or implied, with respect to the material contained herein or for any errors or omissions that may have been made. The publisher remains neutral with regard to jurisdictional claims in published maps and institutional affiliations.

This Palgrave Macmillan imprint is published by the registered company Springer Nature Switzerland AG.
The registered company address is: Gewerbestrasse 11, 6330 Cham, Switzerland

To all the past, present, and future nurses across the world.
Their work is, too, the support for how we live and who we are.

Preface

They seem so far away from us. And, strangely, their ideas have found their way into present-day discussions more than at any time in the past. Nobody is still alive who remembers life in 1900 Chile. To that extent, narratives about that time are not mere chronicles but history proper. After they had recently fought two wars, most Chileans were not entirely sure whether the nineteenth century had closed, stopped, or just adjusted. Their rigid distinctions between civilization and barbarism, their nationalist pride, their worshipping of supernatural power, and their admiration for Europe were the matrix of social imagination.

The wealthy loved France, wanted to live, dress, and eat like the French, and probably felt as if they in fact did. In some ways, Santiago's urban planning imitated that of Paris as politicians prepared for the grand centennial of independence, in 1910. To them, we owe some of the most beautiful architectural works, such as the National Library, the Museum of Fine Arts, the building of the Chilean Architects Association, the Stock Exchange Building, and the Central Railway Station (designed by the very Gustave Eiffel) alongside many impressive structures in *art déco* style that sit in the districts of *Independencia*, *Recoleta*, and *Santiago Centro* albeit often unnoticed. They wore hats. Men had a moustache and preferred tailcoats, and walking canes were in fashion. Women wore long buttoned dresses with long sleeves.

And yet, behind that façade of Frenchness the reality was altogether different by the turn of the century. For today's standards, most houses might look opaque and monochrome. The population was overwhelmingly rural;

many would go in the early morning to sell their produce in the city as horse-drawn carriages circulated on the main cobblestone roads. Although days were long because budlings stuck low to the ground, at night streets were dark—some lightened with gas lamps. Electric lamps had recently made their debut in Santiago's *Plaza de Armas*, while tramways, all the way around the edges of the civic quarter, were the novelty of 1900. Not far, *conventillos* or tenement houses by the outer circle of town served as lodgment for the masses working in the industry. That was a place to stay in, but often to live in: overcrowded, lacking sanitation and even town water—oftentimes entire families with their many children. When they did not prefer the busy streets, the homeless lived packed in almshouses. They ate mostly bread and potatoes, while banquets were a privilege of aristocrats.

Not only might we feel odd traveling back in time. It might even be difficult to have a conversation with 1900s Chileans. They held ideas that we might find strange—senior medics believed that infection and plague were either god-sent or produced by environmental emanations or *miasmas* because disease was common in areas with a foul smell. Like today, casual sexual entertainment was readily available outside marriage, but in public people diverted attention away from the subject. A war on night houses and prostitution indeed intensified toward the turn of the century, mostly resulting in a moral crusade under the disguise of health law. Politicians usually defended a two-class society—a ruling class and a working class—and much as bills may have focused on the public interest, ordinary people were unaware of the debates.

Individuals did not have any welfare, and the poor would rely solely on charitable relief. Even the word "welfare" itself was very far away from the minds of the financial elite. Citizens were convinced that people's ailments could be alleviated by elite philanthropy and that the wealthy's role was indeed that of giving. The poor, on the other hand, were meant to feel fortunate, grateful, and faithful to the donors. Looking at the situation from their perspective, the deprived and the well-off matched each other.

But there is something so intriguing, amusing even, in that their lives are so present in the here and now, though not obvious to the untrained eye. Reading about the past leaves us making realizations about them in the past and ourselves in the present. Like us, they were great consumers of stories in the newspapers and enjoyed gossiping about celebrities. In fact, they made news stories an industry of nationwide reach. That is how a powerful newspaper, *El Mercurio*, came to exist. Younger physicians resorted to science to deal with the problems of the body's health; they consulted celebrity doctors from abroad, visited them, and with some luck could perhaps train in their laboratories. But not everyone believed in science. Not even every educator. Like us today, people refused ideas that contradicted their fundamental beliefs.

As now, back then Chileans worried about the future. That was reflected in the budgets they devoted to education, especially professional training and university—while university itself still smelled of fresh paint—and their taste for science fiction stories that addressed the end of the world. Curiously, we shift our attention to such subjects every time a decade is about to end. Earlier on, both present and future were described as fate, often religiously justified with tales that explained both fortune and misfortune, while one's "flock" exerted great control on individual behavior. But the nineteenth century seemed to have changed the mentality of some. Both nationally and internationally, the boldest of intellectuals even advocated for a religion of humanity, which they dared to call "positivism," as opposed to the negative light in which they saw the dogmatic stance of the church. Their anxieties were not just about the individual but also about the future of society at large. And turning a blind eye to theological explanations had consequences, firstly for the church, secondly for medics in need of alternative theories, like physiology, and thirdly for the planners of social order.

Affluents looked abroad for the modern, the exciting, and the sophisticated, while a cascade of poorer Chileans, fed up with working in the land, underserviced townships, and a lack of opportunities, was flowing into the major cities—very much like in our time.

The ruling class was also the wealthiest. In political parlance, that is known as "plutocracy"—a rule by the rich. A parliamentary system had recently been adopted and that gave more relevance to political parties in lawmaking. In practice, however, differences of opinion across the oligarchy were not very large. Oligarchs bothered with the nation's race to industrialization, the big public works, the roaring exportation of nitrate, the international relations, and the country's spectacular financial recovery from the 1880s onward. Similar to our debates these days, they discussed how social reforms both proposed and enacted might benefit workers but affect production. Criticisms, however, were that economic growth depended on public investment. Moreover, in slightly over a decade Chile's new century experienced economic turmoil. Changing maritime routes, reduced nitrate trade, and a world war led to economic decline, with industrialists looking for other areas for mining operation.

And yet, throughout the first two decades modern thinking began to appear more prominently in public debates. Passing laws was often insufficient to counter the people's precarious housing, poor hygiene, and living conditions. Discussion on sanitation, education, and housing then became dominated by middle-class professionals who centered around social democratic and anti-clerical ideas. Furthermore, the centrality of industrial settlements had fueled working-class activism and the ruling class feared mass political upheaval. Progressivism thus gained momentum. Elsewhere the 1920s roared, and so they did in Chile. As Chilean writer Alberto Blest had noted more than half a century earlier, the rise of a middle class needed a liberal revolution, and that revolution was taking shape.

So, in many ways ideas of early twentieth-century Chileans touch our thoughts repeatedly a century later. It was in that cultural atmosphere that social policy emerged, carrying with it a number of rights for the needy and the workers, which implied more responsibility for the state in the social weal of citizens, as the polemic of the *question sociale* continued to be a hot topic in high politics. Traces of it can be, too, found in today's discussions about social disparities and more specifically public health and staffing policies.

By then, physicians had changed the way they understood illness. Clinical observation and continued laboratory trials in Europe had made it clear that it was germs, not fate or smells, that produced diseases and that germs themselves did not appear by spontaneous generation. This was the cornerstone of a new movement which carried the banner of public sanitation. Aware of the political overtones public problems had, the health movement embraced a threefold approach: controlling disease, reducing poverty, and fighting immorality.

It is debatable to establish as to when exactly nurses entered this new sanitary scene. The problem is one of definition. Many of the convents in post-colonial Chile had an infirmary for the sick, some of which offered shelter and care for seculars, but nuns and friars were unlikely to have physical contact with bodies. As it is today, the term nurse itself was ambiguous. It is just that back then it was more so, ranging from maid (*moza*) to governess (*institutriz*) to chaperon (*tutora*) to sick-carer (*enfermera*). Upper-class families usually had "nurses," from which we can infer they assisted in all types of domestic affairs. However, in the health policy language the term became associated with the care of the sick.

Expectedly, something similar occurred with nursing schools, probably not significant enough for them to write an act of establishment as training is known to have been given by physicians in both hospitals and private facilities from the early 1900s. Regardless of the exact date, while the great paradigm shift took place when training in the principles of modern physiology and hygiene, an institutional shift was to follow with the opening of a secular nursing school in university. Under Riesco's presidency it was decided that the school would operate in one of the leprosy wards (*lazaretos*), a structure next to the Saint Vincent de Paul's Chapel, in the block where today sits the University of Chile Faculty of Medicine, in *Independencia*, strategically located opposite Santiago's general cemetery. More importantly, this training confirmed women as fit for university education in fields other than law, pharmacy, and medicine. This small ward can be regarded as the seed of the mighty oak of university training for non-elite women.

Physicians and surgeons enthusiastically endorsed nursing training. As medicine became "scientificized" and doctors were fascinated by the news about discoveries, instruments, and techniques, they realized that nursing was not only good for the nation. *They needed nurses themselves.*

Modern nursing, in the sociological sense of modernity, grew under a scientific medicine approach. And with that, a powerful device was introduced into nursing teaching: the curriculum. This change was not just about knowledge per se but about political positioning. The rollout of several other training centers took place around the same time, such as in pharmacy and school teaching, a plan probably influenced by President Montt's wife, Sara del Campo, the first First Lady to seek involvement in high politics.

Male doctors soon abandoned nursing training. Throughout most of the century the nursing profession became a subject of reform, but with other stakeholders controlling it externally. How, one may ask, have nurses as women reacted to dissatisfaction and concern with nursing policy and the different policy shifts? How was the monopoly of physicians challenged while shaping health policy? How were the relations between nurses and the state shaped and reshaped across political leanings? How did nurses exert agency in the policies that concerned their own profession? To answer these questions, we took a different approach, not looking at nurses' clinical role, more traditionally researched, but by examining their involvement in social policy, shaping a space where they as professionals, and policies as devices, could more closely interact. Nurses toiled in obscurity. Or rather, obscurity was thrust upon them. This is why we did not aim at assessing the health outcomes of policies, but rather we looked at the political process that policy-making takes, hence the social history approach.

As male authors writing about women, we are aware that we narrate the events using our own internal experiences from the inside out. We could never possibly understand fully lives which are complex and which shaped stories of their own. To the best of our ability, we tried to distance ourselves from the histories we had been used to reading, heroic and biased. This journey has been, after all, a learning process. Writing this book can thus be seen as the result of gender privilege. For female historians, writing is about finally getting, if at all, at least equal time. We hope that in answering the questions we have contributed to correct, at least partly, pervasive historical imbalances in the literature on health policy.

Santiago, Chile — Ricardo A. Ayala

Acknowledgments

I want to thank my wife, Ana, and my children, Sofía and Marcel—you always supported me and gave me strength. My gratitude also goes to Rocío Núñez—you helped me to find the first sources and contacts in Chile. Finally, it was Ricardo who accompanied me during my development as a researcher, writer, and storyteller.

You all are the reason why this book can now convey my passion for nursing history.

Markus

A large portion of this book was written and edited during the 2020–2021 lockdown. I wish to express my sincere gratitude to my brother, Cristián, whose companionship, kindness, and stubbornness have most greatly inspired me, driven me mad, and kept me sane.

Ricardo

Contents

List of Pictures

CHAPTER 1

Background: The Struggle for Public Health and Equality

1 Introduction: Welfare State and the Public Health System

Nursing is, in many ways, a health reform. It grew as the welfare system grew and, as such, its accomplishments reflect broader social and political transformations. By documenting the early beginnings, this chapter provides an overview of the modern Chilean healthcare system's origins, in the 1920s, and its continued development until 1970. Important steps like the implementation of the first national healthcare insurance, in 1924, and the first National Health Service, in 1952, will be analyzed regarding their effects and more importantly their influence on the development of the healthcare professions. Furthermore, the chapter pays particular attention to the influence of international organizations throughout the implementation of a public health concept. The focus on the relation between healthcare institutions and different categories of health staff leads to a more detailed observation of the 1960s. That was the time when the first large strikes would halt the health system and, in response, the Christian Democratic Party (1964–1970) would launch a far-reaching reform, a first major reorganizing process of healthcare since those of 1924 and 1952.

An investigation of nursing in the twentieth century needs to involve more than just the perspective on healthcare. For this reason our approach analyzes the interaction of nursing personnel with other healthcare

© The Author(s), under exclusive license to Springer Nature Switzerland AG 2023
M. Thulin, R. A. Ayala, *Nursing, Policy and Politics in Twentieth-century Chile*,
https://doi.org/10.1007/978-3-030-90835-5_1

providers and state representatives, examining their professional transformation as embedded in Chilean society and politics. In this watershed moment began the adoption of a concept of public health from the US, the formation (1938) of the *Asociación de Enfermeras de Chile* and its institutionalization (1952) as the *Colegio de Enfermeras de Chile* (both referred to as "nursing association"[1]), and the subordination of nursing auxiliaries and untrained health staff. During the 1960s, the nursing profession gained momentum, partly because of its politicization, and partly due to the growing visibility of staffing shortages and poor working conditions in the slums and rural areas.

Explicating the developments of the nursing profession involved the biographies of several nurses, showcasing some of the most influential women of twentieth-century Chile. The commitment of nurses such as Sofía Pincheira and Gladys Peake sheds light on the role of female healthcare professionals in national and international organizations that belonged to a male-dominated world. By this, the history of Chilean nurses is also the history of a group of women who, by using turning points in politics, succeeded in establishing autonomous female spaces in a patriarchal society.

1.1 Processing a Vision: Healthcare for Everyone (1920–1964)

The 1920s marked a turning point for welfare in Chile. The century was still fresh when an urban professional class began to gather around the Radical Party, a force that challenged Liberals' traditional views. Criticisms about the role of the oligarchy grew steadily as major migration into the large cities and mining centers continued to raise issues such as social housing, sanitation, and public instruction. Radicalism gained momentum in 1920, carrying with it an awareness of public weal and social reform.

In a timespan of a mere forty years, by 1920 Chile's working class had grown from 75,000 to 350,000, facing staggering structural marginality.[2] But that was not a single occurrence—throughout the twentieth century the population of Latin American countries ballooned. Santiago alone grew by 40 percent between 1940 and 1980,[3] and was already the largest city in the country. Like all the other governments of 100-year-old countries in the region, the state administration could not manage the structural changes, which sped up in marginalized neighborhoods and rural areas. Health status was the most visible sign of social injustice. Contagious diseases took the lives of countless people in Latin America, especially in the vast periphery and suburbs of the cities.[4] The biggest problem was tuberculosis and the bubonic plague (*peste blanca*), whose contagion extended to more than 50 percent of the Chilean population.[5] The fight against those and other highly infectious diseases such as smallpox, cholera, syphilis, and typhoid was part of the day-to-day life of health personnel. In the slums (*poblaciones*) of the cities and in peripheric villages, malnutrition caused considerable deaths, especially among pregnant women, newborns, and infants.

Yet, following from the fall of oligarchism and the rise of a middle-class consciousness, it was at the beginning of the 1920s that Chilean healthcare would begin to consolidate as a state system.[6] Prior to that although health policies did exist, it was mostly within a whole array of hygiene measures—a network of sanitary stations, public "disinfectories," health visitors, infection control procedures, sewage systems, mandatory vaccination, port quarantine, public baths, and laws that enforced the policies. There were also agreements with other countries to hire specialists and nurses, organized envoys of medical staff to train abroad, notably in the late 1800s, and trade unions' mutual aid societies. However, all this proved completely insufficient due to the lack of a stronger institutional structure. About 40 percent of Chileans did not even have access to care services.[7] Basic measures for controlling endemic diseases, like recognizing and separating septic areas of the home, were rarely observed. In the hospitals, pregnant women had to share beds,[8] while 300 out of 1000 children did not reach one year of age.[9] Initiatives such as the founding of the first children's hospitals intended to counter this trend,[10] and although this had some impact, child mortality remained stubbornly high.[11]

The lack of healthcare derived from a weak state structure. Like Buenos Aires or Lima, Santiago maintained the social, educational, and technical control, meaning healthcare was heavily centralized.[12] All influential professionals in this field graduated from a single institution, the University of Chile, in Santiago.[13] Unlike in federal republics such as the US and Germany, most of the policies and specific measures concerning healthcare work in Chile were centrally decided upon and designed, ruled to be implemented in all regions throughout the 4275 km long country.

During the first twenty years of the twentieth century, Chilean governments did not have a coherent public system,[14] and this was reflected in the big crisis the country was in, a development orchestrated by the economic downturn of the nitrate industry and workers' activism. While the Radicals advocated egalitarianism and, indeed, achieved the end of the oligarchic regime, welfare still seemed more of an "ideal." The great reforming era began only in 1925. The implementation of "social rights" (including healthcare) during President Arturo Alessandri Palma's terms (1920–1925 and 1932–1938) was until then the most far-reaching national policy to tackle serious social ailments and form an institutional infrastructure.[15] Nevertheless, the new legislation could only further welfare to a limited extent.

The 1925 reform would be the turn of the physicians, as scientific medicine—as opposed to the ecclesiastic tradition of the nineteenth century—was gaining increasing respectability and becoming an established institution. Conveniently, it also aligned itself with the reformers' interest. In national conferences, physicians proposed concrete measures like the creation of ministries, think tanks, councils, as well as guidelines for the training and the employment of staff. They were also behind the establishment of training systems of hospital staff that fitted the new scientific medicine. The intertwinement of legislative work with health conferences was politically strategic. Governments changed rapidly, coups followed elections, and the armed forces often disregarded parliamentary rights. However, the political elite and the health professionals had lines of communication open to exchange opinions and information with each other. Argentina and Uruguay had similar social characteristics at the beginning of the twentieth century,[16] but alliances were not always possible. While their political instability interrupted democratic processes, and in Argentina it even disintegrated the homogeneity of the political elite,[17] most of the Chilean healthcare laws were the product of controversial but long-standing discussions both in the parliament and at health conferences.

In the early years of nursing, only male physicians participated in healthcare politics. Until the 1940s, most of them came from or spoke on behalf of the Medical Association of Santiago (*Sociedad Médica de Santiago*).[18] As both politics and medicine were male domains, women, at least not in the public eye, did not have much influence in decision-making. Certainly, the noticeable milestones of the Chilean healthcare conferences, the First and Second Public Charity Congresses (*Congresos de Beneficencia Pública*) in 1917 and 1922 and the Third Congress of Social Assistance (*Tercer Congreso de Asistencia Social*) in 1932/1933,[19] were organized by men, as were the national and international expert conferences. But as we will see, they needed women to implement the decisions they took. That was the reason why female nurses who came as PAHO advisors worked hand in hand with foreign physicians. They became the role models of a new team spirit, this being the reason why Chilean liberal feminists were cautious albeit very active in the 1920s and 1930s, lobbying not only for civil law reform but, importantly, for girls' and women's welfare, relief, and instruction.[20] However, the blurring of this traditional divide started in 1942, when Chile hosted the first Latin American congress of nurses, followed by the earliest meetings of social workers in 1945. By 1969, midwives had, too, organized their own conferences.[21]

Healthcare professions worked effectively when both women and men joined in, but it would take a long time until management level reflected a balanced gender distribution. During the 1920s and 1930s, two male physicians were leading the discussion in the national conferences. They advised politicians on the framing of nascent non-medical professions. These were Alejandro Del Río Soto Aguilar (1867–1937), the first health minister (1924–1925) and one of the pioneers of twentieth-century healthcare,[22] and Sótero Del Río Gundián (1900–1969), who led from 1934 to 1938 the Central Board of Welfare and Social Assistance (*Junta Central de Beneficencia y Asistencia Social*).[23] The Board holds significance here because since 1917 this was the first centralized provider of public healthcare.

Even though the work of Alejandro Del Río should not be underestimated, it was Sótero Del Río who gained more attention during the planning and development of the young healthcare system in the decisive period between 1924 and 1932. This was a moment when the *question sociale* forced the political elite to increase state efforts for the poorer social classes. The democratically elected president Alessandri and the rebelling army generals, especially Carlos Ibáñez del Campo (1927–1931, 1952–1958), faced those demands, and from then on state efforts for the underprivileged increased continuously.

Sótero Del Río's main advisor was the physician John D. Long, an employee of the US Public Health Service and advisor to the Rockefeller Foundation (RF). In 1923, Long was detailed to the Pan American Sanitary Bureau (PASB) to support Latin American health authorities.[24] Under Long's supervision, in 1924, the Alessandri government created the Obligatory Health Insurance Fund (*Caja de Seguro Obligatorio, CSO*), the first of this type within health policy in South America.[25] Conforming to law No. 4054, all blue-collar and white-collar workers who had not been insured yet had to affiliate with an insurance in case of "sickness, invalidity and accidents at work," for themselves and their family members.[26] Today's perception of an "obligation" appears to be mostly negative. Nevertheless, the 1924 law did not aim to eliminate the private insurance companies but to complement them.[27] Passed in the same year, an additional law settled the founding of the Ministry of Hygiene, Social Assistance, Social Welfare and Labor (*Ministerio de Higiene, Asistencia Social, Previsión Social y Trabajo*),[28] from which the contemporary Ministry of Health derived during the 1940s.

The modern nursing profession was distilled into the first public system's framework. Social and healthcare policy became more permanently institutionalized as state affairs, including new areas such as the managing of a state nursing service, the international aid or the supervision of hospitals. Since health became a public concern, words like "assistance" (*asistencia*), "welfare" (*bienestar*), "service" (*servicio*), and "insurance" (*previsión*) were used in collocation with the adjective "social." The goal was to replace the old system of charity (*caridad*) with a North American public health concept (*salud pública*),[29] wherein Long was a key instigator. Long and Del Río wanted to elevate "collective wellbeing" (*bienestar colectivo*) by enhancing the provision of care services and designing a responsible and integrated labor policy.[30]

By the end of the 1920s, the vision of affordable healthcare for everyone had become state law. The pathways to access the services, however, remained unclear. State institutions were weak, underfunded, and fragmented;[31] hospitals did not have enough units or departments;[32] and the lack of good hygiene in residential areas[33] was favorable to the spread of diseases. More than that, the conditions for healthcare workers were precarious as the state provided mostly informal contracts.[34] For these reasons the parliament failed to finalize its socially oriented legislative work in 1924, and as most of its members stood in the Latin American tradition of centralization, during the late 1930s and 1940s, they voted for the merger of the existing health agencies.[35] In doing so, they foreshadowed the 1952 reform which attempted to form a single state institution for healthcare services.

The vision of healthcare for everyone was not only the task of parliamentary decisions. At that time, the political elite was facing the first unions and associations of the healthcare sector, which were lobbying for better working conditions and wages as well as a larger say in shaping policy. A salient group among extra-parliamentary stakeholders was the Chilean Medical Association (*Asociación Médica de Chile*), founded in 1931,[36] generally moved by both public social grievances and monopolistic aspirations of medical practice. However, pharmacists, nurses, midwives, and so on followed their example. Decades later it was these bodies that would become the current professional associations (*colegios profesionales*).

By the end of the 1930s, the health professionals had to deal with the largest reform plans ever, following on from the large-scale reform of the years 1924–1925. It was the Popular Front (*Frente Popular*) of President Pedro Aguirre Cerda (1938–1941) that introduced a bill for a new healthcare structure.[37] However, this was not implemented during his term of office. This was also probably why no resistance movement could form up against his plans or those of his health minister Salvador Allende.[38] The first socialist experiment disappeared as fast as it appeared and the Radical Party returned to power.

The archives of the Ministry of Health during the Radical governments (1942–1952) suggest that the ministry regarded the associations of health professionals with mistrust.[39] But, as in the 1930s, it seems that nurses, physicians, nor midwives (to name only a few of the new modern health professionals) gave any ground for labor disputes. That changed during the second administration of Ibáñez del Campo (1952–1958). From that point on the medical association constantly criticized governmental policies,[40] especially when it came to major healthcare reforms, as was the case in 1952.

The origin of the 1952 healthcare reform dates back to the moment when the war in Europe escalated into an international conflict. For Chile, this meant an aggravation of the existing problems, like the medicine[41] and food[42] shortages. The reform bill was discussed under the pressure of increasing social grievances and without the supervision of the "spiritual fathers," Aguirre Cerda and Allende. The main challenge for the political parties was managing hardship while reaching consensus for a long-term policy, meaning that the healthcare bill was discussed in the parliament over 10 years and across three presidential terms.[43] In the last year of Gabriel González Videla's presidency (1946–1952) the law eventually came into force.

The template for Chile's new health institutionality was the British National Health Service (NHS), beginning in 1948,[44] which consisted of the distribution of the country into so-called health units, which in Chile were known as *unidades sanitarias*.[45] Chile's NHS (*Servicio Nacional de Salud*, *SNS*) merged seven existing public healthcare structures into one agency.[46] After 1924, there came a second stage in the plan to cover prevention, treatment, control of hygiene, and occupational safety by state institutions.[47]

Accounts of the NHS's actual coverage vary significantly, though reporting mostly about doctors' services. Of the medical treatments provided during the 1952–1980 period, between 70 and 90 percent coverage has been reported. This variation responds to the different parameters used in assessing the NHS. When Llambias-Wolff (2013) states 90 percent,[48] he most likely included preventive campaigns in the community, which in South America account for an important part of primary care. Nurse Doris Krebs (1961) and sociologist Clarita Müller-Plantenberg (1972) report the same figure.[49] Yet other assessments state a coverage as low as 70 percent, such as Chanfreau (1979) and Belmar and Sidel (1975).[50]

The NHS was the most comprehensive health service project of the twentieth century, even though it was not a single or unified health service. The public servants and private individuals with high financial resources were successful in defending their independence. Already in 1942, the agencies that were specific to them merged into the National Medical Service of the Employees (*Servicio Médico Nacional de Empleados, SERMENA*).[51] By the time it was founded, *SERMENA* provided services through a few hospitals and healthcare centers. Most of the medical treatments were provided by physicians in either NHS facilities or their own medical practices.[52] But the situation changed rapidly. During the 1950s and 1960s, *SERMENA* attracted most of the well-off patients[53] and lobbying in the parliament assured the expansion of its infrastructure.[54] As a consequence, the success of *SERMENA* was damaging for the NHS. The already existing problems, such as hospitals located only in the big cities, far from *poblaciones*,[55] or healthcare providers who preferred not to work outside the city centers[56], were aggravated by the lack of solidarity within this two-class system. The coexistence of both structures blocked the road to a broader healthcare coverage and more equal treatment.[57]

Nevertheless, across this continued wave of reforms nursing had been virtually neglected, without easily articulating the existing training and staffing for nurses into a larger policy package. UK policy during the inception of the NHS did tackle food rationing and housing shortage, but also the necessary nursing workforce for the reform to work. In Chile, however, this idea arose from a different development, as will be shown in the following section.

1.2 *Sponsoring the Vision and Framing the Nursing Profession: Public Health from North America*

The struggle for healthcare coverage in Chile was inextricably linked with international trade and politics, a development that contributed to the foundations of the current system of nursing and primary care more broadly in the country. At the beginning of the twentieth century, the US was seeking trade expansion overseas, regarding Latin America as its nearest sphere of influence. However, interfering with the expansion of commerce, the vast area from Rio Grande (northern Mexico) to Cape Horn (southern Chile) was an intricate mosaic of various quarantine, inspection, and exclusion regulations, making the free movement of goods very difficult. Besides, eradicating contagious diseases in lagging regions convulsed by political instability became a popular endeavor among US health authorities of the early twentieth century. It was a common fear that "wild" Latin America could infect the US, and the perceived need to protect those areas of the world cemented the plan to extend its economic influence.[58]

The US tactic brought about a noticeable interest in Latin America's health policy and politics. The concept developed for such purpose came to be known as "public health." It spread to Chile in three distinct waves—first, at the beginning of the 1920s; second, during World War II; and third, after the Cuban Revolution. As it would be later with the European-inspired NHS, the North American public health project found supporters in all political camps and became the red line of Chilean healthcare policies during the twentieth century.[59]

Although historically absent from social policy, it was quickly concluded that women were key players in any reform that sought to produce major health improvements. Firstly, the strategy involved enhancing the existing female workforce. The work Dr. Cora Meyers was doing at a nursing school, which by then was affiliated to a university, was known internationally. She specialized in the areas of maternal and childcare, spoke foreign languages, worked closely with health volunteering organizations, and regarded health education as a form of activism by and for women. Meyers and John D. Long met a number of times to discuss the chances to train district nurses at her school. And secondly, new politics of motherhood were crucial to counter sky-rocketing infant mortality. Maternity was considered of utmost relevance in both ensuring the application of the household principles of the hygienist school and inculcating a new set of morally laden concepts.

Likewise, the Pan American Sanitary Bureau (PASB), created in 1902 and serving until the early 1930s as a branch of the US public health service, was one of the organizations with the deepest impact in framing Latin American healthcare.[60] Hygienists like Long were sent to Chile so that the country's healthcare system internalized and adapted to the public health concept. On behalf of the PASB, Long visited no fewer than half of the 33 countries, where he gave his approval to and even made variations to some of their health codes in order that they matched the framing of the Pan American Sanitary Code from 1924.[61] Importantly, as will be shown in detail in the case of nurses and social workers, he negotiated with Mayers the set-up for the caring professions, notably the public health nurse.

The lack of district nurses motivated private international donors, namely the Rockefeller Foundation (RF) and ad hoc state institutions, notably the Institute of Inter-American Affairs (IIAA), to enter the sanitary scene. Chaired by a Rockefeller family member, the IIAA was created to oust European economic powers in the Americas. And they understood that a key outcome of strengthening healthcare and sanitation was a healthy workforce. The decisive moment for Chile to interweave interests with the IIAA took place in 1942–1943 with the signing of an agreement involving primary technical support between the Ministry of Health and the IIAA represented by the US embassy.[62] Between 1943 and 1951, the IIAA subsidized Chile with 5,400,000 USD, a remarkable sum of money considering that in 1950 the country's GDP was 3,827,000 USD. Nine permanent advisors supervised the implementation of the programs, by far the highest number of envoys compared to the other international organizations active in Chilean healthcare at this time (UNICEF had only one and other organizations none).[63]

IIAA's strong involvement came alongside a significant offer of training programs for health professionals by the International Health Commission/Division (IHC/IHD) at Rockefeller.[64] In 1943, the Public Health School (*Escuela de Salubridad*) started operations in Santiago. It was founded by the IHC together with the University of Chile and the Chilean Bacteriological Institute (*Instituto Bacteriológico de Chile*). The aim of the Public Health School was, as the university stated retrospectively, to "increase public health, contributing to the correct assessment of the problems and teaching the way to approach them with the highest efficiency."[65] The school became, too, the most important point of intersection between public health and nursing.

In 1949, the Pan American Sanitary Organization or PASO (wherein PASB was an executive agency) became a regional office of the World Health Organization, WHO.[66] At the beginning of the 1950s, its investment in Chile's healthcare was still small compared to that of the IIAA and Rockefeller.[67] But this would change during that decade.[68] One of the most important steps to increase its engagement was the development of hygiene and vaccination programs.[69] After World War II, tuberculosis, smallpox, and polio were seen as the biggest threat to humankind, and comprehensive immunization as the most suitable, albeit relatively new, artillery. Containment was no longer the task of the IIAA, leaving the healthcare field to international institutions and foundations.

During the 1950s, PAHO's involvement in Chile strengthened and widened as a number of other entities joined, such as the Pan American Medical Confederation, the World Medical Association, the United Nations (notably UNICEF),[70] the Union for International Cancer Control, the Inter-American Children's Institute, and the International Union Against Tuberculosis and Lung Disease.[71] Therefore, the departure of the IIAA caused no harm to the bond between Washington and Latin America. It was only a shift from direct to indirect US influence which took place by the middle of the twentieth century.

Importantly though, this whole array of macro-economic arrangements framed care work in a different way, which was important in national politics and even the branding of politicians. Drawing on earlier strategies, this interlocking would make women—and by extension, nurses—essential to the infrastructure of health policy in the long term.

1.3 One Step Forward and One Step Back: Gender Pay Gap and Healthcare in Times of Christian Democracy (1964–1970)

Contrary to common beliefs, the gender pay gap has been a long-standing concern among nurses, which surfaced during both the unionism era of mid-century and the reconfiguring of political transitions. By mid-century, labor unions had achieved a number of landmarks regarding bargaining power, welfare, wages, relief, and insurance and merged into a powerful federation. However, in several areas the vindication of the unions overlapped with the prerogatives of the professional associations.

Better payment was the most important claim of the healthcare workers and professionals who gathered in 1963 in the hitherto healthcare system's biggest strike.[72] The situation was critical for the government, because the lack of healthcare services produced a general dissatisfaction with its politics. Finally, the most promising candidates of the upcoming elections, Salvador Allende and Eduardo Frei Montalva, successfully mediated between the Confederation of Health Workers (*Confederación de los Trabajadores de Salud*), on the one side, and the government of the conservative president Jorge Alessandri, in office since 1958, on the other side.[73]

Three groups of health professionals did not join the protest in 1963, the physicians, dentists, and pharmacists. They had already stopped working in 1960[74] and 1962,[75] and since then, their wages were determined through a salary scale specific to them, implemented by law No. 15.076.[76] This law consolidated *de facto* privileges on those three professional groups. For the following decades, an overt action against the pay gap, especially of female professionals such as nurses, midwives, and social workers, and the revising of unequal wages within single professions created an atmosphere that seemed to hinder collaboration.

The ephemerality of collective actions became a repeated pattern of the healthcare workers' and professionals' alliances. They were generally weak at the beginning of a presidential term, strengthened up during the reform era, and broke apart when a new government with new faces and promises came to power. While the strikes during Alessandri's presidency served only as the nursery for such an alliance, the successor government had to face its first concerted campaign. It is very likely that nobody had foreseen this development when Eduardo Frei Montalva, leading the Christian Democratic Party, won the 1964 elections.

Frei Montalva was the brother of Irene Frei, a university-trained social worker, well-known within the political socialite, who knew first-hand the work with abandoned and orphan children and hospital patients. She was herself councillor of Santiago. Strategically, Irene was President Frei's closest political associate during the run-up to the election. Unlike his predecessor, Frei had prepared a new model of healthcare policy and started to implement it shortly after he came into office, with Irene likely to have been the mastermind of the social welfare plan. The campaign, indeed, underscored the social issues women were most sensitive to, which at least in part explains why women voters decided the 1964 election—Frei won the votes of 63 percent of women.

In one of their first actions, Frei and his health minister Ramón Valdivieso Delaunay (1964-1970) increased the staff of the NHS. This meant priority of the NHS over other units such as *SERMENA*. Nevertheless, this move did not attempt to remove the private–public dualism.[77] They tried to increase the efficiency of the NHS without having to change *SERMENA*.

Their second move aimed to increase the NHS's coverage in the periphery and the countryside. New healthcare centers with a focus on primary care were built, the public insurance for work accidents was extended to all workers, the immunization program was strengthened, and the distribution of food stuff expanded. Valdivieso took measures to establish a better system for the control of Ministry of Health spending and increased both the working hours for physicians in the NHS and the training hours for all aspiring health professionals.[78] His efforts culminated in 1967 with the reform of the health code, which is still effective today. As we will see in the case of the nurses, the law framed the work area of the profession, and most importantly it guaranteed medical care for pregnant women and children as an undeniable right, exempted of any additional payments.[79]

For the first time since 1952 policies were meant to endure shifts of governments, becoming state policies. Frei's and Valdivieso's idea was to include "sectorial" and "national" actors; that being the reason why they founded the National Advisory Council for Health (*Consejo Nacional Consultivo de Salud*) and the National Office of Planning (*Oficina de Planificación Nacional, ODEPLAN*). The cooperation with the University of Chile was intensified. Women's and children's health, the so-called *materno-infantil* sector, were thus more realistically tackled by focusing on the family. The constantly growing influence of the US in health at policy level aligned Chile with an international system of family planning. In essence, this involved counseling and contraception for overwhelmingly low-income women, who had the highest rates of unwanted or unplanned pregnancy and births. Once the Christian Democrats decided to improve women's and children's living conditions through family planning and methods to control fertility medically,[80] the most important of these initiatives was the Association for the Protection of the Family (*Asociación de Protección de la Familia, APROFA*), founded in 1965.[81]

To finance those efforts in health politics, the Frei administration undertook the biggest budget increase for the NHS since its foundation in 1952. This was expensive. At the beginning of the 1970s, two-thirds of public spending went to social welfare.[82] Nevertheless, even those efforts were not enough to meet people's needs. Like most Latin American countries, Chile continued to depend on international aid in material supplies and staff,[83] which went mostly to *materno-infantil* projects.

Only one measure did not fit into this progressive framework, the Curative Medicine Act (*Ley de Medicina Curativa*) of 1968.[84] This Act drove the Christian Democratic party's "revolution in freedom" into a dead end.[85] However, in defense of the government's position, it ought to be mentioned that a law regulating curative medical services was previously brought before the congress during the period of conservative governments. Because of the conditions laid down by the physicians, and their lobbying in the national parliament, the 1968 curative medicine legislation looked like little more than an upgrade of *SERMENA*. It did introduce a healthcare model based on a psychosocial explanation of diseases, though access depended on the financial situation of the insured,[86] making it difficult for unemployed unmarried women to access. Furthermore, it reorganized and extended the already common practice to pay for treatment out of pocket with borrowed money.[87] For a certain fee, *SERMENA* patients received vouchers to be exchanged for medical services. The physician would then mail the voucher to a *SERMENA* office and receive payment. The Frei government emphasized the expansion of medical care,[88] but even though the Curative Medicine Act benefited employees, it could not solve the inequality in healthcare.

In practice, achieving the goals required strengthening the nursing workforce. Yet, despite its social orientation, the program of the Christian Democrats did not seem to consider caregivers in the betterment of wages, staffing, and working conditions. The health code included, compared to the midwives, only a very general description of the tasks that nurses were required to undertake.[89] This caused a conflict between both professions about the delamination of their work fields in *materno-infantil* starting in the 1970s.[90] Another stumbling block was that non-academically trained women and men, though not nurses, as we will explain hereinafter, remained the most important pillar of personnel policy in healthcare. However, it seems that the exclusion of nurses from the Curative Medicine Act was the main reason why the negotiations between them and the government became hostile.

Nurse Sofía Pincheira, within a working group of other health professionals, proposed an amendment to the Act in 1969.[91] Officially, changes to the curative medicine legislation were still possible to undertake even after enacting it in 1968. The group linked their proposal with the claim to extend Law No. 15.076 to all health professionals. But until the end of the Frei administration, no amendment was achieved. Both laws continued to benefit only physicians, dentists, and pharmacists.[92] The rights granted by Law No. 15.076 also remained a privilege of the three, predominantly male, professions—much as they also felt disadvantaged.

At the end of the decade, the discontent among nurses, midwives, social workers, and other healthcare professionals who did not benefit from the Curative Medicine Act and Law No. 15.076 began to grow. The Confederation of Health Workers, which led the protest in 1963, changed its name to the National Federation of Healthcare Workers (*Federacion Nacional de Trabajadores de Salud*, *FENATS*) and asked for direct negotiations with Frei and Valdivieso.[93] In an internal paper, the Ministry of Health rejected the action in the following words:

> "So far, this group had only unionist goals, threatening with all sorts of work stoppage and strike movements among the NHS staff, which impedes the essence of cooperation."[94]

The medical association, led by Emilio Villarroel, saw an opportunity in the unrest among the healthcare workers to claim for an even bigger cut of the Curative Medicine provisions. They could hide their profession-specific goals, like more influence in the legislation process[95] and rejection of the eight-hours day,[96] behind general claims—like better payment announced by the other healthcare employees—hoping to give their prerogative a more social flavor by carrying the banner of an "integral" and "social" medicine.[97] This was especially useful for the female groups, which in the public imagination were traditionally associated with abnegation and selflessness.

The 1970 strike lasted 22 days.[98] It was the largest display of power of the healthcare workers in Chilean history.[99] Further concessions by the government were unlikely, probably because of the presidential election in that year, which may have caused a new wait-and-see attitude. But conflict was only postponed.

At the end of this whole debate about the healthcare system under the Frei administration, one development merits further reference here, even though its impact became visible only years later. In 1968, many women, farmers, and individuals from the periphery had walked their path to higher education through a church-promoted program. That same year out of this democratic action arose the precursor of a conservative and neoliberal political party in the Chile's second largest and very influential university, the Catholic University in Santiago. Driven by an anti-reform discourse, a rightist political movement known as *gremialismo* won the election of students' representatives in the Catholic University.[100] During the 1970s, its doctrinaire stance would make a great impact not only on the state and the university model but also on the professional associations.

2 The Rise of the Modern Nursing Profession (1906–1970)

2.1 *The Foundation of State Nursing (1906–1926)*

Having reviewed the foundational processes of contemporary welfare, it is necessary to revisit how the nursing profession fitted into and reflected the grand scheme of things. There is a debate about whether the first nursing school in Latin America using a model attributed to Nightingale was founded in Argentina or Chile. How much of that model was really used by reformers remains largely unknown, and so does the actual extent to which Nightingale's ideas were at the foundation of the model. Nevertheless, one can appraise the increasing secularity of the profession and the state sponsorship as decisive in the rise of the nursing profession as we know it today.

Reporting on "the firsts" may sound superfluous nowadays. And yet tracing this training has relevance as to how ground-breaking it was in relation to organization, approach, and mindset. The British Hospital School of Nursing (*Escuela de Enfermeras del Hospital Británico*), founded in 1890 by Isabel Eames, who trained in London, and the School of Nurses of the Argentine Medical Circle (*Escuela de Enfermeras del Circulo Médico Argentino*), launched in 1892 by Cecilia Grierson (the country's first female physician),[101] would inaugurate a new generation of nursing schools in Latin America.[102] Following contemporary author Karina Inés Ramacciotti, Grierson's school became a role model. The school would pass down through generations what she describes as the "English instructive scheme" (*esquema formativo inglés*) for a female job trained in hospital boarding schools (*internados*).[103]

Similarly, in Chile university studies and certificates were provided by a centralized state institution based on newly set scientific principles. What is insightful here is that Argentina and Chile witnessed similar processes of scientification of medicine alongside new ideals of social development (namely "social positivism"), which eventually impacted on the way nursing was thought of. Rosalba Flores, nurse and author of Chile's first nursing history (1965), emphasized the role that the school of nursing located in the University of Chile since 1906 played, and according to her, its relevance for the entire western hemisphere.[104] Much as this period of nursing history in Chile remains largely under-researched, the Nightingalean rhetoric became key to nurses' oral history and identity, holding the status of a creation story which did not re-emerge until mid-century during the associative movements of the unions.

Four years before, the urologist and dermatologist Eduardo Moore (1866–1941) had conducted the first secular training for Chilean nurses at the *San Francisco de Borja Hospital* in Santiago.[105] Moore called it an "experimental" course (he meant "pilot"). His goal was to persuade the Ministry of Health of the importance of state-approved nursing studies as a methodology of ensuring high-quality healthcare,[106] stemming from his interest in war surgery and the ongoing scientific discoveries in Western Europe. Moore's nursing students did not pay tuition fees; nor were they paid a wage during their three-year training. They had to be between 20 and 35 years of age and subordinate to the physician's rules. In the Second Latin American Medical Congress, held in 1904 in Buenos Aires, the Chilean physician Moisés Amaral (1859–1933) described the women to be trained in Moore's school in the following way:

> "We ought to acknowledge that the Public Charity attends to the poor with paternal affection and generosity, and remember that the first assistant in this task is the physician. [...] The Santiago [nursing] school insists with full consistency in penetrating into the mind of the students the conviction to never took over the direction of the patient nor disobey the physician[...]" Citing the physician and specialist in pathologic anatomy, Maurice Letulle, he adds, "The aim is not creating a hybrid type of semi-physicians, semi-surgeons and semi-midwives; but rather training allies for physicians, surgeons and obstetricians."[107]

Probably inspired by a range of different influences, both secular and religious, there appears for the first time the philosophy of uniform dressing for nurses. Amaral's account of Moore's school contains a description of the way students were requested to dress back in 1902:

> "The nurses wear a uniform outfit. It consists of a dress of black fabric, straight cut, wide skirt with no tail, smooth, with no adornment, white neck, black tie, white over sleeves, white apron on the dress and a cap in white muslin."[108]

The lobbying of Moore and Amaral was successful. In 1906, under the supervision of surgeon Francisco Navarro, they opened a nursing school in the St. Vincent of Paul Hospital (*Hospital San Vicente de Paul*) in Santiago's district of *Independencia* aimed at using modern scientific principles.[109] Physicians of the University of Chile's medical faculty took over the teaching in the classrooms, while the practical instruction was provided by the nuns of the St. Vincent of Paul's Sisters of Mercy (*Hermanas de la Caridad de San Vicente de Paul*) who ran the hospital.[110] Despite Moore's plans, studies required only two years and were not free. Interestingly, the requirements for the uniform were optional and less precise, and seemed to better accommodate the physical movements that nursing work demanded, namely a blouse with rollable sleeves.[111]

The most influential director of the first modern nursing school was the pediatric surgeon Eugenio Díaz Lira (1880–1945), who led the institution for 18 of its 23-year existence. In 1929, when it merged with the public health nursing school, he eventually became the first director of the medical school of the Catholic University.[112]

Besides the fruitful establishment of an academic nursing school in the capital in the first decade of the twentieth century, nuns, friars, and traditional healers, as well as families and acquaintances, remained the main, and oftentimes the only, accessible source of care. Research results in Chap. 3–5 suggest that it took 70 more years until the shift toward the university-affiliated model in the frame of Western health[113] took place in the furthest corners of the country. And yet, what had started as an elite group in Santiago would not stop to spread its reforming spirit throughout the entire twentieth century.

As said at the beginning of the book, nursing is, in many ways, a health reform. Contemporary accounts in Chile have shed light only on one aspect, caused by the continued evolution of nursing care on the basis of university-trained personnel. However, they neglect the achievements of other important areas of modern nursing work, such as that of the Red Cross, which was backed by the state and actively supported by the social elite at the same time span.

The Chilean Red Cross trained nursing volunteers, war nurses, and social work volunteers. The reason for neglecting this work could be the smaller impact of this organization on the healthcare and nursing system in Chile compared to Argentina.[114] Besides, Red Cross nurses were systematically excluded from narratives on nursing and professionalization during the twentieth century in Chile, as university-trained nurses dominated those narratives. The little that is known about the women who became Red Cross nurses does not do justice to the impact they made on access to care. Like army nurses, they did not train in university, and this may be another reason it is shrouded in obscurity by common histories. Historian Pilar Morales, in her extensive summary of the institution on occasion of its 100th anniversary in the country, in 2003, shows eloquently that female nurses were the face and the heart of the Red Cross in Chile, and by extension, a part of Chile's institutional healthcare.[115] In fact, the board of the Red Cross was one of the few niches where women operated autonomously and sat on the top of the military-like hierarchy.

Of the Red Cross nursing training much remains under-researched, but decree no. 3347 states it began officially the year WWI broke out.[116] This decree also confirms that the institution was run by a female-only board, which protected zealously institutional autonomy from any ministry. In the early 1920s, the Red Cross issued its own public health journal, and by 1930 female volunteers trained in wartime nursing, health visiting, and social work where they offered care for people who lived until then far away from all professional healthcare facilities. In the very beginning evidence suggests these courses were designed as short training courses, as Ramacciotti described for the Argentine Red Cross.[117] Nevertheless, an extensive handbook for students from 1933 suggests that the contents were not any less than the ones meant for the state schools.[118] The ideal of a healthy nation was, indeed, part of the cultural politics around Chile's centennial independence and modernization, where training nurses through different systems simultaneously seemed key.

Concerning Red Cross nurses, the National Library of Chile provides mostly sources from the 1920s and 1930s. These nurses were instructed to conform to the principles of humanitarian treaties in wartime and assist health professionals in peacetime,[119] but they also had the chance to be recognized for their ordinary and extraordinary services, climb in the hierarchy, and become superintendents of Red Cross centers and nursing schools.[120] Many women entered the public sphere through nursing work, be it for the care of the sick, the care of the wounded, or the care of health.

Interestingly though, in some regions like Rancagua, where volunteers were very respected by citizens, women referred to as "Miss Nurse" (*señorita enfermera*) were allowed to represent and manage a regional division of the Red Cross.

Even though university nursing and Red Cross nursing developed separately, at least two characteristics were similar in the origins of both trajectories. First, the charity circles of upper-class women were used as the primary base to recruit women for modern nursing in Chile, Argentina, and Uruguay;[121] they also attracted volunteers for the nursing section of the Red Cross, framed as a place for women in society, as the original name suggests, Red Cross of Women of Chile (*Cruz Roja de Mujeres de Chile*).[122] Second, apart from the sense of distinction of the new secular nurses, due to their state or university-level status felt as compared to religious nurses, both academic and Red Cross schools kept some of their traditional traits in regard to female vocation. For example, the boarding schools were imbued with the spirit of lifetime devotion[123] as the symbols and mystical rituals of the graduation ceremony enforced a near-religious commitment.[124]

What was the most important common feature of the modern nursing profession? The affiliation to a medical faculty? This would not count for Red Cross nurses. More than that, the short study time and low range of the first academic schools limited the impact of the nascent nursing profession to Chile's metropolitan area. The secularity would serve as a feature in spite of the ever-present powerful position still held by nuns and friars in Latin American healthcare systems. The common features were, however, the spirit of reform and the determined will to challenge the traditions inherited from colonial times. The engagement of elite women was another common feature, as the commitment to nursing required a certain level of education and financial security that most Chilean women were due to economic circumstances unable to attain. Finally, diversity was also a central feature of modern nursing. For the first time since the end of colonialism, new types of caregivers entered the healthcare stage. These women, trained by the Red Cross and state universities, worked to close the gap in medical and social care. However, they did not work alone. The focus on the pay gap in the academic trained healthcare leads to other questions such as, How were auxiliary nurses paid? Did reforms, strikes, and new study schemes also affect their working life?

2.2 *Auxiliary to Health Work, an Appendix of History*

As we have shown, the rise of modern nursing in the first half of the twentieth century turned a small but growing number of women into public health specialists. Their role models, teachers, and donors came from Europe and especially North America, where continuous developments in diagnostic and therapy had led to the differentiation of new medical disciplines. In particular, the increasingly technological hospitals required professionalizing the personnel.[125] It was the birth of the health professions as we know them today, namely a political project attached to specific areas of work within the wider socio-economic order, a notion that grew stronger as Western nations industrialized.

As the work in the new hospitals demanded a higher educational level, the study time and content for health professionals increased, too. Women who succeeded to enter (and afford) one of the few universities had access to very restricted jobs.[126] Taking care of the sick fitted in the frame of submissive dedication in works controlled by men, such as Del Río, Amaral, and Moore, becoming typically midwives or nurses.[127] As was the case elsewhere,[128] trained women were seen as the auxiliary staff of the physician, "completing" or "complementing" his work.[129] In 1925, Del Río described healthcare work as:

> "the combined and harmonic action of two competences, acquired by exhaustive theoretical and practical studies—of the physician, first of all, and of the nurse, his direct assistant."[130]

This framing, submitting to the physician, continued to be the organizing principle of these two professions throughout the first half of the century. In 1919, the Central Board of Welfare and Social Assistance, henceforth referred to as "Welfare Board," founded its own nursing school. As it was accredited two years later by the University of Chile,[131] that was the second school offering academic training for nurses in the country. The top level of the Welfare Board described the purpose of such school as "to prepare subordinate technical staff" (*para la preparación del personal técnico inferior*).[132]

The status of nurses in the healthcare system was as low as that of most women in society. Nevertheless, their professional training, or even university studies, meant an upward move compared to the status of other caregivers like *practicantes* and nursing auxiliaries (*auxiliares de enfermería*). Most of these could not afford academic training and as such were deprived of the opportunity of becoming physicians or nurses.

While the term nursing auxiliary suggests that they undertook care tasks, *practicantes*' work was more difficult to define, albeit widespread, and oscillated between autonomy and assistance, which was probably the main reason why it attracted more men than the more orthodox nursing profession. Quoting F. Puga Borne (1895) and Margaret Yaeger (1999), Zárate and González (2018) describe the *practicantes* in the following way:

> "In the second half of the 19th century, the hospitals and welfare facilities counted on few physicians and a handful of hospital workers. They were mostly men, known as *practicantes*, who fulfilled mainly tasks like washing patients, cleaning floors, making beds and giving cares for the patients' bodies."[133]

The census of 1920 published an estimate of 1430 *practicantes*, 678 male and 752 female.[134] With 1529 registered nurses, this was one of the largest group of caregivers. Surprisingly, they mostly appear in side notes, for example in 1923, when an author of the Public Health Journal (*Revista de Salud Pública*) mentions that nurses "work alongside *practicantes* and physicians."[135] The Welfare Board referred to *practicantes* for the first time in 1932, during a discussion about their status in the city of Curicó, which is located 196 km south of Santiago. Within they were described as technical staff with the title of "medical auxiliary."[136]

In another account, it is stated that the *practicante* was a position similar in scope to the nurse, but one that focused more on surgical matters and had a greater degree of practical knowledge as opposed to academic training,[137] a trait that would gradually make them disappear from the sanitary scene.[138] Yet they continued to exist among the healthcare providers throughout the twentieth and part of the early twenty-first centuries, although mostly working in privately owned offices.

Until the 1960s, the number, work, field, and representation of nursing auxiliaries (today known as *técnicos paramédicos* or *TENS)* also remained on the periphery of historiography. Sometimes their traces were blended into the descriptions of professional nursing,[139] sometimes caught in a small spotlight, as done by Martín in Argentina,[140] González and Zárate in Chile,[141] Sánchez in Uruguay.[142] One exception is a recent piece depicting the cultural tensions between auxiliaries and university-trained nurses in Chile.[143] Curiously, nursing auxiliaries received a passing reference when archives documenting their training programs have been found, but the accounts did not intend to maintain their memory as an inherent part of nursing and healthcare. As such, nursing auxiliaries, despite being a large workforce in nursing care, have become lost to obscurity, an appendix of history, if that, or a mere role, as men like del Río (1923) spoke of them:

> "People of low social extraction [...] poorly paid, without any uniform to wear or not even a collective identity, without any consciousness when their duties are poorly performed; oftentimes they sleep in the same rooms as the sick [...] or in rooms that are filthy."[144]

Even though this description was probably meant to justify the neglect of auxiliary personnel in historiography, it shows us how intensive and unconditional the contact of *practicantes* and nursing auxiliaries with the patients must have been. As our approach aims to cover the history of all types of caregivers, the proceeding summary of milestones in nursing history will put as often as is possible a spotlight on the so-called people of low social extraction. However, many times the obscurity of public records was limiting, which is why the elucidation of public health nursing gives the impression that they did not exist at all.

2.3 *The First Era of Public Health Nursing (1926–1941)*

The founding process of a nursing school in 1906 breathed in the spirit of scientific innovation which came from the large European capitals, such as Paris, Vienna, and London. The second important stage of development was achieved under US influence. On February 28, 1927, Lucas Sierra, Director-General of Health and in this capacity one of the most important implementers of PASB policy in Chile, inaugurated a new type of nursing school. Public health nurse Sarah Adams, one of the first PASB delegates like John D. Long, started training the first 30 women wanting to become public health nurses (*enfermeras sanitarias*).[145]

One of them was Sofía Pincheira, born 1903 in Concepción. In 1925, she was studying medicine in the University of Chile when she heard of this new health profession to be introduced to the medical faculty. She felt drawn to nursing, gave up her medical studies, and passed Adams' admission test, which was much more challenging than the ones in the existing nursing schools.[146]

Like Pincheira, the other 29 women had already joined medical studies, and this is why their training lasted only 12 months.[147] Adams' most prominent teachers were Elianira González and Cora Mayers (1895–1931), the latter being one of the first Chilean females to become a physician.[148]

As an experienced founder of public health nursing schools in Latin America,[149] Adams considered Chilean nursing to be of a low standards. In a 1927 report published in the *American Journal of Nursing*, she primarily pointed to the lack of educational material for nursing training as the reason for this underdevelopment.[150] That report and the knowledge about what she thought were catastrophic conditions of healthcare thwarted the image of Chilean public health nursing as a successful role model for South America since its foundation.[151]

The public health concept for nursing had silted up fast after its implementation.[152] It did not seem to endure after the first cohort. Sierra and Adams failed to expand the study plan to three years and open it up for students without basic education in medicine. In 1928, the University of Chile announced that it could no longer fund two nursing programs at a time, for which reason in March 1929 it merged with the already existing academic institution into a single School of Nursing (*Escuela de Enfermería*).[153] Since then, the concentration in public health was reduced to an optional one-year extension following a three-year basic training in nursing. Most of the students did not sign up for this concentration. By 1950, only 22 percent of the graduates followed the curriculum endorsed by Pincheira to become public health nurses.[154]

And yet, the crises of public health nursing did not affect Pincheira personally. Her career rocketed the moment she finished her basic training. She stayed in school, eventually becoming a teaching practice assistant for hospitals (*ayudante de práctica hospitalaria*). This was at least her position in 1929, when she received a scholarship from the American Association of the University Women (AAUW). It financed Pincheira's bachelor's in nursing at Columbia (1929–1932) and a master's in public health at Yale (1932–1933).[155] The Ministry of Health's archives suggests that she was one of the first nurses, if not the first, to study outside Latin America.

The situation in Chile remained complicated. Adams, the first director of the new School of Nursing,[156] had chosen Mayers as her administrative director[157] and successor, but in 1931 she died unexpectedly. Adams could not find a replacement and apparently did not have the willpower nor the permission to keep the position. Pincheira stayed as an administrative director (*subdirectora técnica*) for two more years, but moved to

Bolivia in 1933. The school then took a U-turn into old role models when a male director was appointed. However, the more pressing problem was the low number of women who wanted to study public health nursing. The new profession risked becoming a brief episode in the history of healthcare.

Pincheira's successors as administrative directors were Teresa Hernández (1934–1936) and Elianira González (1936–1943).[158] Unfortunately, there is no further information about their performance or the shape the school was in during the 1930s.

Meanwhile, the number of the nursing schools managed by the Welfare Board had started to grow. A second school in Santiago was founded, likely in the late 1920s or early 1930s, which merged in 1935 into the existing school.[159] Two years earlier, the Welfare Board in Valparaíso had founded a nursing school in *Carlos Van Buren* hospital.[160] Located next to the most important Chilean harbor, Valparaíso had grown as fast as Santiago by then. As in Santiago, nurses were in short supply for the size of the city. The first to come up with a plan was not the state but Anne Marie Sørensen and her husband, the Swedish-Danish physician Jean Hugo Thierry. In 1922, they founded the first nursing school of Valparaíso, which up until 1932 even had an academic status.[161]

The two nursing schools run by the Welfare Board and the private school of Sørensen and Thierry's provided a three-year-long training but did not offer a concentration in public health nursing. However, a description of the school from 1936 gives insights into the tuition fees and the fees of the boarding school.[162]

Valparaíso reached the highest-level nursing training outside Santiago during this second wave of nursing school foundations in the 1930s. But the available statistics only allow an estimate of fewer than a thousand nurses graduated during the first five years, and the nursing staff numbers remained small in terms of geography and quantity. The absence of trained nurses in most of the towns and regions throughout the vast Chilean territory was evident during the first half of the twentieth century. For most of the needful and the sick, caregivers were still nuns, friars, volunteers, and traditional healers.

The only way how modern nurses could establish a broad coverage for the needful and sick was to connect to the North American public health system. By 1934, when Pincheira returned from the US, the impact of academic and public health nursing on the hospitals and other medical facilities was still very low. Policy-makers on urban nursing and *salud pública*, the Latin American way of public health, all agreed that they were meant to establish a minimal healthcare coverage in undersupplied areas.

Nursing schools played an important role in extending welfare policy. But they were not yet an alternative to self-taught caregivers in entire regions. Nurses only operated in the Santiago-Valparaíso area, and in the case of public health only in the capital. New schools were needed, but the administrative and financial problems affected state-founded nursing. The most important reason was the lack of agreement regarding the length and content of nursing training programs.[163] The two schools in Valparaíso (Welfare Board), for example, had no teaching nurses and education was done (and controlled) by physicians until the late 1930s. Even though this was not the case in Santiago's schools,[164] the progressive public health concept could not avoid that modern nursing did not match with the needs of all who needed care. Women remained not only technically but also ideologically in the territory of a male profession, resulting in that the confines of the patriarchy restricted the public health concept in developing its capacity.

From 1929 to 1941, sources give a clear picture that the economic crisis of 1929 diminished many investment programs aimed at Latin America. Thus, this was perhaps the most important reason why public health nursing was paralyzed. For about one and a half years, Pincheira was the assistant director of the nursing/public health nursing school of the University of Chile during which time she initiated a nationwide reform of the training program.[165] It would appear that one of the reasons why she and her husband decided to leave Chile in 1935 was their disappointment with the state of public health during the period of shrinking US financial assistance in nursing programs and nurses in general. It was only after the attack on Pearl Harbor that foreign engagement rose again and then at a faster rate than had previously been seen mainly in the area of public health nursing.

2.4 *The Semblance of Equality: Women in a Cage*

The National census of 1920 showed that only one percent of the professional workforce was female. In healthcare, only 34 in 800 physicians, 66 in 616 dentists, and 182 in 1172 pharmacists were women. Surprisingly, nursing (in a broad sense) was in those days a gender-balanced grouping: 606 men and 923 women were labeled under the heading *enfermeros*.[166] But this does not mean it was a model for equality.

First, it is important not to see nursing in those early stages of development as a unified women's sector in politics and society. Women and men performed as caregivers, the Welfare Board and the University of Chile were involved, some had connections to inter-American cooperation, some did not, there were still a considerable number of Red Cross nurses, etc. Men could be involved in different positions like trainers, deans, ministers, and co-workers in mobile healthcare. But what they all had in common, including the area of public health in both Chile and the US, was their adherence to and promotion of conservative views on gender roles. Nursing was reduced to minor competences and still perceived as a female job.

Public health had the first entirely feminized nursing profile. Zárate (2021) outlines the importance Doctors Mayers, Amaral, and A. Del Río furnished in closing off enrolment in nursing to male students.[167] Although existing male nurses did not disappear, their number shrank constantly. In 1950, only 27 percent of all registered nurses (628 of 1619) were males, likely resulting from the restriction policy and a discourse aimed at the general public depicting nursing work as better fitting for women.[168] Nevertheless, it should be noted that the reduction of university places for men did not affect men with higher administrative responsibilities. As physicians, men could perfectly sit in leading positions in the nursing schools. Until the mid-1940s, those appointed in the headships in Santiago and Valparaíso were, in fact, men. For example, Pincheira and González could aspire to administrative directorships as their only opportunity for promotion.[169] This principle of submission in the public sphere is illustrative of gender relations in all aspects of healthcare. During the first half of the twentieth century, decisions on national and international levels were exclusively undertaken by men; they were the ones who held and represented power, could sit in the highest-ranking posts,[170] and were paid homage through honorary titles and appointments in different societies.

Contemporary discourses of gender disparities in the workplace contrasts to the self-interpretation of nurses working in the early twentieth century. Pincheira, in one of her first articles on behalf of the nursing school of the University of Chile (1934), backed the employment of women in nursing and justified it with an argument that was common back then: "tradition."[171] Similarly, Elianira González's description of nursing was "an interesting profession, feminine par excellence".[172]

In retrospect, nurses were confined in their work in what can be interpreted as a symbolic cage. And although the cage became more spacious, it was a cage nonetheless. Thus, protecting an occupation for women working outside of the home could secure female professionals some financial autonomy. The following passage from the Nursing Association of Chile from 1942 seems to reinforce this view:

> "You are a woman; you can shape the man. When you are a mother. When you are a girlfriend. When you are a wife."[173]

Obviously, though, women in general, including the professionally trained ones, were affected by this scheme of gender relations at the workplace. Midwifery was for González and Zárate (2018) the "oldest female health job" (*más antiguo oficio profesional sanitario femenino*).[174] Since the earliest of days, women helped each other to give birth, a process that is often attached to a mystical connotation. But during midwifery's own institutionalization process, male obstetricians had the last say when it came to giving trained midwives a voice, as scientific medicine expanded into and dominated pregnancy and delivery.

Nursing, medicine, and midwifery were, regarding their preliminary stages, the professions with the longest traditions. However, they took their modern shape during the course of the 1920s, when another healthcare profession was born, the social worker (*asistente social*). This job profile also located social workers in the same symbolic cage. The shift from the old model of charity to the welfare state policy was as modern but also as conservative as the public health model because it consolidated the submission of women.

Until today, two groups of women do not appear in health workforce descriptions. Nursing auxiliaries and female *practicantes*, the most ubiquitous health personnel in Chile, together with physicians, tend not to appear in the literature, as discussed above. Gender-neutral titles like *auxiliar de enfermería* and *practicante* do not enable disaggregating the composition of these large categories. Only in the notes of physicians and nurses, when it came to giving orders to subordinates, either the word "women" or a female ending of a Spanish word would slip out from time to time.[175]

What gender relations, then, did nurses have with auxiliaries and *practicantes*? Based on the archives alone, this question is likely to remain unanswered. Their exchanges were mostly oral; that is, information was disseminated by word of mouth in the wards and classrooms, and quite a few workers may have been illiterate. Primary education became compulsory only in 1920 as the economy industrialized. However, judging by the available descriptions the relationship of nurses to the auxiliary staff mirrored the submission professional nurses experienced in relation to their superiors.

Most of the female professionals did not see auxiliary staff as caregivers but as cleaning staff, and by this, auxiliaries were not supposed to have a say in patients' assessment, planning, or therapy. In practice, though, auxiliaries far outnumbered trained nurses in hospitals, which suggests they performed a large number of clinical tasks, either alone or alongside a nurse or a physician. Even though the subordinate staff represented a majority, university nurses, even being a strong minority, had, too, placed them in another symbolic cage.

As scientific approaches expanded, female work expanded, too. But the process did not evolve just by virtue of scientific discoveries or health policy alone. Rethinking and reshaping, delegating and supervising, and planning and controlling nursing work was thus an area where gender relations and class relations intersected.

2.5 *The Rockefeller Foundation and the Second Era of Public Health Nursing (1941–1952)*

The time between World War II and the Cold War would become a decisive period in Chilean nursing. In the early 1940s, however, this development was not foreseeable. Academically trained nurses represented only a minority among all the institutional caregivers across the country with an average of 315 nurses for 4.9 million inhabitants in 1942.[176] The University of Chile and the schools of the Welfare Board constantly increased the professional workforce from the 1930s on,[177] but nurses were still too few to provide sufficient care, especially according to public health standards.[178] In 1941, a mere 79 nurses graduated from nursing schools;[179] a rather modest figure for a growing and industrializing society, highlighting the subsequent demand for nurses, midwives, and auxiliaries in all areas of healthcare.[180]

Away since 1935, Pincheira's return from Bolivia was long awaited. The first bulletin of the Nursing Association of Chile from 1938 announced that her grand comeback was due to take place in June 1941. Until 1942, however, she divided her time between Bolivia and Chile. Nevertheless, her appointment as the Chilean representative before the International Council of Nurses (ICN) and her ties with the Rockefeller office in

Santiago suggest that there was a strong desire and need to return to her home country.[181] Eventually, family reasons brought her definitively back to Chile, in 1942, as her husband fell sick and she had to resume working to maintain her family.[182]

That was the time the war in Europe escalated and affected both world politics and the world economy. The documentation of the Ministry of Health suggests an expectation of worsening healthcare services as a direct consequence of this for the Americas.[183] Thus, the need for healthcare professionals continued to grow. The international reach of the war sped up the internationalization of healthcare and thus of the academic women who felt they could be important actors in this struggle for public health and hospital nursing.[184] Officers at Rockefeller became the most influential co-operators.[185] Its IHC started projects with universities and healthcare providers in Argentina, Chile, Uruguay, Paraguay, Peru, Ecuador, and Bolivia,[186] assigning to Chile a key role in the region.

Pincheira was one of the 10 to 20 Chilean nurses who, by then, had graduated in public health training programs from Johns Hopkins, Yale, Columbia, Harvard, and Toronto.[187] Through exchange programs subsidized by US foundations, notably Rockefeller,[188] she became the ideal contact partner for international projects. They were not long in appearing. Soon after the US entered the war, IHC advisors visited Chile to start a permanent cooperation in order to promote public health nursing.

Mary Elizabeth Tennant[189] coordinated the nursing department of the IHC. In December 1941, she visited Chile together with Rockefeller's Head of the Andean region, Lewis Hackett, and his wife. Throughout 11 days, they did field observations in various hospitals and the four nursing schools.[190] They heard about poor standards of hygiene in medical facilities, the unwillingness of Chilean women to work as public health nurses, and nurses' complete subservience to physicians.

Six months later, Tennant sent another nursing consultant, Elizabeth W. Brackett (graduate of the universities of Columbia and Johns Hopkins), to the Southern region of Latin America. Brackett's task was to prepare a detailed plan for cooperation with the nursing schools, the universities, and the Welfare Board.[191]

Brackett, who previously worked in the slums of Harlem, NY City, described the situation in Chile worse than anything she had ever seen.[192] Soon after, she canceled her plans to sojourn for a longer time in the other four countries she was in charge of. Hackett agreed that Brackett stayed working mostly in Santiago during the following two years.[193] There, she reinforced the IHC team of John H. Janney (Johns Hopkins University) who had arrived shortly before her. Together, they set up the first IHC office in South America in Santiago. Their task was to open a public health school and a public health unit (*unidad sanitaria*) in the suburbs of Santiago,[194] meant to be the ports of entry of a public health system, which in the first place would serve neighborhoods barely covered by medical care.

Together with the directorate of the Welfare Board, they chose *Quinta Normal*, one of the poorest boroughs in Santiago, as the place for a pilot project for the subcontinent.[195] Brackett and Janney put a group of five public health nurses together to run the health unit of *Quinta Normal* in 1943. On her return from Bolivia, Pincheira was the most obvious choice for the post of head nurse.[196]

In the first two years, Pincheira and Brackett worked closely together. They did a door-to-door survey in the whole district and planned the education and care of the inhabitants based on the gathered data. Co-financed by the Welfare Board and the IHC,[197] the health unit provided services in the *materno-infantil* area and educational work about sexually transmitted diseases, set up new health units, and ran vaccination programs.[198]

The most prominent feature of the public health nurse in *Quinta Normal* was the *maletín sanitario*, the leather bag of supplies that nurses carried during each visit.[199] In her dissertation about Chilean nursing in the first half of the twentieth century, nurse-historian Jeannine Uribe (2008) described the use of the bag as follows:

> "The technique involved keeping the inside of the bag and its contents as clean as possible even when things such as thermometers, soap, and dressings were removed from it for use on the patient. The lack of disposable items meant everything had to be cleaned before being replaced in the bag and going on to the next visit. The technique was judged especially important because of the sanitary problems in the homes of the poor and the need to prevent the spread of communicable diseases. Brackett used the bag technique as a measure of how quickly a Chilean nurse grasped public health nursing."[200]

In an interview for a recent study on nursing history in Chile, a former nursing student described the procedures they used to teach patients and their families how to stop the spread of diseases through droplets, as follows:

"They taught me how to get to the houses, how to hush the dogs [...] never do this or that, and to prepare a clean workplace, aseptic to put the nursing briefcase, to show them [patient and family] how to wash their hands, because there was no town water in most of the houses. All those things of that time. I think that we, as nurses, were marked by that experience."[201]

Public health nursing was even wider in scope than its description of mostly technical tasks. The unmeasured and unrecorded emotional work public health nurses did in the homes inevitably became the biggest challenge for women like Pincheira. In an interview with researchers Núñez et al., a nurse recalled:

"They told me that the husbands not only bate their wives, that they were even sexually abused by the husband... Horrible! Because I'd never heard of this part. Back then, these things were not spoken of. Nurses never talked about that. It was a delicate subject, until we grew and understood."[202]

Social work was the third important task for the women who decided to take on the challenge and follow on from the example of Pincheira and Brackett. Its combination of medicine and nursing, theoretical and practical, connected to the needs of the patients and rooted in North American standards, was the reason why the *Quinta Normal* project became a lighthouse project in national healthcare. Students of different health professions, female and male, received their practical training in *Quinta Normal*. While in hospitals equality was still at premium in administrative ranks, the project of sanitary units was of cultural significance as it was a system where women helped other women, which remained the most common way for them to receive care. Students and professionals alike learned from women-led organizational models. In the slums of Santiago, the pragmatic approach of *salud pública* thus helped overcome conservative gender roles.

The success and the comparatively well-documented international project in Santiago's suburbs was probably why Chile would become the standard bearer of public health nursing in Latin America, which obscured eventual drawbacks in common narratives. Since its start in 1942, nurses from several South American countries came to visit the project.[203] Within two years the system of the health units had been fully established. Brackett had succeeded with her pilot project and returned to New York.[204] However, it was only another step on the way to a full healthcare coverage for everyone. Health units remained rare exceptions in undersupplied regions.

In June 1944, Pincheira spoke in a conference organized by the IHC-founded Public Health School (*Escuela de Salubridad*) about the role of the nurse in *salud pública*. The numbers she presented showed that Chile was still far from the gold standard set for national public health nursing. Understaffing indeed undermined the project. Since 1906, from the 1038 nurses who had graduated, only 204 specialized in this area.[205] Consequently, many dedicated positions had to be allocated to interim personnel,[206] likely *practicantes* and nursing auxiliaries. Regarding this, Pincheira's description of the major tasks in public health nursing for the entire country appears to be more like a "vision," rather than a road map.[207]

The year Pincheira took over the lead of the *Quinta Normal* unit, Gladys Peake—also a fellow but seven years her younger—left for Canada to undertake master's studies in Toronto (1942–1944).[208] She entered this through the selective circle of Chilean nurses who studied abroad.[209] Born in 1910 near the Peruvian border, Peake moved with her family to Valparaíso, where she went to school and trained as a nurse. She was one of the first graduates of the Carlos Van Buren Nursing School in 1937, becoming its director in the same year.[210] In one of her first published essays, Peake agreed with Pincheira's vision and pictured the public health nurse, referring to her as *enfermera visitadora*, as evidence for nurses' claims to be the most important caregiver of 1940s Chile.[211]

In contrast to Pincheira, commitment to party politics would become an essential and constant factor in Peake's career. Before moving to Canada, she had been a candidate for the Socialist Party[212] in Valparaíso, a reason for several physicians to dissuade the IHC to hire her as the head nurse for the *Quinta Normal* health unit in 1942.[213] While in North America, Peake went through an astonishing change of her political persuasions and upon return became an influential rightist woman.[214] No other nurse had, or showed, such a strong relationship with the RF/IHC and the dedication to anti-Marxism and anti-Communism, all at the same time, and the determination of a political life after her stay in North America.[215] It is possible that other nurses were also enthused by this political influence, although those who appeared in written sources, most importantly Pincheira, did not disclose their political views explicitly nor tried to climb in the political party system, as did Peake. This shows that North American scholarships brought Latin American nurses into contact with ideologies and discourses that were common in US society during the Cold War era.

Chile became a major location for projects, although the IHC also managed to educate several other Latin American nurses into leaders in schools and political representatives. During the 1940s, the council with its headquarters in Santiago implemented at least the basic elements of public health in most of the nursing programs in the Americas.[216] This was done in collaboration with the already introduced IIAA, as a direct aid by the US government, the US-dominated PAHO, and the Kellogg Foundation, also specializing in public health nursing.[217]

In comparison with international developments, the narrow country on the *Cono Sur* became a blueprint for the development policy of the US. The Chilean health policy with its focus on nursing was extraordinary as a tryout for the rest of South America, and the impact of the IHC in Chile lasted longer than it did in Argentina,[218] Uruguay, and Paraguay.[219]

Accommodating public health nurses with North American degrees came along with new developments in self-organization of Chilean nurses, a process induced by a growing culture of associationism in the country. The nursing association was founded in 1938, and in June 1941 the association published the first issue of its bulletin[220] propagating the public health nurse as the role model for the profession.[221] However, as in the case of the Quinta Normal Health Unit, which started four years later, the effort extended only to the outer limits of Santiago. In the first half of the 1940s, during the presidency of Graciela Arcaya, Luisa Arcaya, Hilda Lozier, [222] and Luisa Instroza,[223] the impact of public health on national nursing policy was not measurable, the reasons for which seem to be at least partly political.

At the beginning of the 1940s, Chile was politically unstable. Nurses had to adapt to the left-wing government of the Popular Front (*Frente Popular*). As Aguirre held power for such a short time (1938–1941) he and his team could not introduce any new nursing policy. At least, like its planned national health service, the law was not passed at the congress. Then, as already mentioned, the Radical Party (*Partido Radical*) won the 1942 elections. The previous ten years had brought the stability for nurses to organize a national network and an international network.

In 1942, the University of Chile celebrated its centennial. The nursing association took advantage of the international attention this attracted and organized simultaneously the First Pan American Nursing Congress (*Primer Congreso Panamericano de Enfermería*).[224] Hilda Lozier invited her colleagues to Santiago. The start of the war was still fresh, but the Latin American nurses, probably inspired by the cooperation with advisors like Brackett, used the international stage to promote confidence in the US leadership. Ana Maria Dias, representative of the Brazilian nursing association, first related to the generalized fear of the fast-spreading warfare but finished her speech with the following words: "God save Chile! God save the united American nations! God save the Americas!"[225] On the same note, the author of an article in the Bulletin of the Nursing Association of Chile (1943) called all nurses to their posts (*¡Ocupa tu puesto!*) and emphasized it with another appeal:

> "We live the hardest and strangest period humanity has ever experienced. We are heading into the unknown. Woman, get ready! Be a nurse and understand better those around you. Understanding is a synonym of love, and that is what we need. Get to know each other that much. The following generations, which are training today, will need tomorrow a guide, and that guide will be you, nurse [...] your intelligence, your love as a mother, your spirit of sacrifice, your unquestionable kindness."[226]

In 1944, Peake moved back to Valparaíso, possibly resuming the directorate of the nursing school. She published several articles to further publicize the nursing profession and eventually became the president of the regional branch of the nursing association.[227] There, she also started her career as an author in what would later become some form of nursing scholarship. Along with her colleagues, she proposed a study plan of 4 years of university education for all the existing nursing schools and a 10-month training program for nursing auxiliaries. Both were designed for nationwide implementation.[228]

Peake's closest partner in the nursing association was Rosalba Flores.[229] Like Peake, Flores had worked as a head nurse and gained her master's degree in Toronto. Once back in Chile, she became a nursing teacher in the University of Chile.[230] Having campaigned actively within the women's suffrage movement of 1947,[231] she led one year thereafter the organization of the first Chilean nursing congress in Concepción.

As units had until then operated in isolation from each other, the 1948 gathering of representatives of the operating nursing units was a skillful and strategic maneuver of Flores and Peake, together with other organizers like Elianira González, Garciela Arcaya, Luisa Arcaya, and Hilda Lozier. They planned the event to be held in Concepción. Their guests of honor, the provosts of the University of Chile and the University of Concepción, valued the initiative and the outcome, and they were members of the accreditation body of the new nursing school. The presence of international delegations, consisting of Janney, Tennant, and Hirst representing the IHC, and Theodore Gandy for the IIAA,[232] would amplify the attention the "Chilean role model in nursing" was having internationally.

The nursing congress was a bright but short beacon, and the founding of a new Welfare Board nursing school in the same year and the same town produced a longer-term impact.[233] After a break of 13 years,[234] the expansion of academic nursing continued, but this time right from the beginning in the garb of public health and led by a woman. These improvements are attributable to Peake, the founding director.[235] With almost a decade of experience as the head of the equivalent institution in Valparaíso, in the following years she would elevate Concepción to the second rung of academic nursing with a focus on public health in Chile.

At first glance, the school in Concepción stood exclusively in the tradition of the foundations of the Welfare Board in Santiago (1919 and 1935) and Valparaíso (1933). It sent four physicians and only three nurses to set up the new school.[236] But this was the first and last time physicians were mentioned in the context of this institution. It would seem that Peake took control right from the beginning. Even though the male-dominated medical profession was involved, Concepción became, after the *Quinta Normal*, the second lighthouse project of female nurses.

Another achievement of Chilean nurses as a female collective was the complete takeover of the nursing school of the University of Chile by female faculties during the mid-1940s. Contradictory accounts about the exact year (from 1944 to 1947) and the name of the first director (probably Flores) lead to the conjecture that it needed a long transition period until the university authorities finally decided to hand over the school from male physicians' control.[237] Nevertheless, that was only the second step on the long way toward female emancipation and self-determination within the academic system. For the school was but a division of the medical faculty, and thus led overall by male physicians.

Flores was then leading the most prestigious nursing institution in the country. Even though it is not clear when precisely she started to chair it, be it 1944, 1947, or 1957,[238] it is clear that from 1943 her powers extended so prominently not only in nursing education but also in the nursing association and the government. Except in the area of international relations, where Pincheira and Peake were representatives,[239] Flores crafted the public image of Chile's nurses for about 30 years. Ultimately, in 1965, she enshrined her own memories and the memory of other nurses in such a rapidly changing society by publishing a book on nursing history.[240]

It was also in the mid-1960s that nurses' lobbying reached its highest display of power. Nursing, alongside its professionalizing project, was then an inherent part of the growing public health system. Parallel to the increasing US engagement, the university degree program became part of all major academic institutions throughout the country. In 1950, Brackett supervised the founding of a nursing school at the Catholic Church's university in Santiago.[241] One year later, the government finally approved a nationwide study plan drafted in 1947, edited by Peake, and implemented it in the four nursing schools. From then on, the studies increased to four years, with three years of basic education and a one-year qualification in public health. Midwives entertained this increase, too, although it took longer for them to see actual changes. Similarly, the training of nursing auxiliaries was set to 10 months, with an optional extension of three to four months to train in public health as well.[242]

Unlike Peake, it would seem that Pincheira was not interested in developing a nationwide curriculum, not even in the affairs of the nursing association. Her focus was much wider and concerned establishing professional nursing in other Spanish-speaking countries, many of which had cooperation agreements with PAHO, right after Rockefeller's support ended in the early 1950s. As the health units proliferated in Chile,[243] Pincheira wanted to implement the same principle in other countries. For example, Pincheira advised María Elena Ramos Mejía, whose school pioneered the introduction of academic training for nurses in Argentina.[244]

Pincheira and Lozier promoted PAHO's nursing division in several Latin American countries during the 1940s, 1950s, and 1960s.[245] Begun 20 years earlier by Long and Adams, spreading the PAHO nursing policy took Chilean nursing and nurses to a whole new level of female networking in the subcontinent. For the first time, nurses and international advisors belonged to the same cultural area.

2.6 All Goals Achieved? The Nursing Law of 1953

For nursing policy and politics, 1953 was a crucial year. Until then, all proposed approaches in public or private health as well as the organizations and conferences, national and international, of women who worked in this profession developed in separate ways. The transition of the association into a *colegio profesional*, a parastatal authority, canalized all efforts to create an equivalent to the medical profession by unifying the elite nurses in a national council.

The national congress of nurses and the foundation of the nursing school in Concepción seemed to have increased the credibility and authority of Chile's international role in the academic nursing networks of the Americas. In 1951, its nursing association took the lead by hosting a six-week PAHO workshop. They met in Viña del Mar with nurses from Argentina, Brazil, Colombia, Panama, Uruguay, and Peru.[246] The system of the public health units, even on a very low level compared to the auxiliary workforce, had been established, and nurses like Pincheira, Peake, or Lozier were very keen on forwarding stable female work relations.

In 1953, the nursing elite founded the *Colegio de Enfermeras de Chile* (*CECh*), which replaced the former association.[247] Its legal basis was public law. It defined nursing standards, established that the Ministry of Health and the council of the nursing association would be the main nursing policy-makers, and confirmed the university examination and membership in the association as the prerequisites to enter the public healthcare system. From then on, and up until 1980, nursing bodies became legally bound to both the state administration and the NHS.

Although similar nursing associations appeared in other South American countries during the same time span, for example 1954 in Brazil[248] and 1957 in Argentina,[249] Chilean law laid the foundations of the most far-reaching cooperation of nurses with state authorities. State collaboration embedded nursing views and lobbying in health policy-making in many governmental institutions. Yet, nowhere was nurses' influence as strong in daily politics as it was in the NHS Nursing Division (*Sección de Enfermería*), where Peake was sitting as the founding director.[250] Although easy to miss in current accounts, from a gender perspective the law enabled for the first time a public entity that was fully independent from male control. Nurses represented other nurses on a governmental level. Pincheira became the first president of the *CECh*,[251] but due to her commitment to PAHO, she only remained in office for a short time.

However, this new institutionality of the nursing profession still lacked an important component—a staffing policy. Even though the number of graduates nationwide rose from 79 to 133 per year between 1941 and 1950,[252] this was still insignificant for the 181 NHS facilities in need of nurses.[253] Equally critical in the project, and despite nursing leaders' praise, the scant number of public health nurses for the entire country (113 by 1952)[254] suggests that the *CECh* represented only a minority of caregivers. The reasons for this may have been a persistent shortage of nurses, but also strict requirements to apply for a place in university, the unattractive working conditions, or the conservative attitudes toward women working outside the home.

On the other hand, the 1950s would witness Peake's fast gain in power. She was representing Chile on an international stage as a PAHO advisor.[255] Much as she never led long-term projects abroad like Pincheira, Peake's high-profile persona and her engagement in a number of committees and bodies of the *CECh* were probably why senior nurses still refer to her as *la jefa* or "the boss" of the nursing profession.[256] It is not clear in which year Peake rose as the director of the *CECh*, and in which other capacities she represented the association until the 1970s,[257] when she would become its general secretary. But as she was also the first and only person to lead the NHS Nursing division and the education program for nursing auxiliaries,[258] she was able to shape the nursing legislature more than any other nurse before her.

Most of the other caring professions followed nurses' example. Social workers (1955),[259] midwives (1962),[260] laboratory technicians,[261] and physical therapists (1970)[262] were also able to influence lawmaking for their associations' statutes. One noticeable outcome was that the academic institutions delivered the diplomas together with membership cards for the respective professional associations to the graduates. In order to be eligible for a position within the NHS or *SERMENA*, membership was mandatory, too—the state was by far the largest employer in healthcare.

The new status of the *CECh* was perceived as a recognition from the state and represented an important part of nurses' lives and thus key to their shared memory. And, in spite of that, the figure of minister Allende as an instigator of the NHS law and the governments of the Radical Party as supporters of nursing within that ideal quickly faded away. What remained in their collective memory is that nurses could make a significant advancement in the direction of vindication and social equality. Nurses, as many other women, had voted for Ibáñez, and it was under his government when they could shape for the first time the authority they had been granted. This was an important reason for their leaders to refuse to cooperate with the Socialist and Radical parties when they came back to power in 1970.

Important for cross-national policy analysis, university-trained nurses benefitted from the new institutional arrangements, but they were a small elite within the larger set of nursing caregivers, which makes comparison difficult by language usage alone. In 1960, the health system counted upon some 1299 active nurses and about 11,000 nursing auxiliaries,[263] where auxiliaries received little or no attention from politicians. Mostly training in practical matters, women who became auxiliaries were kept in a status of servant-like workers and subject to the NHS Nursing division.[264]

Born to a modest family in Santiago, Ivette Cap de Ville was a nursing auxiliary who started off in the 1950s. Her parents sometimes could not even cover their daily expenses, let alone provide their daughter with a university education. She faced not just structural obstacles like economic hardship and traditional gender roles, but also struggled to finish secondary school and manage personal life and family obligations. And so, care work would allow her to find jobs right away. In 1957, she joined a hospital in Santiago. By the age of eighteen she worked in the pediatric unit, before even having any relevant training—oftentimes, in a job like that, women like her learned by watching others. Nurses would rarely make an appearance in the wards, and instead, coordinated work from an office desk.[265] This was typical of the Taylorist model of management—not only the nurse-to-auxiliary ratio would explain this "distancing," but also nurses' efforts to achieve industry-like efficiency. What Cap de Ville's story illustrates though is how the institutionalization of nursing within the health system reflected wider dynamics of the sector as well as structural social divides, both of which turned nursing into a disjointed field.

All in all, by the time nurses had reached a peak of political influence, in 1953, this was felt like a mission accomplished. Ever since their association came to exist, the work done at strengthening the profession's institutional form seemed to have paid off. Maturity and consolidation would henceforth be needed. Rockefeller started to withdraw its nursing program from Chile,[266] moving its focus to Peru and Europe.[267] Losing such a key player was to be compensated by the engagement of PAHO and the UN.[268] In retrospect, this transition left no mark. Chilean nursing was in control of what, in the oral tradition, is still remembered as the "golden age of nursing."

2.7 *The "Golden Age" of Nursing? 1960s Policy and Politics*

Historical accounts on nursing in Chile have been strongly influenced by the reflections of men and women who experienced the political and social upheaval of the 1970s. In retrospect, most of them refer to the preceding years as the "golden age" of Chilean nursing.[269] Even though this optimism would match perfectly the reforming spirit of the Christian Democratic government, the following analysis will show that the key developments, most importantly the becoming of a nationwide established profession, had already begun when Frei came to power.

The 1960s started with the most extensive study about education and employment of nurses, written by Doris Krebs Wilkens. In 1961, the NHS and the PAHO published the resulting report titled "Needs and Resources of Nursing in Chile" (*Necesidades y Recursos de Enfermería en Chile*).[270]

Like Lozier and Peake, Krebs completed her master's degree in public health in Canada, and pursued another master's in nursing education at Columbia, and eventually became Chile's first nurse to hold a PhD degree. After returning to Chile, she was promoted to the position of head nurse.[271] While other nurses used similar career paths to reduce their scope of duties to a regional level, Krebs always tried to look at the larger picture. She maintained her contacts with the PAHO to fulfill her project of a national nursing poll. It was a tragic coincidence that helped her to attract the attention of the world to the focus of her investigation, the nursing situation outside of Santiago.

In 1960, the earth trembled in the southern city of Valdivia. Essential infrastructures such as hospitals, universities, health centers, schools, and roads were either severely damaged or rendered inoperable throughout the entirety of two neighbor regions. Even the nursing school in Concepción was affected by the event.[272] Overnight, state and private organizations worldwide set out to help the people affected by the most powerful earthquake in recorded history. It was the first time large foreign aid went far from the capital. But the aid was not enough. Soon, the need for more nurses to work in the field became apparent.

In 1963, the nursing school of Austral University of Chile was founded out of a pilot project after the quake.[273] The curriculum was drafted by Krebs and implemented together with the PAHO study board.[274] The Valdivia earthquake had turned out to be the last step to establishing the academic model of nursing in all major universities. [275] The founding of nursing schools expanded soon after to the University of Chile's branches in Temuco (1963), Antofagasta (1964), La Serena (1964), and Talca (1966).[276] It is unknown whether the study plan was implemented in all the new schools. But it would seem that the school boards worked independently of the central administration during the 1960s and 1970s.[277]

Krebs' poll also pushed for movements in nursing scholarship. Since 1960, the University of Chile awarded the first degree in administration of public health nursing (*licenciado en administración de enfermería de salud pública*). In 1962, members of the *CECh* founded the Chilean Association for Nursing Education (*Asociación Chilena de Educación en Enfermería, ACHIEEN*). Its pro bono members, like those at *CECh*, wanted to adopt the proposed curriculum. They anticipated a growing number of nursing students[278] and new developments in the nursing discipline. In fact, a peak in the local nursing literature was reached in 1965.[279] And with that, a graduate program in nursing was established for the first time in South America.

At that time, a new generation of nurses became rather active in the public sphere and their names began to resonate more widely. Perhaps, it was believed, they could gradually replace the nursing "pioneers" someday. In 1962, Patricia Talloni finished training at the University of Chile and was granted *CECh* membership, by which time she had already met Pincheira and Peake. During the 1950s and 1960s, both of them, alongside other elite nurses, had visited the nursing schools in order to promote the association's work. Talloni found her first job in the city of La Serena. From 1963 to 1970, she worked in one of the few *SERMENA* facilities in this area. She simultaneously began teaching at the local branch of the University of Chile, where she also gained her master's degree in public health.[280]

During the 1960s, women like Talloni, who devoted their lives to nursing, indeed studied and worked in one of the few female-dominated sectors. Unlike a couple of decades earlier, a hundred percent of the nurses who took Krebs' poll were women,[281] and according to her analysis, all of them had been taught by other females.[282] With this, the training seemed to complete the transition to women-only teaching staff. Likewise, the nursing association was one of the few bodies of political representation for women. By this, the *CECh* created a microcosm for middle-class women where they could speak for themselves and take a stance for their collective interests.[283]

The *CECh* was the political circle and space of the nursing elite. As explained, since the early 1950s it was controlled by Peake.[284] Together with Flores and Nora Fardella, both in the directorate of the University of Chile nursing school,[285] and Krebs as the most prominent nursing researcher,[286] Peake used the association to demand better wages and working conditions. Those were goals younger colleagues like Talloni agreed on. But they had different ideas about the type of society they wanted, for the association, for nurses, and for other fellow Chileans.

Different from the US-inspired anti-Communist sentiment, many younger nursing leaders felt attracted to the growing left-wing movements and parties in Latin America that arose after the Cuban revolution. One's political positioning, like Marxism, Catholicism, or, in the specific case of Chile, *gremialismo*, would become significant at work as well as in social life, especially during Frei's presidency.

After beginning on a high note, the linkages between nurses' plans and the policies of the Christian Democrats soon deteriorated. Policies started with the old vision of a health system that was universally accessible. As we have seen, Frei and health minister Valdivieso did introduce reforms, but they also backed the existing state institutions. Accordingly, a central point of nurses' strategy was cooperating with the conservative elites, mostly graduates from the University of Chile and the Catholic University.

Following the advice of his late sister Irene, Frei achieved concrete results where general staffing policy is concerned. In the first half of the term, the administration had secured additional jobs for some 272 nursing auxiliaries, 24 midwives, and 118 nurses.[287] However, this measure was not enough to satisfy the need for care in the country—the fast-growing population surpassed the services any health center could provide.[288]

By the beginning of the Christian Democratic government, Pincheira had 45 years of work experience and was one of the oldest nurses still in service in the country. But her engagement in the *CECh* was marginal compared to the work of Flores, Peake, Fardella, and Lozier. Pincheira's main attainment was a still functioning international network. In 1967, she joined the circle of founders of the Pan American Federation of Nursing Professionals (*Federación Panamericana de Profesionales de Enfermería, FEPPEN*).[289]

Pincheira's project was intended to intensify international networking that had started in 1942 with the first Latin American congress of nurses.[290] But just like 15 years earlier, the South American nursing organization was still in its early stages, primarily becoming a bilateral project between Argentina and Chile[291] with Pincheira as the lead.[292] The national network of academic nurses was better developed but not as well documented. A continuous reporting was needed to unify the widespread nursing centers and promote the public health concept.

The year of 1965 saw the issuing of a permanent publication, *Enfermería* (Nursing), which was edited by the *CECh*. Since the July edition of 1966, Peake was the editor-in-chief.[293] Even though Pincheira authored the editorials, *Enfermería* was first and foremost Peake's top career ladder. She coordinated the nursing section of the NHS, decisively contributed to the work of the nursing association, and then also became the most important voice in academic nursing.

The improvements for the *CECh*, and for nursing and other female health professions during the Christian Democratic administration,[294] were unmistakable. Since 1967, the *CECh* joined the advisory body of the health minister,[295] increased its influence over the nursing auxiliaries,[296] and backed advanced training in pediatrics.[297] Its involvement furthered the development of the national study plan[298] and improved the settings for teachers in the nursing schools.[299] Like never before, nurses organized various scientific groups, congresses, and conventions.[300] The involvement in international organizations led to regular attendance to nursing conferences in the Americas and Europe by *CECh* representatives.[301]

Nevertheless, the nursing association continued to fail in one very key project: establishing fees for nurses' services within the *Medicina Curativa* plan. In 1968, *CECh* president Marilia Fonseca was little more than an observer of the law enactment and implementation.[302] The nurses were invited to watch and discuss,[303] but did not reach better service fees or a higher tariff scale (i.e., Law No. 15.076).

Negotiations were almost at a standstill, and the success of another female profession would lower the spirits even more. In 1968, the midwifery profession eventually extended the studies from three to four years. During the first two years, students attended the same courses as nursing students.[304] Under obstetricians' rule for so long, midwifery was back then a young profession in terms of professional training, but it would soon be granted access to the benefits of Law No. 15.076. With that, nursing leaders lost their trust in the government. Even though they kept polite relations with political authorities,[305] they no longer saw the parliamentarians as trustworthy stakeholders.[306]

Another problem for the nursing leads grew from bottom-up. Since 1964, nursing students grew ever more indifferent toward the *CECh*,[307] which is to say some 1725 nurses and 1084 nursing students drifting apart.[308] Many students resented the inability of senior nurses to move the association further forward, which turned this high reputation institution into a tired, static one. Young, politically active nurses, like Talloni, did not see the association as a place for self-realization as women in Chilean society. Even less so in national politics. However, during the 1960s, the unrest among the younger nurses remained under the façade of a united profession.[309] One likely reason being the upcoming atmosphere of strikes and protests by the end of Frei's government.

The participation of nurses in the 1963 health worker strike and their reaction toward the government during the physicians' strike in 1970 are not well documented. However, it is very likely that nurses were directly involved in broader activism and work stoppages. And the effect on nurses' demands appears to be minor. Further agendas and outcomes in nursing policy are not evident, mediated by a wait-and-see attitude after the 1970 election.

Whether the 1960s were the "golden age" of nursing remains open to interpretation. Before the 1960s, the shortage and maldistribution of nurses, especially public health nurses, and after the 1960s the violent confrontations in the streets, may have well influenced a perception of a prosperous era for nurses in between two difficult periods. Understabdably, history has shown that disheartening events for the nation's morale, like the year 1973 in Chile, are likely to shape a narrative of a golden age. One such event can divide an entire nation just like it can divide the nurses, where preceding epochs feel more comfortable if looked upon with rose-tinted glasses.

3 Conclusion

During the first 70 years of the twentieth century, Chile was affected by contagious diseases, most tragically tuberculosis, and respiratory and gastrointestinal infections.[310] Even influenza viruses and coliform bacteria took the lives of hundreds of thousands of people in Latin America, most commonly women of childbearing age and children. Malnutrition, lack of education, and political as well as social conflicts caused by the economic downturn during World War II and the early Cold War were part of the backdrop of healthcare policy, with nursing becoming a health reform in its own right.

What can we learn from this history today? Over 100 years after the *question sociale* and the setting up of the modern health institutions, the question of how healthcare and professions as collectives are connected within national politics through wider societal issues, such as gender and class relations, still bears unique significance for policy-making. Despite common beliefs, the idea of developing the institutionality of health as monopolized by male physicians is highly debatable, as this research demonstrates.

Nurses were not mere recipients or executors of a model of public health. They actively sought training for themselves, gave training for other nurses, organized primary care units, proposed and lobbied for an appropriate salary structure to attract nurses, and advocated for a suitable staffing policy across the country both nationally and internationally. They also crafted an image of nursing as a suitable place for women in society, and as such defined, protected, and promoted an area where women could have financial autonomy. By this, they called into question a patriarchal decision-making tradition.

While university-trained nursing grew socially detached from a very large workforce of uneducated auxiliaries doing nursing work, nurses' development relied on that work, and this development intertwined class and gender relations that mirrored broader social dynamics. Similarly, the work in the community intersected with volunteer women working in, for example, the Red Cross, while female volunteering became an integral part of Chile's welfare state project. Importantly, female work was not a provisory strategy to just reduce infections; it set the foundations of a contemporary system aiming to provide an equal and affordable healthcare, where long-term education and healthcare staffing policies were as key as it was placing the new health professions, like public health nurses and social workers, in strategically chosen places. Any nursing policy today might thus consider this systemic perspective.

On a macro level, other developments facilitated the centrality of female work in healthcare policy. The two most important ones were Chile's cultural ambience wherein a middle-class consciousness challenged the old charity model of welfare of the nineteenth century, and increasing international trade that enabled policy transfer and cultural expansionism from the Anglo-Saxon world to Chile. This also framed Chile as a developing economy, compared to Bolivia or Haiti, for instance, and by extension, fed the reputation of its healthcare and nursing systems. But more importantly, the case highlights the co-dependence of systems where health and social equality are concerned.

Notes

1. In this publication, the entity that represented nurses' collective interests is generally refered to as nurses' association, *colegio professional, Colegio de Enfermeras de Chile*, or simply *CECh*.
2. Barr-Melej, Patrick. Reforming Chile: Cultural politics, nationalism, and the rise of the middle class. Univ of North Carolina Press, 2002.

In 1970, 58 percent of Chileans were younger than 25 years old. Santiago was and is by far the largest Chilean city. In 1970, 3.4 million lived in the capital, 9.7 million in the entire country. Instituto Nacional de Estadísticas: Censos 1970–1982.

3. Still during the 1960s, 100 out of 1000 babies died before they reached six months of age, in: Thibaut, Bernhard: Soziale Entwicklung und Demokratie in Lateinamerika zu Beginn der neunziger Jahre, in: Lateinamerika am Ende des 20. Jahrhunderts [Ed. Junker, Detlef; Nohlen, Dieter; Sangmeister, Hartmut], München [C.H. Beck] 1994, p. 124-148, 139.

   Ramacciotti describes the disastrous impact of contagious diseases in Argentina, in: Ramacciotti, Karina Inés: El cuidado sanitario. Hacia una historia de la enfermería en Argentina, in: Historias de la enfermería en Argentina. Pasado y presente de una profesión [Ed. Ramacciotti, Karina Inés], Buenos Aires [EDUNPAZ] 2020, p. 29-66, 45.
4. Almandoz, Arturo: Modernización urbana en América Latina. De las grandes aldeas a las metrópolis masificadas, Santiago [Ril] 2018, p. 160-161.
5. The bubonic plague in Latin America, in: Armus, Diego: Disease in the History of Modern Latin America: From Malaria to AIDS, New York [Duke University Press] 2003.
6. Regarding the disastrous health conditions, Chile was not a particular case in Latin America, in: Armus (2003).

   In 1922, even the Ministry of Health described the provision of healthcare in Chile as "precarious," in: Dirección General de Sanidad: Informes de la comisión designada por el gobierno para estudiar los servicios sanitarios, Santiago 1922, http://www.memoriachilena.gob.cl/archivos2/pdfs/MC0027674.pdf [05.05.2022].
7. Behn Theune, Verónica; Ortiz Rebolledo, Nestor; Valenzuela Suazo, Sandra: Nursing in Chile, in: Nursing and Globalization in the Americas. A Critical Perspective. [Ed. Karen Lucas Breda; Ray Elling], Amityville, N.Y. [Baywood Pub. Co.] 2009, p. 55-98, 73.

   Cruz-Coke painted a more positive picture, stating that by the end of the 1920s, the number of beds offered in the hospitals was sufficient, in: Cruz-Coke Madrid, Ricardo: Historia de la Medicina Chilena, Santiago [Ed. Andrés Bello] 1995, p. 531.
8. Interview with the midwives Ernestina Valdebenito Lizama and María Inés Zavala Lehuede, Santiago, February 2017.
9. Desarrollo y dinámica de la población en el siglo XX: Baja de las tasas de mortalidad infantil, http://www.memoriachilena.gob.cl/602/w3-article-93237.html [05.05.2022].
10. Cruz-Coke (1995), p. 532.

11. In 1940, 200 out of 1000 newborn babies died. After 1950, that fugure lowered to around 40 of 1000, in: Ibid.
12. Díaz-Cayeros, Alberto: Federalism, Fiscal Authority, and Centralization in Latin America, Cambridge [Cambridge University Press] 2006, p. 233.
13. Letter of the Intendant of Valdivia from 1935. Only the University of Chile was entitled to issue the professional degree of a midwife, in: Ministerio de Salubridad Pública: Oficio No. 167, 167-84-1935, 16.03.1935, 1-1 [1/3].
14. Political instability was a general trait of Latin American countries until the 1990s. Mauricio Cárdenas from the Brookings Institution (Washington, D.C.) defined it as a "generally low state capacity," in: Cárdenas, Mauricio: State capacity in Latin America, in: *Economía*, Vol. 10, No. 2, 2010, p. 1-45, 33.
15. One important step before the 1920s constitutional and health reforms was the first Sanitary Code from 1890, in: Raczynski, Dagmar: Social policies in Chile. Origin, transformations and perspectives, in: Democracy and social policy series, Working Paper No. 4, Santiago [CIEPLAN] 1994, p. 7.

    González and Zárate state that the ideas for those laws were promoted for the first time by the political "conservatives," especially the physician Exequiel González Cortés, in: González Moya, Maricela; Zárate Campos, María Soledad: Profesionales modernas y carismáticas: enfermeras y visitadoras sociales en la construcción del Estado Asistencial en Chile, 1900-1930, in: Niterói, V. 24, No. 2, 2018, p. 369-387, 374.
16. Nohlen used the term "middle class" to describe a similar element of Argentinean, Uruguayan, and Chilean societies, in: Nohlen, Dieter: Lateinamerika zwischen Diktatur und Demokratie, in: Lateinamerika am Ende des 20. Jahrhunderts [Ed. Junker et al.], München [C.H. Beck] 1994, p. 12-26.
17. Noemi Girbal-Blacha (1998) describes the situation in Argentina as a "restricted democracy," in: Girbal-Blache, Noemi M.: Política, Economía y Sociedad en la Argentina del Siglo XX. Una Aproximación Histórica a sus Continuidades y Cambios., in: CUYO. Anuario de Filosofía Argentina y Americana, No. 15, 1998, p. 11-22, 13.
18. More information about the national congresses, in: Zárate, María Soledad: Formar enfermeras, no empleadas domésticas. Profesionalización del cuidado sanitario en Chile, 1930-1950 in: *Dynamics*, Vol. 37, No. 2, 2017, p. 317-343, 319, 326.

    Sumary of the international congresses, in: 1945 Primer Congreso Panamericano de Servicio Social in Santiago, in: Castañeda Meneses, Patricia; Salamé Coulon, Ana María: 90 años de Trabajo Social en Chile.

apuntes para una cronología, in: Revista Cuarderno de Trabajo Social, Vol. 1, No. 7, [Ediciones Universidad Tecnológica Metropolitana] 2015, p. 25-49, 32, https://sitios.vtte.utem.cl/cuadernots/wp-content/uploads/sites/10/2017/08/CUADERNO_TRABAJO_SOCIAL_2015.pdf [05.05.2022].

19. Tercer Congreso de Asistencia Social, in: Zárate, María Soledad: Formar enfermeras, no empleadas domésticas. Profesionalización del cuidado sanitario en Chile, 1930-1950 in: *Dynamics*, Vol. 37, No. 2, 2017, p. 317-343, 319, 326.
20. Milanich, N. B.: Children of Fate: Childhood, Class, and the State in Chile, 1850–1930. Ebook [Duke University Press] 2009.
21. For the first time, from November 15 to 22, 1969, Santiago hosted the 15th World Congress of Midwives (*XV Congreso Mundial de Matronas*). It was also the first time the congress did not take place in Europe, in: Cogreso Mundial, in: Consejo General del Colegio de Matronas: Boletín de la Matrona, Año 1, 07-1969, No. 1.
22. In 1911, Del Río launched the Foundation for Public Assistance (*Fundación de la Asistencia Pública*) in Santiago. He was also the co-founder of the Ministry of Health and of the School of Social Work School (*Escuela de Trabajo Social*), in: Biblioteca del Ministerio de Salud: Dr. Bogoslav Juricic Turina, http://www.bibliotecaminsal.cl/wp/wp-content/uploads/2011/09/Biografia-Dr-Alejandro-del-Rio-Soto-Aguilar.pdf [05.05.2022].
23. Sótero Del Rio studied medicine in the University of Chile, was president of the medical association, and was until 1961 Minister of Health, in: Tobar Guerra, Iris; Godoy Fuenzalida, María: Aporte al estudio comparativo de las Escuelas de Enfermeras, in: Primer Congreso Panamericano de Enfermería, Santiago 1942, p. 133-148, 136;

    The origins of the Welfare Board date back to the last decade of the nineteenth century, in: González; Zárate (2018), p. 373.
24. Greve, Karin: Die öffentlich-staatliche Gesundheitsversorgung in Chile, Marburg [Tectum Verlag] 2001;

    John D. Long worked for several employers, sometimes even at the same time, which is why he is referred to in different roles, for example:

    1. According to Maria E. Labra, John D. Long was an advisor to the RF, in: Labra, Maria Eliana: La reinvención neoliberal de la inequidad en Chile. El caso de la salud, in: Cad. Saúde Pública, Rio de Janeiro, Vol. 18, No. 4, 2002, p. 1041-1052, 1042;

    2. González and Zárate describe Long as an employee of the RF, in: González; Zárate (2018), p. 381;

3. Patricio Hevia describes Long as an advisor of the US government, in: Hevia, Patricio: Los inicios de la Escuela de Salubridad de Chile: 1943-1957, in: *Rev Chil Salud Pública*, Vol. 10, No. 3, 2016, p. 170-176;

4. Cueto (2006) describes him as an employee of the US Public Health Service, in: Cueto, Marcos: The value of health. A history of the Pan American Health Organization, in: Scientific and Technical Publication No. 600, Washington (PAHO) 2006, p. 54, https://gato-docs.its.txstate.edu/department-of-history/people/faculty/delapuente/other-links/History_of_PAHO.pdf [05.05.2022].

Ministerio del Interior: Ley No. 4.054, 26.09.1924.

25. Zárate (2018), p. 323.
26. Ministerio del Interior: Ley No. 4.054, 26.09.1924.
27. Yáñez Andrade, Juan Carlos: La intervención social en Chile y el nacimiento de la sociedad salarial, Santiago [RIL] 2008, p. 257.
28. Del Río led the departments of Social Assistance (*Asistencia Social*) and Public Charity (*Beneficiencia Pública*). He was also the president of the High Council of Public Hygiene (*Consejo Superior de Higiene Pública*), in: Yáñez (2008), p. 256.
29. Raczynski (1994), p. 3.
30. Yáñez Andrade (2008), p. 257.
31. An internal paper of the Welfare Board from 1932 gives information about the "difficult situation which the welfare and asistance services undergo" and about a "constant demand for free services." That is why its directorate asks for more funding from the Ministry of Health, in: Servicios de Beneficiencia y Asistencia Social: Oficio No. 3171, Demanda por un mejor financamiento, 3171-12-1932, 14.07.1932, p. 1-1 [5/8].
32. An internal report (1943) from the Ministry of Health describes the deficits: Insufficient hospital beds, notorious shortage of beds for patients with tuberculosis, chronic and mental diseases, in: Ministerio de Salubridad Previsión y Asistencia Social: Oficio No. 1491, 1491-475-1943, 27.12.1943, p. 1-3 [2-4/4].
33. Ministerio de Salubridad Previsión y Asistencia Social: Oficio No. 788, Proyecto de extensión de alcantarillado para Santiago, 788-407-1942, 15.09.1942, p. 1-2 [14-15/19].
34. For example, in 1929 many employees of the San Juan de Dios hospital were not listed in the yearly financial plan, in: Junta Central de Beneficencia: Decreto No. 1725, Empleados del Hospital San Juan de Dios, 1725-1-1929, 11.09.1929, p. 1-2 [15-16/25];

    In 1952, the medical association stated that many dental treatments were provided by self-taught individuals, in: Ministerio de Salubridad Previsión y Asistencia Social: Oficio No. 489, Solicita del Ministerio del

Interior retirar Proyecto de Ley del H. Congreso Nacional, a petición del Colegio Médico de Chile, 489-203-1952, 26.04.1952, p. 1-1 [3/3].

35. The first steps to unify the system were undertaken in the late 1930s. Most important was the fusion of the Welfare Board with the Obligatory Health Insurance (*Caja Seguro Obligatorio y Sanidad*), in: Ministerio de Salubridad Previsión y Asistencia Social: Oficio No. 724, Servicios de Salubridad Fusionados - Organización del Sistema Público, 724-407-1942, 31.08.1942, p. 1-9 [5-13/19].
36. Molina Bustos, Carlos: Orígenes de la Asociación Médica de Chile: Una mirada crítica, in: *Polis*, 12-2005, https://journals.openedition.org/polis/5663 [06.04.2022].
37. Llambias-Wolff, Jaime: The Rise and the Fall of Welfare Health Legislation in 20th Century Chile: A Case Study in Political Economy of Law, York (Canada) 2013, p. 221.
38. A source from July 1941 suggests that the Ministry of Health under Salvador Allende increased the salaries for employees. This indicates a good relationship with the health professionals, in: Ministerio de Salubridad Pública, Previsión y Asistencia Social: Oficio No. 550, Proyecto Ley Aumento de sueldos para los empleados particulares, 550-346-1941, 01.07.1941, p. 1-10 [13/16].
39. Ministerio de Salubridad Previsión y Asistencia Social: Oficio No. 703, Aprobación de la personalidad jurídica de 15 sindicatos, 703-474-1943, 01.07.1943, p. 1-2 [3-4/8].
40. In 1954, various physicians announced their resignation. They protested against the shrinking autonomy of the NHS, in: Regional de Valparaíso: Entrego 283 renuncias, in: *Vida Médica*, Vol. VI, No. 8, 12-1954, p. 4.
41. Alarming internal report about the urgent need for medication supply, in: Ministerio de Salubridad Previsión y Asistencia Social: Oficio No. 13, paralización en la importación de numerosos artículos que provienen de países de guerra, 13-406-1942, 09.01.1942, p. 1-1 [1/8].
42. Ministerio de Salubridad Previsión y Asistencia Social: Oficio No. 614, Protesta de parte de los consumidores de leche en polvo en Santiago [working title], 614-347-1941, 15.07.1941, p. 1-1 [1/11].
43. Llambias-Wolff (2013), p. 78.
44. Behn et al. (2009), p. 60, 64.
45. Ramacciotti, Karina Inés: La internacionalización de salud pública. La Fundación Rockefeller y su mirada sobre la región andina y el Río de la Plata (1941-1950), in: A conexão OIT - América Latina [Ed. Ferreras, Stagnaro, Caruso], Rio de Janeiro [MAUAD] 2018, p. 141-162, 147.
46. The following public institutions merged into the NHS: Dirección General de Beneficencia y Asistencia Social, Servicio Médico de la Caja de

Seguro Obrero, Servicio Nacional de Salubridad (Higiene), Sección Técnica de Higiene y Seguridad Industrial de la Dirección General de Trabajo, Instituto Bacteriológico de Chile, Servicios de Salud y Medicina de las Ciudades and *PROTOFINA*, in: Llambias-Wolff (2013), p. 112.

47. Llambias-Wolff (2013), p. 98.
48. Ibid., p. 134.
49. Krebs W., Doris: Necesidades y recursos de enfermería en Chile, Santiago 1961, p. 7;
    Müller-Plantenberg stated that 100 percent of medical check-ups and 75 percent of treatments were assured by the NHS, in: Müller-Plantenberg, Clarita: Frauen und Familie im gesellschaftlichen Befreiungsprozeß, Drei Analysen zur chilenischen Situation zwischen 1964 und 1982, Frankfurt am Main [Vervuert] 1983, p. 94.
50. Chanfreau, Diana: Professional Ideology and the Healthcare System in Chile, in: *International Journal of Health Services*, Vol. 9, No. 1, 1979, p. 87-105, 91;
    Belmar, Roberto E.; Sidel, Victor W.: An international perspective on strikes and strike threats by physicians: The case of Chile, in: *International Journal of Health Services*, Vol. 5, No. 1, 1975, p. 56-64, 57.
51. Law No. 16.781, 02.05.1968, Otorga Asistencia médica y dental a los Imponentes Activos y Jubilados de los Organismos que señala;
    The most important joining agencies were the *Caja de Previsión de Empleados Particulares* and the *Caja Nacional de Empleados Públicos y Periodistas*, in: Ministerio de Salubridad Pública, Subsecretaría: Oficio No. 660, Coordinación de los Servicios Médicos de las Cajas de Previsión de Empleados Particulares y Nacional de Empleados Públicas y Periodistas, 660-474-1943, 22.06.1943, p. 1-2 [2-3/8].
52. According to Müller-Plantenberg, *SERMENA* received in absolute numbers more funding than the NHS considering that it covered only 10 to 15 percent of the population, in: Müller-Plantenberg (1983), p. 90, 92;
    Greve confirms this statement, in: Greve (2001), p. 88.
53. Greve (2001), p. 86.
54. The *SERMENA* directorate constantly requested a higher funding from the Ministry of Health, as seen for example in 1952, in: Ministerio de Salubridad Previsión y Asistencia Social: Oficio No. 1148, Locales para el Servicio Médico en provincias, 1148-204-1952, 23.09.1952, p. 1-1 [3/5];
    In 1954, health minister Sergio Altamirano Pinto (office term: 05.06.1954-03.01.1955) claimed for the expansion of *SERMENA*, in: Dice el Dr. Sergio Altamirano: "Es indispensable la armonía entre el Gobierno y Servicios de Salud," in: Vida Médica, Vol. VI, No. 4, 08-1954.
55. In communities without access to public healthcare, people practiced naturopathy, in: Del Pilar Campaña, Carmen: Participación comunitaria y

salud rural en Chile, in: Salud rural, Santiago [Ed. grupo de investigadores agrarias, Academia de Humanismo Cristiano] 1988, p. 42.

56. In 1954, health minister Altamirano tried to implement an obligatory assignment to a health center in rural areas or in the *poblaciones* for all health professionals, in: Dice el Dr. Sergio Altamirano: "Es indispensable la armonía entre el Gobierno y Servicios de Salud," in: *Vida Médica*, Vol. VI, No. 4, 08-1954.
57. Llambias-Wolff (2013), p. 113.
58. Cueto, Marco: The cycles of eradication: the Rockefeller Foundation and Latin American public health, 1918-1940, in: International health organisations and movements, 1918-1939 [Ed. Weindling, Paul], Cambridge [Cambridge University Press] 1995, p. 222-243, 222.
59. For example, in 1941, Salvador Allende signed a cooperation agreement with the Pan American Association of Public Health, in: Ministerio de Salubridad Previsión y Asistencia Social: Oficio No. 918, Allende en la Reunión Annual de la Asociación Panamericana de Salud Pública, 918-347-1941, 09.10.1941, p. 1-1 [8/11]
60. Cueto, Marco (1995), p. 222.
61. Long was described as the first "traveling representative" of the PAHO, in: Kiernan, James Patrick: 1902 - 2002: 100 Years of Pan-Americanism, https://www.paho.org/en/who-we-are/history-paho/1902-2002-100-years-pan-americanism [06.04.2022].
62. Prutsch, Ursula; Cramer, Gisela: Nelson A. Rockefeller's Office of Inter-American Affairs and the Quest for Pan-American Unity: An Introductory Essay, in: *Hispanic American Historical Review*, Vol. 86, No. 4, 2012, p. 785-806, 793.
63. Ministerio de Salubridad Previsión y Asistencia Social: Oficio No. 220, Contesta Oficio No. 980 del Ministerio de Relaciones Exteriores sobre consulta del Consejo Económico para América Latina, 220-202-1952, 19.02.1952, p. 1-5 [1-5/14].
64. The RF was also cooperating with the IIAA in Chile, for example, in 1943 when both organizations together with the NHS set up a fund for a higher payment for employees in the public health service, in: Ministerio de Salubridad Pública: Oficio No. 238, Remite proyecto de reestructuración del Servicio Nacional de Salubridad, 238-202-1952, 20.02.1952, p. 1-9 [6-14/14].
65. Escuela de Salud Pública: Historia, http://saludpublica.uchile.cl/escuela/escuela/historia [06.04.2022].
66. De Lima, Liliana; Bruera, Eduardo: The Pan American Health Organization: Its Structure and Role in the Development of a Palliative Care Program for Latin America and the Caribbean, in: *Journal of Pain and Symptom Management*, Vol. 20, No. 6, 2000, p. 440-448.

67. Ministerio de Salubridad, Previsión y Asistencia Social: Oficio No. 220, Contesta Oficio No. 980 del Ministerio de Relaciones Exteriores sobre consulta del Consejo Económico para América Latina, 220-202-1952, 19.02.1952, p. 1-5 [1-5/14].
68. There were various job changes from the RF to the PASB, like in the case of Fred Lowe Soper, graduate of the Johns Hopkins School of Public Health. Since 1927, he held several posts in the Latina American Department of the IHC. From 1947 to 1959, he was the director of the Pan American Sanitary Organization, PASB, in: PAHO's former directors, https://www.paho.org/en/who-we-are/pahos-former-directors [06.04.2022]
69. Ministerio de Salubridad Previsión y Asistencia Social: Oficio No. 220, Contesta Oficio No. 980 del Ministerio de Relaciones Exteriores sobre consulta del Consejo Económico para América Latina, 220-202-1952, 19.02.1952, p. 1-5 [1-5/14];

    The Americas was one of the first regions to eradicate polio, in: Tambina, Gina et al.: Regional immunization programs as a model for strengthening cooperation among nations, in: *Revista Panamericana Salud Pública*, Vol. 20, No. 1, 2006, p. 54-59, 55.
70. Ministerio de Salubridad Previsión y Asistencia Social: Oficio No. 220, Contesta Oficio No. 980 del Ministerio de Relaciones Exteriores sobre consulta del Consejo Económico para América Latina, 220-202-1952, 19.02.1952, p. 1-5 [1-5/14].
71. Considering the UN, especially the United Nations Children's Fund (*Fondo Internacional de Socorro a la Infancia de las Naciones Unidas*), in: Ministerio de Salud Pública: Oficio No. 842, Solicita inclusión en Presupuesto de 1961 del Ministerio de Relaciones Exteriores cuotas para Organismos Internacionales que indica. Ministerio de Salud Pública, 842-1526-1960, 20.10.1960, p. 1-2 [1-2/5].
72. The strike was aginst the new tariff scale from 1962, in: Law No. 14.904, 14.09.1962, Fija normas para encasillar al personal del Servicio Nacional de Salud, in: Ministerio de Salud Pública: Oficio No. 1111, Imparte instrucciones para encasillamiento personal Servicio Nacional de Salud, 1111-1558-1962, 26.10.1962, p. 1-12 [1-12/12].

    Description of the strike, in: Morales, Eduardo: Sistema político, planificación y políticas públicas. La política de salud, Chile 1964-1978, No. 110, Santiago [FLACSO] 1981, p. 57.
73. Attempt of the medical association to mediate between the government and the striking professional associations, in: Colegio Médico procuró solución en el conflicto de trabajadores del SNS, in: *Vida Médica*, Vol. XV, No. 9, 09-1963, p. 8-9;

    Morales confirmed that the 1963 strike lasted 25 days, in: Morales (1981), p. 57.

74. Evidence for the 1960 strike of physicians, dentists, and pharmacists, in: Se logró solución en grave conflicto del SNS, in: *Vida Médica*, Vol. XII, No. 8, 08-1960, p. 8-9.
75. The strike of the physicians, dentists, and pharmacists in 1962 took 16 days, in: Ministerio de Salud Pública: Oficio No. 654, Conflicto Profesionales del Servicio Nacional de Salud, 654-1555-1962, 12.07.1962, p. 1-1 [3/7].
76. Ley No. 15.076, 13.12.1962, Fija el texto refundido estatuto para los Médico-Cirujanos, Farmacéuticos o Químicos-Farmacéuticos, Bio-Químicos y Cirujanos Dentistas;

    Molina describes Law No. 15076 as a success for the physicians in "keeping their privileges and improving economic incentives," in: Molina (2010), p. 140.
77. Jiménez de la Jara, Salud en tiempos de Frei Montalva, 2014, p. 7-8, 20.
78. Zárate, María Soledad; González, Maricela: Planificación familiar en la guerra fría chilena: política sanitaria y cooperación internacional, 1960-1973, in Historia Crítica, Nr. 55, 2015, p. 207-230.
79. Including health and safety regulations for pregnant women in the workplace, in: Decreto Ley No. 725, 11.12.1967, Código Sanitario.
80. Paredes M., Pamela; Rivas R., Edith: Historia del Ejercicio Profesional de Enfermeras Hospitalarias del Sur de Chile (1940-1980), in: *Ciencia y Enfermería*, Vol. XX, No. 1, 2014, p. 9-21.
81. Subsidized by the International Planned Parenthood Foundation (IPPF), in: Pieper Mooney, The Politics of Motherhood, Pittsburgh [Univ. of Pittsburgh Press] 2009, p. 120.
82. Thibaut Bernhard: Soziale Entwicklung und Demokratie in Lateinamerika zu Beginn der neunziger Jahre, in: [Hrsg. Junker, Detlef, Nohlen, Dieter, Sangmeister, Hartmut], München (Beck) 1994, p. 124-148.
83. The most prominent example is the so-called Basic Plan of Basis Rural Sanitation (*Plan Primitivo de Saneamiento Básico Rural*) from 1962. To implement the plan, the Interamerican Development Bank assured the transfer of 2.5 million USD in two years. The most important goal of the cooperation was to assure drinking water in rural areas, in: Ministerio de Salud Pública: Oficio No. 456, Remite copia "Plan Bienal de Saneamiento Básico Rural," 456-1554-1962, 15.05.1962, p. 1-1 [2/4].
84. Ley 16.781, 28.03.1969, Otrorga asistencia médica y dental a los imponentes activos y jubilados de los organismos que señala.
85. Biblioteca del Congreso Nacional: Eduardo Frei Montalva: Fe, política y cambio social, Santiago [Ed, Biblioteca del Congreso] 2013.
86. Molina (2010), p. 152.
87. *SERMENA* had to pay at least 70 percent for a medical treatment. The insured were charged with the remaining cost, in: Law No. 16.781, Medicina Curativa, Article No. 4.

88. Valdivieso D., Dres. Ramón; Juricic T., Bogoslav: El sistema nacional de salud en Chile, in: Boletín de la Oficina Sanitaria Panamericana (OSP), Vol. 68, No. 6, pp. 478-485, 479; Valdivieso praised the achievements of the law. He stated that together with Law No. 10.383 (foundation of the NHS), the *Medicina Curativa* assured the health coverage for 92 percent of the population, in: Discurso del Ministro de Salud Pública, Dr. Ramón Valdivieso Delaunay, in: *Vida Médica*, Vol. XXI, No. 6, 06-1969, pp. 10-14.
89. Decreto con Fuerza de Ley No. 725, Código Sanitario, 31.01.1968.
90. Zárate, María Soledad: Formar enfermeras, no empleadas domésticas. Profesionalización del cuidado sanitario en Chile, 1930-1950, in: *Dynamics*, Vol. 37, No. 2, 2017, p. 317-343, 319.
91. Memoria Anual del Consejo General del Colegio de Enfermeras. Periodo 1 de Junio de 1977 a 31 de Mayo de 1978, in: *Enfermería*, No. 58, 10-11-12-1978, p. 31–40
92. Since March 26,1968, midwives had entered the bill-for-service system of the *Medicina Curativa*, in: Comisón Medicina Curativa para empleados, in: Consejo General del Colegio de Matronas: *Boletín de la Matrona*, Año 1, 07-1969, No. 1.
93. Belmar et al. (1975), p. 57.
94. Quote: "esta agrupación hasta la fecha tiene fines estrictamente sindicales, promoviendo toda clase de paros y movimientos huelguísticos del personal del Servicio Nacional de Salud, lo que va contra la esencia misma de toda corporación," in: Ministerio de Salud Pública: Oficio No. 412, Personalidad jurídica a entidad denominada "Federación Nacional de Trabajadores de la Salud," "FENATS," 412-1686-1968, 30.02.1968, p. 1-1 [9/20].
95. Dr. Emilio Villarroel González: "Deseamos conclusiones objetivas y realistas que señalen camino firme," in: *Vida Médica*, Vol. XXII, No. 8, 08-1970, p. 10-11.
96. H. Consejo General del Colegio Médico de Chile: El Colegio Médico a la opinión pública, in: Vida Médica, Vol. XXII, No. 8, 08-1970, p. 11.
97. Conclusiones y propósitos, in: *Vida Médica*, Vol. XXII, No. 8, 08-1970, p. 5;

    Santiago physicians intended to devote only 15 percent of their work time to patients who could afford *SERMENA* services, in: Discurso del Dr. Olav Olsen P.: El Gremio Médico frente a la Ley de Medicina Curativa, in: Vida Médica, Vol. XXII, No. 8, 08-1970, p. 12-14;

    In retrospect, the medical association published a critical statement about the association's behavior during the time of political confrontations, stating that in 2018 members had been forced to obey to the political opinion of the board members, in: Colegio Médico de Chile: Memoria 70 Años, Con la Salud de Chile [Ed. Izkia Siches Pastén et al.], Santiago 2018, p. 44.

98. Molina (2010), p. 160;
    Belmar et al. (1975), p. 57.
99. The medical association reports about 30 healthcare centers on strike, in: H. Consejo General del Colegio Médico de Chile: El Colegio Médico a la opinión pública, in: *Vida Médica*, No. 8, V XXII, 08-1970, p. 11.
100. Amplio triunfo de gremialistas en U. Católica, in: Mercurio, 13.-19.11.1972, p. 7, [1/5].
101. Velandia (2016), p. 1622-1653;
    Ramacciotti refers to the *Hospital Británico* running a nursing school in 1890. But she accorded more importance to Grierson, who founded the School of Nurses, Male Nurses and Masseurs of the City of Buenos Aires (*Escuela de Enfermeras, Enfermeros y Masajistas de la Ciudad de Buenos Aires*) in 1892, in: Ramacciotti (2020), p. 37-39;
102. Braga do Espírito Santo et al. (2011) date the foundation of the first Brazilian nursing school (without claiming it has been the first in South America) for 1890, in: Braga do Espírito Santo, Tiago; Oguisso, Taka; Godoy Serpa de Fonseca, Rosa María: La Profesionalización de la Enfermería Brasileña en los Medios de Comunicación Escrita de Final del Siglo XIX: un análisis de género, in: *Revista Latinoamericana Enfermagem*, Vol. 19, No. 5, p. 1-7, 6.
103. Martín, Ana Laura: Trayectorias que se cruzan. Cecilia Grierson y María Elena Ramos Mejía, in: Historias de la Enfermería en Argentina (2020), p. 80-81.
104. Flores, Rosalba: Historia de la Enfermería en Chile. Síntesis de su Evolución Educacional, Santiago 1965, p. 48.
105. Zárate, María Soledad: Al Cuidado Femenino, Mujeres y Profesiones Sanitarias, Chile, 1889-1950, in: Historia de las mujeres en Chile, Tomo 2 [Ed. Ana María Stuven-Joaquín Fermandois], Santiago 2013, p. 119-156, 130.
106. Rotario Internacional: XXIX Conferencia Tridistrital de los Rotary Clubes de Chile, Osorno 1955;
    Biblioteca Nacional de Chile: Enfermería y Servicio Social, http://www.memoriachilena.gob.cl/602/w3-article-96243.html [06.04.2022].
107. Quote: "En la escuela de Santiago se insiste con toda constancia en hacer penetrar en la mente de las discípulas la convicción de que en ningún caso pueden atribuirse la dirección del enfermo, ni desobedecer al médico sino quieren desprestijiar su profesión i esponer la salud i la vida de los pacientes con gran riesgo de incurrir en los severos castigos que las leyes tienen establecidas. [...] Debemos reconocer que la caridad pública atiende a los pobres con paternal cariño i munificencia, i recordar con satisfacción que su primer auxiliar en esas tareas es el médico [...] No crear una clase híbrida de semi-médicos, semi-cirujano ni semi-matronas; sino que formar, allado de los médicos, de los cirujanos i de los tocólogos," in: Amaral (1904), p. 20-21.

108. Ibid, p. 20-21.
109. Muñoz et al. (1999), p. 48.
110. Zárate (2013), p. 130.
111. Uniform requirements. Once the students graduated, they received a nursing case, in: Prospecto de la Escuela de Enfermeras, Santiago [Imprenta Barcelona] 1914, http://www.memoriachilena.gob.cl/archivos2/pdfs/MC0065706.pdf [06.04.2022].
112. The Medical Faculty of the Universidad de Chile was founded in 1929, in: Escuela de Medicina: En 1929 se fundó la Facultad de Medicina, https://medicina.uc.cl/noticias/en-1929-se-fundo-la-facultad-de-medicina/ [06.04.2022].
113. Zárate (2017), p. 321.
114. Ramaciotti describes the role of Red Cross nurses in Santa Fe, Rosario, and La Plata as "outstanding," in: Ramacciotti (2020), p. 41-42;
    About Red Cross nurses in Uruguay, in: Sánchez (2002), p. 87.
115. Revista de Salud Pública de la Cruz Roja Chilena, Vol. 4-6, 1923, p. 256.
116. Secretaría General de la Cruz Roja Chilena: Reseña Histórica de la Cruz Roja Chilena, 1963, p. 4, http://www.memoriachilena.gob.cl/archivos2/pdfs/MC0056277.pdf [06.04.2022].
117. Ramacciotti (2020), p. 41.
118. In 1923, for the first time a nursing handbook (*manual de enfermeras*) for Red Cross nurses was mentioned, in: *Revista de Salud Pública de la Cruz Roja Chilena*, Vol. 4-6, 1923, p. 290, 299;
    The first edited version we found of this book is from 1933, in: Cruz Roja Chilena: Manual de instrucción para sus enfermeras, Vol. 1, Santiago 1933, http://www.memoriachilena.gob.cl/archivos2/pdfs/MC0056317.pdf [06.04.2022].
119. *Revista de Salud Pública de la Cruz Roja Chilena*, Vol. 4-6, 1923, p. 279.
120. Quote: "Como superintendente de hospital o escuela de enfermeras, como jefe de enfermeras en salas de hospital o salas quirúrgicas, y como supervigilante de dispensario o clínica, siempre hay oportunidades para un rápido ascenso," in: Minnigerode, Lucy E.: La Profesión de Enfermera, in: *Revista de Salud Pública de la Cruz Roja Chilena*, Vol. 4-6, 1923, p. 354-362, 356, 361.
121. Ayala, Ricardo A.; Gerard M. Fealy, Raf Vanderstraeten, Piet Bracke: Academisation of nursing: An ethnography of social transformations in Chile, in: *International Journal of Nursing Studies*, No. 51, 2014, p. 603-611, 604-605.
122. La Cruz Roja Chilena (1903): Cruz Roja de las Mujeres de Chile, in: http://www.memoriachilena.gob.cl/602/w3-article-93115.html [06.04.2022].

123. In 1943, the nurses association justified a boarding school on the grounds of ethical and intellectual education of the profesional nurse, in: Reparticiones y servicios donde desempeñan cargos la enfermeras y enfermeras visitadoras, in: *Boletín de la Asociación de Enfermeras de Chile*, Vol. 2, No. 10, 12-1942-01-1943, p. 50-53, 53.
124. Ramacciotti: "Durante gran parte del siglo XX, el vestido blanco y la cofia se constituyeron en el paradigma del cuidado y del prestigio profesional. La capa se ligaba con un ritual que de por vida les haría recordar a las enfermeras el peso de la responsabilidad que había contraído con la sociedad. La cofia estaba considerada como un elemento de distinción social y reconocimiento," in: Ramacciotti (2020), p. 43.
125. Ayala et al. (2014), p. 604.
126. At the beginning of the twentieth century, only 40 percent of the population knew how to read and write, in: Census from 1907, quoted in: González et al. (2018), p. 380.
127. Ayala, Ricardo A.; Gerard M. Fealy, Raf Vanderstraeten, Piet Bracke: Academisation of Nursing: An Ethnography of Social Transformations in Chile, in: *International Journal of Nursing Studies*, No. 51, 2014, p. 603-611, 604-605.
128. Müller Plantenberg stated that only 25 percent of women who could work had a job, in: Müller-Plantenberg (1983), p. 27, 47.
129. Power, Margaret: Right-Wing Women in Chile, Feminine Power and the Struggle Against Allende, 1964–1973, Pennsylvania [Pennsylvania State University Press] 2002.
130. Quote: "la acción combinada y armónica de dos competencias, adquiridas por detenidos estudios teóricos y prácticos, la del médico en primer término, la de la enfermera, su auxiliar inmediato, en segundo," in: Del Río, Alejandro: Consideraciones sobre el personal auxiliar del médico, de la sanidad y del servicio social, in: *Revista de Beneficencia Pública*, Vol. 9, No. 3, 09-1925, p. 396-411.
131. Collao Avilés, Carmen; Osorio Spuler, Ximena: Acontecimientos Históricos en la Formación Académica de los Profesionales de Enfermería en Chile, in: Historia de la Enfermería en Chile [Ed. Rivas Riveros, Edith], Santiago [Universidad de La Frontera] 2019, p. 29-62, 34, 36.
132. Junta Central de Beneficencia: Decreto No. 1602, Plan de Clasificación, Ubicación y Dotación de los Servicios Hospitalarios, 1602-1-1929, 27.08.1929, 1-6 [6-11/25].
133. Quote: "En la segunda mitad del siglo XIX, los hospitales y otras obras asistenciales contaban con un escaso número de médicos y con un puñado de trabajadores hospitalarios, mayoritariamente hombres, conocidos como 'practicantes,' que cumplían principalmente funciones de aseo, limpieza de pisos, mantención de camas y cuidados corporales de los enfermos," in: González; Zárate (2018), p. 379.

134. Dirección General de Estadísticas: Censo de población de la República de Chile 1920, Santiago de Chile 1925, p. 407.
135. Revista de Salud Pública de la Cruz Roja Chilena, V. 4-6, 1923, p. 256.
136. Oficina Central de Beneficiencia: Oficio No. 3781, Estatuto de los Enfermeros Practicantes de Curicó [working title], 3781-12-1932, 12.08.1932, 1-2 [7-8/8].
137. In 1943, the Ministry of Health considered the possibility of founding a school for (male) *practicantes*, in: Ministerio de Salubridad Previsión y Asistencia Social: Oficio No. 758, Ejercicio de la profesión de enfermeros-practicantes—creación de una escuela de practicantes, 758-474-1943, 15.07.1943, 1-1 [6/8];

    We found no trace that this school actually opened.
138. Ayala et al., 2014.
139. Ramacciotti interprets the nursing ratio considering professional nurses alone. "El ideal pautado por el secretario de Salud Ramón Carrillo, quien retomaba tendencias internacionales sobre la materia, era que una enfermera atendiera cuatro camas, por lo que un hospital de 100 camas necesitaría un mínimo de 25 enfermeras," in: Ramacciotti (2020), p. 50.
140. In 1935, only 24 percent of nurses in Buenos Aires were professionally trained (Memoria del Departamento Ejecutivo de la Municipalidad de la Ciudad de Buenos Aires, 1936), in: Martín (2020), p. 86.
141. Zárate; González (2021).
142. Sánchez actually offers more information about the *auxiliares de enfermería*. Nevertheless, this type of memory fades out in her historiography after the 1970s, in: Sánchez (2002), p. 117.
143. Ayala et al. (2014).
144. Quote: "personas de baja extracción social [...] mal pagados, sin uniforme ni espíritu de cuerpo, sin conciencia de las funciones que tan malamente desempeñan, alojados en la misma sala de los enfermos [...] o en habitaciones con frecuencia antihigiénicas," in: Del Río, 1923, p. 225-233, quoted in: González; Zárate (2018), p. 376.
145. Nüñez, Elizabeth; Jana, Alejandra: El legado de las enfermeras sanitarias en el cuidado de la salud chilena, in: Ciencia y enfermería, Vol. 23, No. 3, 2017, p. 113-124.
146. González and Zárate quote Adams when they describe a "rigorous physical, mental and professional examen," in: González et al. (2018), p. 382.
147. *Bulletin of the Pan American Union*, Vol. 61, 1927, p. 622.
148. Mayers studied in Paris, London, and Berlin, in: Zárate (2013), p. 131.
149. Until October 1926, she had been the head nurse of the *Hospital Santo Tomás* of Panama City, in: *Bulletin of the Pan American Union*, Vol. 60, 1926, p. 100.

150. For her courses, Adams used teaching material from the US, in: Adams, Sara E.: A School of Nurses in Chile, in: *American Journal of Nursing*, Vol. 27, No. 12, 1927, p. 1029-1030, 1029.
151. Various contemporary descriptions of Chilean public health nursing give the impression of a continuous story of success, for example Núñez et al. (2017), p. 116-117.
152. In 1951, nurses María Godoy, Yolanda Ortiz, and Nora Fardella, all of them close to the Nursing Association of Chile, founded in 1938, described that period as a time of "hesitancy," "lack of discipline," and "disorder," in: Godoy, María; Ortiz, Yolanda; Fardella, Nora: Desarollo y perpectiva de la enfermería sanitaria en Chile, in: *Boletín de la Oficina Sanitaria Panamericana*, Año 30, Vol. XXXI, No. 2, Washington 1951, p. 158-164.
153. Sierra, Lucas: Cien años de enseñanza de la medicina en Chile, Santiago 1934, p. 318, https://libros.uchile.cl/680 [06.04.2022].
154. Ugarte, José Manuel: Balance de las necesidades y disponibilidades de enfermeras en Chile, in: *Revista Chilena de Higiene y Medicina Preventiva*, Vol. 14, No. 1, 1952, S. 53-56., quoted by Zárate (2017), p. 325.
155. Dirección General de Sanidad: Oficio No. 2205, Beca de estudios en Estados Unidos para Sofía Pincheira, 2205-12-1932, 18.06.1932, p. 1-2 [1-2/8].
156. There is no exact information about the year she took on this position, but we know when she ended, in 1933, in: Adams, Sara; de Bray, Leo: Cómo dignificar la profesión de enfermera, in: *Revista de Asistencia Social*, Tomo II, No. 1, Santiago 1933, p. 76-85.
157. Zárate quotes that Mayers was the nursing schools' director in 1930, in: Zárate (2013), p. 134.
158. Tobar Guerra et al. (1942), p. 136-137.
159. An enthusiastic instigator of this process was Sótero del Río, in: Ibid, p. 136;

     The schools belonged to the hospitals *Roberto del Río* and *Manuel Arriarán*, in: Biblioteca Nacional de Chile: Primeras escuelas de enfermería, http://www.memoriachilena.gob.cl/602/w3-article-96996.html [06.04.2022].
160. de la Fuente, Rudecindo: Escuelas de Enfermeras, in: *Revista de Asistencia Social*, Vol. 2, No. 1, 1934, p. 70-75;

     The school in Valparaíso would seem to be the second oldest nursing school of Chile, in: Escuela de Enfermería es reconocida como Patrimonio de la ciudad, in: Universidad de Valparaíso 2013, https://pdn.uv.cl/?id=5465 [06.04.2022];

     The Chilean National Library states that the Welfare Board school in Valparaíso belonged to the *Hospital San Agustín*, in: Primeras escuelas de enfermería [Biblioteca Nacional de Chile].

161. Thierry founded the school in 1918. In 1922, it was affiliated to the University of Chile, but lost this accredition in 1932, in: Biblioteca Ministerio de Salud: "Dr. Bogoslav Juricic Turina": Historia Hospital de Niños "Jean y Marie Thierry" de Valparaíso, http://www.bibliotecaminsal.cl/wp/wp-content/uploads/2011/09/Historia-Hospital-de-ninos-Jean-and-Marie-Thierry-de-Valparaiso.pdf [06.04.2022];

    In 1943, the nursing association counted four nursing schools, in: Escuelas de Enfermeras de Chile, in: *Boletín de la Asociación de Enfermeras de Chile*, Vol. 2, No. 10, 12-1942-01-1943, p. 48-49, 48;

    In 1942, four schools confirmed by Tobar Guerra and Godoy Fuenzalida: one of the University of Chile, two of the Welfare Board and Thierry's school in Valparaíso, in: Tobar et al. (1942), p. 134;

    Two nursing schools of the Welfare Board, confirmed by the Ministry of Health in 1942, in: Ministerio de Salubridad Previsión y Asistencia Social: Oficio No. 960, Dos escuelas de enfermería bajo control del sistema público [working title], 960-407-1942, 23.10.1942, p. 1-1 [17/19];
162. The students had to pay tuition fees and buy their own education material and working clothes, in: Ivovich, Esteban: Reglamento de las Escuelas de Enfermeras de la Junta Central de Beneficencia y Asistencia Social, Servicios de Beneficencia y Asistencia Social, Santiago 1936, http://www.memoriachilena.gob.cl/archivos2/pdfs/MC0065707.pdf [06.04.2022].
163. González et al. describe a regulation project for nursing schools in 1921 and the creation of a High Council of the Nursing Service (*Consejo Superior del Servicio de Enfermeras*) in 1924, in: González; Zárate (2018), p. 381.
164. Tobar et al. (1942), p. 146.
165. During her short term as the management director of the university school, Pincheira published in 1934 an article in the most important medium for publication of professional healthcare, the Journal of Social Assistance (*Revista de Asistencia Social*). There, she criticized that Chilean hospitals did not provide enough personnel to impart the theoretical content in practice. For her, this was the most important reason why the nursing profession was not very popular among school graduates. Pincheira proposed to offer more seminars and courses to complement, specialize, and refresh the knowledge of students and professionals, in: Pincheira O., Sofía: Especialización en las enfermeras, in: *Revista de Asistencia Social*, Vol. 3, No. 2, 1934, p. 132-139, 134-135.
166. Census 1920 (1925), p. 407.
167. For example: González et al. (2021), p. 88;

Amaral and Del Río Soto also co-founded the Social Work School (*Escuela de Trabajo Social*). Since 1924, Del Río Soto was also the Minister of Hygiene, Social Assistance and Welfare (*Ministro de Higiene, Asistencia y Previsión Social*). He was responsible for the administration of the work of the healthcare workers, in: Biblioteca Ministerio de Salud: Alejandro del Río Soto Aguilar, http://www.bibliotecaminsal.cl/wp/wp-content/uploads/2011/09/Biografia-Dr-Alejandro-del-Rio-Soto-Aguilar.pdf [06.04.2022].

168. Huaiquián-Silva et al. (2013) confirm the use of male nurses;

In 1954, the nursing school of Valparaíso opened the enrolment procedure also for men, in: Acreditadora de Chile: Acuerdo de Acreditación No. 283, Santiago 2014, http://www.acreditadoradechile.cl/wp-content/uploads/2015/04/Acuerdo-N%C2%BA283.pdf [06.04.2022];

Mayers was against the hiring of men as nurses, in: Zárate (2013), p. 134;

Ramacciotti states that by the beginning of the twentieth century, more than 50 percent of Argentine caregivers were men, in: Ramacciotti (2020), p. 41;

Sánchez, in her book about the history of Uruguayan nurses, did not mention gender policy and cultural politics. Nevertheless, her historiography suggests that percentage of men shrank throughout the course of the twentieth century.

169. de la Fuente, Rudecindo: Escuelas de Enfermeras, in: *Revista de Asistencia Social*, Vol. 2, No. 1, 1934, p. 70-75;

The absence of women in high-ranking positions did not change during the 1930s, in: *Boletín de la Asociación de Enfermeras de Chile*, Vol. 2, No. 10, 12-1942-01-1943, p. 58;

We found less information about the directorates of other nursing schools. Only one example came to light. In 1941, the director of Valparaíso's nursing school was a man, in: Cocktail al Señor Ministro de Salubridad, in: *Boletín de la Asociación de Enfermeras de Chile*, Vol. 1, No. 1, 06-1941, p. 8.

170. For example, the Interamerican Conference of Social Welfare *(Conferencia Interamericana de Previsión Social*) in 1942. It was only attended by men, in: Ministerio de Salubridad Previsión y Asistencia Social: Oficio No. 697, Delegación Chilena para la Conferencia Interamericana de Previsión Social [working title], 697-407-1942, 27.08.1942, p. 1-2 [3-4/19].

171. Pincheira O., Sofía: Contribución al estudio de la organización de escuelas de enfermeras en Chile, in: *Revista de Asistencia Social*, Vol. 3, No. 1, 1934, p. 1-46, 45.

172. González, E.: La subdirectora de la Escuela de Enfermeras de la U. de Chile, dice, in: *Boletín de la Asociación de Enfermeras de Chile*, Vol. 1, No. 1, 06-1941, p. 4.
173. Quote: "Tú eres mujer, puedes formar al hombre. Cuando eres madre. Cuando eres novia. Cuando eres esposa," in: Ocupa tu puesto, in: *Boletín de la Asociación de Enfermeras de Chile*, Vol. 2, No. 10, 12-1942-01-1943, p. 55.
174. Since the foundation of the Universidad de Chile in 1842, midwifery was a graduate profession, in: González et al. (2018), p. 380.
175. Only a few times, but Peake did not talk about auxiliaries but about women, in: Peake, Gladys: Formación de la Enfermera y Auxiliares de Enfermería, in: Actas de las Segundas Jornadas Chilenas de Salubridad, Santiago 1953, p. 84-114;

     The medical association, in 1962, also refers to auxiliaries as female workers, in: Solo personal entrenado podrá ingresar al S.N.S., in: Vida Médica, Vol. XV, No. 11, 11-1963, p. 13.
176. Reparticiones y servicios donde desempeñan cargos la enfermeras y enfermeras visitadoras, in: *Boletín de la Asociación de Enfermeras de Chile*, Vol. 2, No. 10, 12-1942-01-1943, p. 50-53, 51.
177. 56 graduates of the University of Chile, 23 of the Welfare Board nursing school in Santiago, and 19 of the Welfare Board nursing school in Valparaíso, in: Paredes et al. (2014), p. 18.
178. Between 1926 and 1936, the University of Chile had trained 142 nurses. From 1936 to 1941, 122 more would graduate from here, in: Tobar et al. (1942), p. 147.
179. The documentation of the Ministry of Health suggets that in 1943 only 30 public health nurses worked in Chile, in: Ministerio de Salubridad Previsión y Asistencia Social: Oficio No. 1031, Grado 12 para 30 enfermeras sanitarias, 1031-475-1943, 13.09.1943, p. 1-1 [1/4].
180. Between 1938 and 1941 the number of hospital beds increased from 1871 to 2111. In the same period, the number of vaccinations rose from 10,550 to 35,889 and the medical consultations from 286,035 to 762,561, in: Ministerio de Salubridad Previsión y Asistencia Social: Oficio No. 724, Servicios de Salubridad Fusionados - Organización del Sistema Público, 724-407-1942, 31.08.1942, p. 1-9 [5-13/19].
181. Noticias, in: *Boletín de la Asociación de Enfermeras de Chile*, Vol. 1, No. 1, 06-1941, p. 8.
182. Ibid., p. 153.
183. The new nursing association assured a temporary "civil defense seminars" for its members, in: Tobar et al. (1942), p. 138.

184. For example, the first sign of an official training for Red Cross nurses we found dates back to 1942, in: Morales Alliende, Pilar: Cien Años de la Cruz Roja Chilena, Santiago 2004, p. 63, 101.
185. Ramacciotti (2020), p. 35.
186. Ramacciotti (2018), p. 141.
187. Ramacciotti (2020), p. 45-46.
188. Labra stated that there was a strong influence of the RF on the Chilean healthcare system since the 1920s, in: Labra, María Eliana: La Reinvención Neoliberal de la Inequidad en Chile. El Caso de la Salud, in: *Cad. Saúde Pública*, Rio de Janeiro, Vol. 18, No. 4, 2002, p. 1041-1052, 1042.
189. Tennant was in charge of the IHC's nursing programs and had worked before as a head nurse in Colorado and New York, at the beginning for the public system and then for a private insurance company, in: De Chesnay, Mary: Nursing research using grounded theory, New York [Springer Publishing Company] 2014.
190. Uribe (2008), p. 116.
191. Rivas Riveros, Carmen; Catalán Melinao, Yaqueline: Patrón sociocrítico en la formación de enfermeras y enfermeros. Historiar conflictos y legitimidades en torno al pasado reciente, in: Historia de la enfermería en Chile [Ed. Rivas Riveros, Edith], Santiago [Ufro] 2019, p. 187-210, 197.
192. Her successor in Chile was Yale graduate Esther Mary Hirst, whose term lasted until 1952, in: Ibid, p. 192.
193. Black, Victoria Lynn: Taking care of baby: Chilean state-making, international relations and the gendered body politic, 1912-1970, University of Arizona 2002, p. 40.
194. Uribe (2008), p. 140.
195. John H. Janney, in: The online collections and Catalog of the Rockefeller Archive Center, https://dimes.rockarch.org/collections/fmKqCqH-nARFtdF8Xi2tfcv [07.04.2022].
196. Uribe (2008), p. 147.
197. Ibid., p. 154.
198. Ibid., p. 150.
199. The government's priority was the control of tuberculosis, in: Ramacciotti (2020), p. 147.
200. Uribe (2008), p. 155-156;
201. Quote: "ella me enseñó cómo llegar a las casas, de cómo hacerle el quite a los perros [...] nunca hacer tal cosa y preparar un lugar limpio, aséptico para poner el maletín, para enseñar a lavarse las manos, porque no había agua potable en la mayoría de las casas... todas esas cosas de ese período. Yo creo que a las enfermeras de esa época nos marca esa huella (relato de vida)," in: Núñez et al. (2017), p. 118.

202. Quote: “me contaban [...] que los maridos no solamente les pegaban a las mujeres sino que sufrían abuso sexual por parte del marido...terrible!, porque yo nunca había escuchado esa parte. En ese tiempo no se hablaba de eso. La enfermería no hablaba de esas cosas. Era delicado, hasta que uno fue madurando (Relato de Vida, Enfermera D),” in: Núñez et al. (2017), p. 119.
203. Godoy, María; Ortiz, Yolanda; Fardella, Nora: Desarollo y perpectiva de la enfermería sanitaria en Chile, in: *Boletín de la Oficina Sanitaria Panamericana*, Año 30, Vol. XXXI, No. 2, Washington 1951, p. 158-164, 159.
204. Her successor in Chile was Yale graduate Esther Mary Hirst, whose term lasted until 1952, in: Historia de la enfermería en Chile (2019), p. 192.
205. Pincheira Oyarzún, Sofía: La Enfermera Sanitaria en los Servicios de Salud Pública, Santiago 1944, p. 1-15, 5, 13.
206. The public health facilities hired mostly hospital nurses (*enfermeras hospitalarias*) to fill the positions originally planned for public health nurses, in: Ministerio de Salubridad Previsión y Asistencia Social: Oficio No. 634, Enfermeras sanitarias, 634-347-1941, 18.07.1941, p. 1-2 [2-3/11].
207. The public health nurses had to provide the following benefits for the population: health education, maternal and antenatal hygiene, school hygiene, prevention of contagious diseases, prevention of sexually transmitted diseases, mental hygiene, workplace safety, in: Pincheira (1944).
208. Leal Román, Valentina: Lo que pueden estudiar las mujeres en Valparaíso de Gladys Peake. Análisis de habla de un documento de época, in: *Ciencia y Enfermería*, Vol. XX, No. 2, 2014, p. 9-15, 10.
209. 35.3 per cent of the nurses surveyed by Krebs in 1961 had studied abroad, in: Krebs (1961), p. 13.
210. Gratz, Alejandro: Gladys Peake Guevara, in: Diario Concepción, 02.09.2018.
211. Peake G., Gladys: Reorganización de la enfermería en Chile: Carrera única, in: *Revista de Asistencia Social*, Vol IX, No. 1, Santiago 1940.
212. Hackett, June 26, 1941, Diaries.
213. Uribe (2008), p. 152;

     The Socialist Party was founded in Valparaíso, in: Quiroga Zamora, Patricio: La Dignidad de América—El retorno Histórico a Salvador Allende, Santiago [Ediciones Escaparate] 2016, p. 75.
214. Ayala, Ricardo; Thulin, Markus; Núñez, Rocío: Cold Interests, Hot Conflicts: How a Professional Association Responded to a Change in Political Regimes, in: *Nursing History Review*, Vol. 27, No. 1, 2018, p. 56-87.
215. Behn et al. (2009), p. 85.

216. Velandia Mora, Ana Luisa: Helen Howitt: Una semilla canadiense en la enfermería latinoamericana, in: *Avances en Enfermería*, Vol. XXVII, No. 1, 2009, p. 93-101, 93.

 In Argentina, for example, the RF had a powerful influence on the foundation of the first academic nursing school in 1940, associated with the Medical Faculty of the *Universidad Nacional del Litoral*, in: Ramacciotti (2020), p. 46.

217. Flores de Fernández (1965), p. 23;

 Behn et al. describe the Kellog Foundation as the most important donor of grants for Chilean nurses, in: Behn et al. (2009), p. 56.

218. Ramacciotti described the political changes in her home country as the "revolution of 1943." It caused the end of the cooperation of the state with the RF, in: Ramacciotti (2018), p. 148.

219. Ramacciotti states that RF's engagement was not sustainable because of the lack of local support and skilled health professionals, in: Ramacciotti (2018), p. 142-143.

220. *Boletín de la Asociación de Enfermeras de Chile*, Vol. 1, No. 1, 06-1941, http://www.memoriachilena.gob.cl/archivos2/pdfs/MC0065760.pdf [07.04.2022].

221. Reparticiones y servicios donde desempeñan cargos la enfermeras y enfermeras visitadoras, in: *Boletín de la Asociación de Enfermeras de Chile*, Vol. 2, No. 10, 12-1942-01-1943, p. 50-53.

222. Zárate, María Soledad; González, Maricela: ¿Qué hacemos las enfermeras? Profesionalización, autonomía y asociatividad de la enfermería chilena, 1940-1960, in: Enfermería e historia: Género y Estado en América Latina Siglo XX, [Ed. Zárate Campos] 2019, p. 5.

223. Instroza became president in 1943, in: *Boletín de la Asociación de Enfermeras de Chile*, Vol. 2, No. 10, 12-1942-01-1943, p. 58.

224. The Congress took place from December 14 to 20, 1942. Pincheira spoke about the organization of nursing schools, in: Primer Centenario Universidad de Chile - Primer Congreso Panamericano de Enfermería, in: *Boletín de la Asociación de Enfermeras de Chile*, Vol. 2, No. 10, 12-1942-01-1943, p. 44-46;

 Participants were nurses of the American Nurses Association and the American Red Cross as well as nurses from Bolivia, Argentina, Peru, Brasil, Ecuador, Colombia, and Paraguay, in: Primer Centenario de la Universidad de Chile: Primer Congreso Panamericano de Enfermería, Santiago 1942, http://www.memoriachilena.gob.cl/archivos2/pdfs/MC0065726.pdf [07.04.2022];

 For details about the participation of Argentinean nurses in the congress, see Martín (2020), p. 86.

225. Quote: "¡Salva Chile! ¡Salva a las naciones americanas unidas! ¡Salva a las Américas!," in: Dias, Ana Maria: Mensaje de las enfermeras brasileras a sus colegas de América, in: *Boletín de la Asociación de Enfermeras de Chile*, Vol. 2, No. 10, 12-1942-01-1943, p. 47.
226. Quote: "Vivimos la época más dura y más extraña que jamás ha vivido la humanidad. Vamos hacio lo desconocido. Mujer, prepárate, sé Enfermera, y comprenderas major tus semejantes. Comprender es sinómino de Querer, y es eso los que necesitamos. Conocernos hasta ese punto. Las generaciones que se están gestando hoy, necesitarán mañana de una guía y ese guías serás tu, enfermera.[…] tu inteligencia, tu amor de madre, tu espíritu de sacrificio, Tu bondad jamás discutida," in: Ocupa tu puesto, in: *Boletín de la Asociación de Enfermeras de Chile*, Vol. 2, No. 10, 12-1942-01-1943, p. 55.
227. The most quoted article Peake published was "Lo que pueden estudiar las mujeres en Valparaíso" from 1945, in: Leal (2014).
228. Peake, Gladys: Formación de la Enfermera y Auxiliares de Enfermería, in: Actas de las Segundas Jornadas Chilenas de Salubridad, Santiago 1953, p. 84-114, 90, 98-99, 107.
229. No sources found about her biography before the 1940s.
230. The nursing association described her in 1943 as a head nurse (*enfermera jefe*) but did not provide information about the hospital where she worked and how long she was in this position, in: *Boletín de la Asociación de Enfermeras de Chile*, Vol. 2, No. 10, 12-1942-01-1943, p. 58.
231. Zárate (2013), p. 120;

    The first time women were entitled to vote in national elections was in 1949, in: Klimpel: La mujer chilena, Santiago [Ed. Andrés Bello] 1962, p. 94.
232. Asociación Nacional de Enfermeras Universitaria 1948, quoted in: Zárate (2019), p. 5;

    Theodore Candy was the director of the Cooperative Inter American Department of Salubrity Projects (*Departamento Cooperativo Interamericano de Obras de Salubridad*), the right arm of the US Office of the Coordinator of Inter-American Affairs, in: Suárez, Eugenio: La Sanidad en Chile, in: *Boletín de la Oficina Sanitaria Panamericana*, Vol. 23, No. 11, 1944, p. 961-966, 962.
233. Zárate (2019), p. 7.
234. Collao Avilés et al. dated the foundation to 1947, in: Collao Avilés et al. (2019), p. 44.

    Zárate dates the foundation of the school to April 1948, in: Zárate (2019), p. 7.
235. Gratz, Alejandro: Gladys Peake Guevara, in: *Diario Concepción*, 02.09.2018.

236. Collao Avilés et al. (2019), p. 44.
237. Collao Avilés et al. state that it was in 1944, but did not name the first director, in: Collao et al. (2019), p. 43;

   Rivas Riveros et al. are not specific about this, but their formulation suggests that the first female director was Flores, in: Rivas et al. (2019), p. 196;

   In doing so, they agreed with the committee which organized the celebrations of the first centenary of Universidad de Chile's nursing school, honoring Flores as the first director, but without giving an exact date when she took on this position, in: Universidad de Chile: Escuela de enfermería cumple un siglo, https://www.uchile.cl/noticias/39486/escuela-de-enfermeria-cumple-un-siglo [07.04.2022];

   Campos Harriet (1960) listed Elianira González as the first female director in 1947, followed by Flores in 1957, in: Campos Harriet, Fernando: Desarollo educacional 1810-1960, Santiago [Editorial Andrés Bello] 1960, p. 151;
238. In 1950, Flores was the administrative director of the University of Chile's nursing school, in: Sociedad Chilena de Salubridad y Medicina Pública: Actas de las primeras jornadas chilenas de salubridad, Santiago 1952, p. 35, https://obtienearchivo.bcn.cl/obtienearchivo?id=documentos/10221.1/57860/2/75958.pdf&origen=BDigital [07.04.2022].
239. In 1949, on the occasion of the Second Regional Nursing Congress in Lima, Flores represented the Chilean nurses alongside Pincheira and Peake, in: Segundo Congreso Regional de Enfermería 20.09.1949-02.10.1949: Informe final, https://iris.paho.org/bitstream/handle/10665.2/11840/v29n1p94.pdf?sequence=1&isAllowed=y [07.04.2022];

   In 1951, it was only Peake who integrated the Chilean delegation in the WHO executive board alongside two physicians, in: WHO: Appointments to expert advisory panels and committees, Eighth Session, 01.06.1951, https://apps.who.int/iris/bitstream/handle/10665/132863/EB8_16_fre.pdf?sequence=1&isAllowed=y [07.04.2022].
240. Flores (1965).
241. Uribe, Jeannine: Nurses, Philanthropies, and Governments: The Public Mission of Chilean Nursing 1900—1945, Philadelphia [University of Pennsylvania Press] 2008, p. 189;

   The school was named "Isidora Lyon Cousiño Nursing School" after its benefactor, in: Rivas (2019), p. 44.
242. Women who wanted to become nursing auxiliaries had to accomplish at least a few years of secondary education, in: Peake, Gladys: Formación de la Enfermera y Auxiliares de Enfermería, in: *Actas de las Segundas Jornadas Chilenas de Salubridad*, Santiago 1953, p. 84-114, 107.

243. The system of the health units expanded. Until the end of the 1940s, 18 of them existed throughout the country. This was probably the reason why Pincheira could hand the administration over to her colleagues and increase her commitment as a PAHO advisor in Latin America, in: Romero et al.: Unidades Sanitarias de Chile, in: *Boletín de la Oficina Sanitaria Panamericana*, Vol. 13, No. 1, 07-1952, p. 11-17, 16, https://iris.paho.org/bitstream/handle/10665.2/11942/v33n1p11.pdf?sequence=1&isAllowed=y [07.04.2022].
244. Martín (2020), p. 94.
245. Zárate relies on the information of Klimpel, in: Zárate (2013), p. 151;
 Klimpel (1962) listed Pincheira and Lozier as the two Chilean nursing advisors of the WHO in 1962, in: Klimpel (1962), p. 164;
 In 1952, Lozier helped to establish postgraduate studies in nursing at the *Universidad Nacional Autónoma de México*, in: Castañeda Godínez, María Cristina et al.: Formación profesional de enfermería durante la primera mitad del Siglo XX en la UNAM, in: Revista Enfermería Universitaria ENEO-UNAM, Vol. 7, No. Special, 2010, p. 25-33, 32;
 In 1965, Lozier visited Rio de Janeiro as a PAHO advisor, in: Instituto Latinoamericano y del Caribe de Planificación Económica y Social: Quinto curso de capacitación en planificación de salud, Santiago 1966, p. 3
 Zárate also awards to Amanda Parada an important share in transplanting US-American ideas to Latin America, in: Zárate (2013), p. 150.
246. White, Verna; Waddell Chagas, Agnes: A Workshop Experiment in Latin America, in: *American Journal of Nursing*, Vol. 51, No. 6, 1951, p. 374-77.
247. Law No. 11.161, 20.02.1953, Crea el Colegio de Enfermeras y fija las disposiciones por las que regirá;
 Founded in 1888, the British Nurses Association became a role model for similar organizations worldwide, in: Velandia (2016), p. 892
248. More details about the foundation of the Brazilian nursing association, in: Miotto Wright, María da Gloria; Puntel de Almeida, Maria Cecília; Coelho de Souza Padhila, Maria Itayra; Leal David, Helena M.S.; de Albuquerque, Gelson; Da Silva, Jaqueline: Nursing in Brazil, in: Nursing and Globalization in the Americas (2009), p. 99-135, 131.
249. More information about the Argentinean Association of Diploma Holding Nurses, in: Chervo, María Alejandra; Arzani, Eduardo Miguel; Micozzi, Teresa Isabel: Nursing in Argentina, in: Ibid., p. 104-105;
 In 1967, the first nursing law was implemented in Argentina, in: Ibid, p. 128.
250. Flores de Fernández (1965), p. 23.
251. Záarate (2017).

252. Tobar et al. (1942), p. 133-148, 147.
253. In 1961 existed 181 NHS facilities, in: Krebs (1961), p. 8.
254. Ministerio de Salubridad Pública: Oficio No. 238, Remite proyecto de reestructuración del Servicio Nacional de Salubridad, 238-202-1952, 20.02.1952, 1-9 [6-14/14].
255. Leal (2014), p. 10.
256. Núñez Carrasco, E. Rocío: Enfermería chilena 1970-1980: Dos décadas de transformación de la identidad, una revisión desde la memoria colectiva de la enfermería, Santiago 2012.
257. Zárate stated that Peake had also been the *CECh*'s president, in: Zárate (2013), p. 151.
258. In 1956, Peake presented a training course for auxiliary workers to the US ambassador, in: International Cooperation Administration: Health summary 1955-1956, Chile. Monthly activities, p. 14.
259. Law No. 11.934, 27.10.1955, Crea Colegio de Asistentes Sociales.
260. Law No. 14.895, 11.09.1962, Crea la institución con personalidad jurídica denominada Colegio de Matronas.
261. Law No. 17.164, 02.08.1969, Crea el Colegio de Tecnólogos Médicos de Chile.
262. Decree Law No. 1, 17.01.1970, Estatutos del Colegio de Kinesiólogos.
263. Krebs (1961), p. 7.
264. Flores (1965), p. 23;
265. Interviews with Ivette Cap de Ville and Teresa Aburto, Santiago, 2015 and 2017.
266. During the 1960s, the RF invested personnel and financial aid mostly in Mexico, but continued to work with Chilean universities, in: The Rockefeller Foundation: Our history, https://www.rockefellerfoundation.org/about-us/our-history/ [22.05.2022].
267. Schleiermacher, Sabine: Die Rockefeller Foundation und ihr Engagement bei einer Neuorientierung von Medizin und Public Health in Deutschland in den 1950er Jahren / The Rockefeller Foundation and its efforts toward a reorientation of German medicine and public health in the 1950s, in: *Medizinisches Journal*, Vol 45, No. 1, 2010, p. 43-65.
268. Contracts with the UN, in: 15.01.1957 Ministerio de Salud, Asesoría Jurídica, Dr. Givovich Mercier, Ministro de Salud, Subrogante: Ord Nr. 152 A.J./Nr. 1523 Carta Convenio Nr. 1375 para curso Enfermería-Obstetricia en Salud Materno-Infantil, 1990-1523, 17.06.1975;

    Contract with the PAHO, in: Flores de Fernández (1965), p. 22.
269. Interview with Patricia Talloni, Santiago 2017;

    Contemporary researchers in Chilean nursing history like Chuaqui-Kettlun (2014) and Zárate (2019) use the term "golden age of nursing" without defining it.

270. Krebs, Doris: Necesidades y recursos de enfermería en Chile, Santiago [Imprenta de la Central de Talleres del S.N.S.] 1961.
271. International Council of Nurses: Desarollo de mesas de trabajo celebradas durante los días 15, 16 y 17 de enero, con motivo de la visita de miss Doris Krebs, in: Boletín Cultural e Informativo, p. 7.
272. Lazo Hinrichs, Roberto Germán: Estudio de los daños de los terremotos del 21 y 22 de mayo de 1960, Santiago 2008, p. 128, http://www.tesis.uchile.cl/tesis/uchile/2008/lazo_rh/sources/lazo_rh.pdf [12.04.2022].
273. Lehmann, Paulo: Escuela de Enfermería UACh celebra sus 50 Años de existencia,19/20.04.2013,http://noticias.uach.cl/principal.php?pag=noticia-externo&cod=57788 [22.05.2022].
274. Paredes; Rivas (2014), p. 11.
275. Up until 1980, the University of Chile had faculties in all large cities of the country. There also existed two technical universities in Punta Arenas and Santiago, two Catholic universities in Santiago and in Valparaíso, and the two semi-public universities *Universidad de Concepción* and *Universidad Austral*, in: Esfera de Acción de la *Enfermera* en Chile, in: *Enfermería*, No. 55, 01-02-03-1978, p. 7–11, 10.
276. Monsálvez; Valdés (2016), in: Rivas (2019).
277. Paredes et al. (2014), p. 11.
278. Castellano Salas; Tagle Vargas, Cristina; Galdames, Luz; Riquelme, Náyade: Examen Nacional de Enfermería en Chile: Importancia y Desafíos, in: Ciencia y Enfermería, Vol. 17, No. 1, (2011) p. 27-36, S. 28.
279. Ministerio de Salud Pública, Oficina de Asuntos Internacionales: Oficio No. 1466, Convalidación de títulos de post-grado en Enfermería, 1466-1819-1972, 17.08.1972, 1–2.
280. Interview with Patricia Talloni, Santiago, March 2017.
281. Krebs does not mention the nursing auxiliaries, in: Krebs (1961), p. 36.
282. The study listed only nurses as members of the teaching staff. Krebs called them instructors (*instructoras*). They spent one-third of their working time in classes and two-thirds in supervising the clinical preparation of the students, in: Krebs (1961), p. 26.
283. Ibid, p. 36.
284. Peake as the president of the *CECh* in 1962, in: Klimpel (1962).
285. Fardella was the director at least until 1971, in: Fardella N., Directora Departamento de *Enfermería*, U. de Chile: Atención de Enfermería Proporcionada a los pacientes del Servicio de Cirugía Hospital San Fernando, in: Enfermería, No. 29, 07-08-09-1971, p. 48–51.
286. Krebs was one of the founders and the first director of the nursing school in Valdivia (*Universidad Austral*), in: Paredes et al. (2014) , p. 11;
287. Ministerio de Salud Pública: Oficio No. 974, Comunica autorización de Dirección de Presupuesto para contratar funcionarios del Servicio Nacional de Salud, 974-1686-1968, 01.06.1968, p. 1-4 [16-19/20].

288. This is suggested by an NHS report from 1972. The number of nurses and midwives did not grow in the 15 preceding years, in: Informe de la Comisión investigadora del Servicio Nacional de Salud, in: Camara de Diputados: Sesión 10a, 19.04.1972, https://www.bcn.cl/laborparlamentaria/wsgi/consulta/verDiarioDeSesion.py?id=583523. [07.04.2022].
289. Colegio de Enfermeras de Chile: Memoria Anual (Junio 1967-Junio 1968), in: *Enfermería*, No. 17, 07-08-09-1968.
290. Primer Congreso Panamericano de Enfermería, Santiago 1942.
291. The foundation took place on October 26, 1967, in Mendoza, Argentina. Members of the *CECh* integrated the first board. Only representatives from Chile and Argentina participated in the Congress, in: *Colegio de Enfermeras de Chile: Memoria Anual* (Junio 1967-Junio 1968), in: Enfermería, No. 17, 07-08-09-1968.
292. The *CECh* led the first provisory board of the *FEPPEN*, until the foundation process finally ended in 1970.
293. From July 1965 to July 1966, the journal was monthly published, in: Pincheira: Editorial, in: *Enfermería*, No. 43-44, 01-06-1975, p. 3;

     The *CECh* council in Santiago, notably president Sonia Garrido Ballerino, encouraged the foundation of the journal, in: Ibid., p. 3;
294. In 1969, the association of midwives published for the first time a bulletin. A group of midwives, most of them working in the hospitals Del Salvador and San Borja, had recently started to build an organization similar to the already existing associations of nurses and social workers. The midwives also wanted to publish a journal like *Enfermería*, but they had no financial resources for such a project, in: Consejo General del Colegio de Matronas: *Boletín de la Matrona*, Año 1, 07-1969, No. 1.
295. Decree Law No. 217, 03.06.1967, in: Colegio de Enfermeras de Chile: Memoria Anual (Junio 1967-Junio 1968), in: *Enfermería*, No. 17, 07-08-09-1968, p. 7.
296. In September 1967, *CECh* president Marilia Fonseca participated in the Second Congress of Nursing Auxiliaries (*Segundo Congreso Nacional de Auxiliares de Enfermería*), in: ibid, p. 2.
297. The foundation process took more than two years, in: La Sociedad Chilena de Enfermería Pediátrica esta en marcha, in: *Enfermería*, No. 29, 07-08-09-1971, p. 28.
298. The first sign of a governmental nursing policy can be verified only for the second half of the term. In June 1968, Valdivieso claimed for the harmonization of the NHS schools with the academic standards of the University of Chile's nursing school. The health minister formed a commission directed by Juan Hepp Dubiau, the General Health Director, and Guillermo Adriasola Espejo representing the Medical Faculty. For the

first time, such a committee included also nurses Alicia Letelier, administrative director, and Blaza Nahum Iturregui, deputy board member of the of the Carlos Van Buren school, in: Ministerio de Salud Pública: Oficio No. 055, Nombra comisión estudio problemas escuelas dependientes del Servicio Nacional de Salud, 055-1685-1968, 14.06.1968, p. 1-2 [1-2/2];

299. Colegio de Enfermeras de Chile: Memoria Anual (Junio 1967-Junio 1968), in: *Enfermería*, No. 17, 07-08-09-1968, p. 7.
300. Ejercicio Profesional como tema Central en el V Congreso Nacional de Enfermería, in: *Enfermería*, No. 16, 04-05-06-1968.
    The national convention of nursing teachers took place in November 1968, in: Convención Nacional de Docentes, in: *Enfermería*, No. 18, 10-11-12-1968, p. 13–14.
301. Octavo Congreso Interamericano de Enfermeras en Guatemala, in: Colegio de Enfermeras de Chile: Memoria Anual (Junio 1967-Junio 1968), in: *Enfermería*, No. 17, 07-08-09-1968, p. 10.
    In 1968, *CECh* president Fonseca took part in the Fourth Argentinean Nursing Congress (*IV Congreso Argentino de Enfermeras*), in: Ibid, p.2.
    An unknown number of Chilean nurses participated 1969 in the ICN congress in Montreal, Canada, in: Ibid, p. 12.
302. In 1968, Fonseca assisted the celebration on the occasion of the *Medicina Curativa* implementation, in: Colegio de Enfermeras de Chile: Memoria Anual (Junio 1967-Junio 1968), in: *Enfermería*, No. 17, 07-08-09-1968, p. 2.
303. In 1968 or 1969, an academic commission to analyze the *Medicina Curativa* act was founded. The *CECh* was one of the co-founders, in: Informe de la Comisión "Ley de Medicina Curativa," in: *Enfermería*, No. 18, 10-11-12-1968, p. 12.
304. Quote: "se aprobó la duración de 4 años para la Carrera, correspondiendo el 4° año a internado. Que el 1er Año las carreras de obstetricia y enfermería tuvieran los ramos básicos [...] común en 2 años y de ahí se diversificara," in: Duración Carrera obstetricia, in: Consejo General del Colegio de Matronas: *Boletín de la Matrona*, Año 1, 07-1969, No. 1.
305. Colegio de Enfermeras de Chile: Memoria Anual (Junio 1967-Junio 1968), in: *Enfermería*, No. 17, 07-08-09-1968.
306. Ibid.
307. The earliest reference to dissatisfaction among younger colleagues was mentioned in 1977 in *Enfermería*, in: Memoria Anual del Consejo General del Colegio de Enfermeras de Chile, Periodo 18 de mayo de 1975 al 30 de Abril de 1976, in: *Enfermería*, No. 51, 01-02-03-1977, p. 34–43, 34.

308. Flores (1965), p. 20.
309. The documentation of the 6th National Congress celebrated in October 1970 in Santiago suggests extensive attendance to the general council, in: Krebs Wilkens et al.: Relatos y Correlatos del VI Congreso Nacional de Enfermeras, in: *Enfermería*, No. 26, 10-11-12-1970, p. 15–18;

    The attendees formulated the goals for the following years. They voted for closer cooperation with the physicians, dentists, pharmacists, midwives, and other health professions. On a legislative level, once again they claimed for a new career scheme and the inclusion of their services to the *Medicina Curativa* act, in: Colegio de Enfermeras: Plan de Trabajo para 1971, in: *Enfermería*, No. 26, 10-11-12-1970, p. 79–80.
310. Leonardo Bravo, Alfredo: Prologo, in: Krebs W., Doris: Necesidades y recursos de enfermería en Chile, Santiago 1961, p. V.

CHAPTER 2

Nursing in Times of Socialism (1970–1973)

1 Introduction

The 1970 election was decisive for Chilean nursing. Not only did national politics gain momentum for fundamental social reforms but also political and social conflict quickly escalated to radicalization resulting in a steady weakening of the state's Keynesian approach. However, although the history of nursing under socialism, and especially public health nursing, seemed to have continuity from the Frei era but without many new developments. After the "revolution in freedom," Allende's Popular Unity (*Unidad Popular, UP*) continued to work with community health councils (*consejos comunitarios de salud*) and expanded them with socialist-inspired groups called health brigades (*brigadas de salud*). These were state funded in order to help bridge the gap in healthcare coverage. On that same note, a unified health system was to be created. That plan, however, failed due to the physicians, dentists, pharmacists, and nurses' rejection of the changes to worktime, payment schemes, and the additional health services being requested of them.

UP's lack of an integrated healthcare reform gained notoriety when increasingly polarized fronts would avoid all governmental measures that had a socialist bent. Until 1972, strikes sabotaged intended reforms so that *UP* Ministry of Health could only carry on with plans from the Frei administration. One of them was a strong focus on *materno-infantil* problems, financed and advised by international aid organizations.

© The Author(s), under exclusive license to Springer Nature Switzerland AG 2023

M. Thulin, R. A. Ayala, *Nursing, Policy and Politics in Twentieth-century Chile*,
https://doi.org/10.1007/978-3-030-90835-5_2

Initially, nurses tolerated the governmental measures, although their institutionalization and academization continued to grow. However, as in the years before, the nursing association sought to benefit from a specific health insurance for public employees and an improved position on the salary scale. The nurses' association board backed the physicians to block all governmental measures except those which could open up bargaining for better payment terms. Most importantly, nurses refused the expansion of volunteer organizations and the expansion of the auxiliary workforce in care services.

Noticeably, at the beginning and the end of political mobilization in Chile stands the involvement of women. Their workforce and political behavior were decisive when the male leaders of the country (i.e., government, Armed Forces, parliament, or social movement spokesmen) needed to strengthen their power base. Nevertheless, the outcome for the female professionals remained modest compared to the goals they had for themselves; for nurses these involved more staff, equal pay, and a better standing in the bureaucratic hierarchy. The largest group of women in healthcare, the nursing auxiliaries, was given no voice in the political process and, likely because of their social origin, continued to be oppressed by male and female professionals alike. One might argue that the "working class" was Allende's main constituency base. And yet, the intersection with gender can explain why excluding nursing auxiliaries from high politics continued in times of socialism.

However, this rejection by professionally trained nurses of the government's key plans marked the high point of their political power within the profession since the early 1950s. While there is a common assumption that nurses as women remained strictly apolitical during state reforms, this chapter supports the increasing argument of nurses' political agency in the defense of their collective interests, even if they were unable to actually turn prerogatives into gains.

2 Politics Without Policies: The Popular Unity's Vision of an Equal Healthcare Provision

Shortly after rising to power, in 1970, the Popular Unity announced an ambitious plan to expand the provision of healthcare services for all Chileans within the next six years (*Plan Sexenal de Salud*).[1] As other coalition partners disagreed about the measures leading up effectively to this goal, and with the opposition dominating the parliament,[2] Allende and his cabinet made use of decrees to implement at least some of its elements. They ordered an increase of salaries, the recruitment of volunteers, a control mechanism for physicians' work hours, and the expansion of the already existing *Medicina Curativa* Act (see Chap. 1). Several interpretations suggest that beneath those measures lay the intention to merge the NHS and *SERMENA* into a unified health system (*sistema único de salud*).[3] The government's range of decrees, and even the power it held, would prove insufficient to make such a change in the system.

Nevertheless, the start was promising. Measure number one, the pay rise in the public system, in March 1971, was gladly welcomed,[4] and with that the government thought the associations would bear, and even endorse, the measures to follow.[5] It appeared to be the right moment to introduce socialist-inspired volunteer groups as part of the masterplan for enhancing care services.

In September 1971, health minister Juan Carlos Concha (1971–1972) decreed the statutes for founding what came to be known as health councils (*consejos de salud*) and health brigades (*brigadas de salud*). In doing that, Concha wanted to reinforce Frei's system of neighborhood committees (*juntas de vecinos*), mothers' centers (*centros de madres*), and community health councils (*consejos comunitarios de salud*).[6] The new arrangement integrating health brigades doing self-taught work was meant to expand the area of responsibility and the workflow of the healthcare staff.[7]

Concha praised the program and labeled it "a success."[8] But the study of the German researcher Müller-Plantenberg suggests that by March 1973 only 45 percent of the councils had been formed. According to her study, the still effective Law No. 15.076 and the authoritarian management style of the physicians greatly hindered cooperation between volunteers and the professional staff.[9] Archives documenting the work of the brigades and councils are rare. Even if they may have meant some improvement, any trace of them had disappeared during the coup d'état. In May 1972, Concha himself admitted "multiple difficulties" which shrank the possibilities of implementing volunteer work smoothly.[10]

In the few cases Müller-Plantenberg described effective cooperation between health volunteers and staff, she referred only to technical and "social" workshops. The participants of the volunteer program mostly helped to promote education campaigns to limit the spread of contagious diseases like diarrhea and pneumonia, and improved hygiene measures. Some of the volunteers were referred to by Müller-Plantenberg as "participants" (*Teilnehmer*), adding that by being trained by health professionals they could even become *Krankenpflegerinnen* (nurses). As nursing services were provided by both self-taught and trained staff, working together often led to overlapping tasks between groups.

Müller-Plantenberg did not seem pessimistic about the overall success of such a strategy, but she pointed out how, instead of actually addressing Chile's gaps in coverage, the *UP* volunteer system had failed.[11] Health brigades and councils did not have any legal status or regulation[12] as the political polarization of the country hindered any eventual agreement on the backing of their work. Women did not lead those councils, which is why using volunteers can be interpreted as an ideological device within the fight between males, socialists, conservatives or otherwise. In this respect, the nursing association also became a battleground of the medical association.

Resistance against volunteer work in health had grown progressively since the outset, but it was only at its peak during the 1972 strike that it appeared for the first time in the newspapers. The rejection of the brigades and councils was evident on an extensive list of professional associations' complaints. The nurses, physicians, dentists, and pharmacists called the volunteer groups the "frontline brigades" (*brigadas de choque*), but these were "only implemented to cause ideological discord without any real intent toward improving the health care coverage."[13] What was initially meant to be a technical solution was then taken by the professional establishment as a rather political intervention.

For the *UP* the road ahead would be uphill. This became evident when Concha attempted to increase the level of control over the physicians' work time[14] and expand *Medicina Curativa* to all NHS insured. Physicians who treated *SERMENA* patients feared the end of their privileges, with the medical association organizing a resistance movement.[15] At first glance, nurses had no reasons to join them, but as we will see nationalist feelings overshadowed interprofessional conflicts.

A new conflict surfaced between the medical association and the government in a moment when the NHS announced that it would need to hire a further 4500 physicians and 3000 university-trained nurses to guarantee full healthcare coverage.[16] *UP* leaders decided to intensify the hiring of health professionals from abroad, especially Cuba, to solve this issue.[17] In doing so, Allende and Concha gave the medical association a good reason to convince health professionals like nurses to turn against the government.[18] Nurses joined the resistance movement when the rhetoric that

Cubans would deprive nationals of the already scant job offers came to surface.[19] However, before describing the confrontations that arose, we will highlight some of the other measures the *UP* tried to implement to improve public health in the *materno-infantil* sector.

As illustrated in Chap. 1, governmental health policies were assessed by the services provided to women and children. Such policies also received the highest amount of international attention. During the 1970s and 1980s, Chilean authors like Chanfreau and Belmar or US researchers like the physician Victor Sidel, nurse Hillary Modell, and sociologist Howard Waitzkin praised the achievements of the Popular Unity in the area of public health and the *materno-infantil* area. They highlighted especially the launching of brand-new children's hospitals.[20] Statements of the Ministry of Health confirmed this perception.[21] But all those sources failed to provide evidence for the real estate projects for healthcare facilities, not continued but started by the Allende administration. This leads us to the view that the measurable positive effect in the *materno-infantil* area, especially in the reduction of child mortality and the growth of university-trained nursing, was not prompted by the Popular Unity and did not significantly expand the health coverage as compared to the previous administration.[22] Healthcare coverage did expand, mainly due to public health becoming an integral part of the system, but despite increasing efforts, the process remained just as slow as in the preceeding fifty years.

But the need was urgent. The Ministry of Health's hotline went almost into meltdown with calls from all over the country. One case within the long, narrow Chilean geography was the town of Coyhaique, 1700 km south of Santiago. In March 1972, the ministry rejected the local authority's request to hire a gynecologist onto an NHS facility. Some 1200 inhabitants and 70 births per year did not seem high enough a workload to spare a professional in one of the rare specialities. Instead, the ministry sent a *practicante* to support the two nursing auxiliaries working there.[23] But this was not the kind of collaboration the government hoped to perform with the volunteers and self-taught staff. Political issues, however, took the focus away from practical solutions, a result of which being that professional representatives often could not come through.

Inevitably, the Popular Unity began to lose its initial spark as the insufficient healthcare coverage, among other things, lowered people's trust in the government. Often, municipalities had only half of the necessary health staff.[24] In August 1973, three weeks before the coup d'état, in six out of the 26 provinces of the region of Maule not a single health professional or nursing auxiliary was available to monitor labor and delivery.[25] Plus, the intensively propagated campaign of milk distribution stagnated,[26] and as a consequence a number of cities and villages had no formal access to healthcare or foodstuffs.

Despite this, not all health professionals responded to the emergency with rejection and protest. One case of a volunteering project managed by physicians, dentists, nurses, and midwives adherent to the Popular Unity can be traced back to 1972. Modell and Waitzkin described the achievements of the health train (*tren de salud*), according to whom 30,000 Chileans received nursing and medical care from this type of vehicles, meant to serve as health centers on wheels.[27] An yet as in the case of information campaigns about addictive behavior and hygiene improvement,[28] its impact is difficult to assess.[29]

It would seem that most of the nurses who were active in the association board did not believe in the socialist-inspired volunteer work, in collaborating with health professionals from Cuba, or even in an egalitarian healthcare system. The absence of nursing in the government plans and the strong focus on medical care may explain their aversion to these policies. Concha and Allende barely knew about the nurses' claims and aspirations, which in essence were not politically motivated. As will be shown, in October 1972 when the board led by Gladys Peake positioned itself against the government, it was the first time that nurses' claims appeared in the headlines. This decision was more an outcry for recognition of equal status in healthcare policies, and thus why nurses decided to distance themselves from the traditional ways of doing political work and called for a systemic change.

3 Dependence on International Aid

As we have seen, during the twentieth century, Chile's healthcare was poor, especially when judged within the context of international standards. A significant number of Chileans had no access to medical care or could not afford the entirety of the necessary professional services. Only large international investments in finance, technology, and staffing avoided a complete breakdown of the healthcare system. These investments also enabled the country's geographical growth and steady population growth. The consequence was a greater dependence on North America and Europe. Chilean governments were framed as mere recipients, and by this it was meant that the nation was in a weak position for negotiations with foreign companies, institutes, foundations, and NGOs about how healthcare would be managed.

Since World War II, the US made the largest investments. Their national advisors, their NGOs, aid programs, and universities provided help and set the basis of Chile's modern healthcare administration. Most importantly, until 1950 the IHC—and since then PAHO as well as US American foundations, NGOs, and universities—trained, advised, and supported several generations of professionals and workers in health and other related areas. US professionals in health, administration, finance, and education were substantially involved when it came to designing and promoting health plans recommended by PAHO/WHO and the UN. Therefore, it was not only one of the state's responsibilities to cure the injured or look after the sick, pregnant women, and children, but also to plan the population growth and create appropriate remedies to ensure the healthcare system was suitable and up to date to match with the expanding population. Foreign actors either implemented entire processes in healthcare or monitored them closely.

Chile during the Cold War provides a prime example of the Western World's growing philanthropic engagement in Latin America.[30] The intentions of foreign supporters were, however, far from selfless. Health and medicine were decisive in ensuring support for a specific political system. Since the growth of Soviet influence and the Cuban Revolution, North American and Western European governments acknowledged that the decision to either support or fight an ideology was not only taken in party headquarters. Hospitals and health centers were also important battlegrounds of the so-called "third world" during the Cold War. For many, the best presidential candidate would not be the one who could fix and expand healthcare but, very important, the one who crafted the best political program ideologically.

The third special meeting of Latin American health ministers and the governing board of PAHO, held in Santiago in 1972, was one of the most prestigious international achievements of Allende's presidency.[31] PAHO had become the most important donor for the Chilean healthcare system. In 1972 alone, it co-financed 30 projects in Chile totaling some 926,751 USD.[32] That was about 37 percent of the state's yearly budget for healthcare.[33] PAHO classified the projects into six categories:

- Control of sexually transmitted diseases
- Clinical and community pediatrics

- Training in nutrition and body development
- Medical care
- Water supply
- Tuberculosis control

Foreign help covered primarily the first three categories, meaning public health and hospital services in the *materno-infantil* area. Framed as a priority area, it seems that on the eve of Allende's fall, gynecology and pediatrics were assigned more than two-thirds of the entire NHS and PAHO funding.[34] Still in the planning phase were "health services" and "rehabilitation" as well as a cooperation with the Chilean Bacteriological Institute.[35]

The PAHO projects were co-financed, which in practice meant that the government had to invest about a half million USD in order to receive about the same amount of money. Like most other poor countries, Chile could not cover such expenses and as a result the PAHO had to abate part of the country's share on several occasions.[36]

The second important foreign donor was the United Nations, which was the most active in two of the programs. In 1972, the World Food Programme (WFP) provided funding of 335,111 USD and UNICEF another 556,000.[37] In June of the same year, the United Nations Population Fund (UNFPA) announced to endow the amount of 3.1 million USD in the next four years. The goal was to finance universities and training centers as well as scholarships for health professionals to specialize abroad.[38] Yet what may sound like a great success of the Popular Unity was, like in most foreign-supported policy, a result of projects started during the Frei administration.[39]

For the purpose of this chapter, as the ministry did not detail resource allocation, one might wonder how much of the PAHO funding really reached healthcare staffing schemes. The new deal with UNFPA suggests that the agreements focused on the alignment of Chilean health professionals with international standards. Nevertheless, the impact seems limited. In 1972, some 98 (0.58 percent) of the 16,681 health professionals working in the NHS received a scholarship to have specialized training abroad or attend international workshops or conferences.[40] Once again, the auxiliary personnel did not appear on the records for any kind of scholarships.

Staff shortages were a major problem Allende's health ministers faced, and in the early 1970s the lack of a national pharmaceutical industry became apparent. In February 1972, undersecretary of health Carlos

Molina Bustos (1970–1973) visited seven countries in North America and Europe. His interest was to convince potential partners to help him bridge the gap in the distribution of pharmaceutical products and medical supplies.[41] Despite the growth in foreign aid, shortages and delivery problems increased constantly during the course of 1972. Finally, political confrontations between right- and left-wing groups from October 1972 complicated, and in some cases even blocked, several projects with international partners.[42] While a shortage of medical supplies was critical in medical services, nursing care was equally dependent on the availability of stocks, which added to the demoralizing atmosphere. While the nurses' association board was dominated by an anti-Allende sentiment, structural problems hindered any policy in the terms nurses were calling for.

4 Continuities in Nursing Practice and Standstill in Nursing Politics

It would seem that the measures of the previous governments to increase the availability of nursing professionals continued during the Popular Unity government. The number of study places for students in nursing schools increased significantly. At the University of Chile, the number of places being offered quadrupled within a two-year span, rising from 50 in 1970 to 200 in 1972,[43] taking into consideration only the Santiago branches. The same upward development was mirrored in the academization of the profession. After the nursing schools in Santiago, the NHS schools in Valparaíso and Concepción tightened collaborations with the local medical faculties and the public sector.[44] This development can be regarded as further academization of female health professions, as more students of midwifery, laboratory technology, dietetics, and social work were too enabled to enter university.[45] The existence of a Chilean Association of Nursing Schools (*Asociación de Escuelas de Enfermería de Chile*) and the launching of various master's programs in nursing reflect the ever-expanding university-based nature of this profession during this era. This reality took place alongside the evolution of national standards of practice and the adoption of international ones.[46]

The most influential nursing school, both in size and research orientation, was located in the University of Chile in the north of Santiago. During the 1960s, it was chaired by Iris Monardez and Doris Krebs, who trained most of the new generation of nurses and published frequently in

Peake's trade magazine, Nursing (*Enfermería*).[47] This was mirrored by the expansion of similar nursing schools housed in various universities, which had started in the decade before and continued developing. It is not clear how many new schools opened between 1970 and 1973, but it becomes evident that this process stopped abruptly due to the political climate that emerged from the July 1972 events.[48]

Although the Popular Unity supported the academic institutionalization of nursing, as the government did not last for a long time, it could not develop a nursing policy of its own, and most of the projects being run were passed down from the Christian Democratic administration. The archives of the Ministry of Health show that the then ministers Jirón and Concha did not even know about recurrent subjects nurses tried to vindicate, such as the salary scale comprised in Law No. 15.076.[49] Concha met Peake and Garrido, who were sitting on the *CECh* board since July 1971,[50] at events like the National Congress of Nurses in May 1972.[51] One would expect he was aware that the nurses' association could become an oppositional front were the salary affair to worsen. However, he confirmed to us in an interview in 2017 that he only learned about this after his term of office.[52]

The efforts undertaken by the socialist government benefited nurses in the first place. What was not foreseen though was a move to partly cover the shortage of nurses, and partly be on good terms with the midwifery association, by creating the "nurse-midwife" profession or *enfermera-matrona*. Nevertheless, the Ministry of Health's policies were not stringent. One sign of this was nurses' unsuccessful struggle to climb in the *Medicina Curativa* plan (fee-for-service scheme), whereas Jirón permitted midwives to do so.[53]

Nurses generally perceive the 1970s as a "bad" decade, possibly idealizing their institutional achievements in the decades before. However, on closer inspection one can find important continuities. Chilean nurses greatly benefited from the tight cooperation between the governments and PAHO. The most important subject in their correspondence was the Program of Education for Chilean Nursing (*Programa de Educación de Enfermería en Chile*).[54] One of its most applauded parts was the constant delivery of educational literature for healthcare professionals, beginning in 1968, a subsidy totaling 3 million USD in 1972. The nurses' association together with the NHS oversaw the allocation of the budget for nursing students.[55]

Another important field of philanthropic funds was the allocation of scholarships for health professionals, including nurses. Stays abroad and visits of foreign consultants in Chile are the best-documented aspects of the cooperation with PAHO. Archives show that, among all the female health professions, nurses were by far the main recipients.[56] Even though their number was small, the destination choice for the grantees was impressive: in 1972, nurses undertook training in Cuba, Puerto Rico, Peru, Argentina, and Colombia.[57] In the same year, the North American nurses Carolyn Williams (University of North Carolina) and Margaret Cammaert (University of Alberta) visited Chile at the request of PAHO to advise the nurses' association board as well as the government and an undetermined number of medical faculties and NHS directors. Cammaert represented the organization in South America and the Caribbean, eventually becoming the Chief Nurse for the Region of the Americas.[58]

Contacts with the Soviet Union and Cuba remained limited. However, in 1972 nurses took part in an NHS mission to Cuba, albeit this time not overseen by PAHO, in order to establish future partnerships.[59] Equally, it is most likely that the Popular Unity was generally willing to employ foreign nurses. A 1972 guideline of the Ministry of Health addressed foreign nurses looking for jobs in NHS and *SERMENA* facilities. According to the guideline, they could work in Chile so long as they held a certification from the home country's nursing association, among other requirements. Preferences for particular countries or blacklisted countries were not specified.[60]

The early 1970s saw a peak of state funding for health professionals. Nurses became again a role model for other professions in using those new possibilities for further studies. But the increasing spending for nursing training was not sufficient to bridge the multiple gaps of the system. The range of grant recipients was limited to an elite group of nurses. However, this was not the only limitation caregivers experienced. As in the years before, the nurse–auxiliary relationship mirrored the domineering rule of their male supervisors. Even if the term "nurse" involved a large array of nursing staff in the US, local interpretations in Chile deemed nursing auxiliaries as unfitting of the professional workforce, excluding them from most of the projects financed and run by foreign organizations. Health policy thus captured and reproduced both gender and class asymmetries.

Furthermore, the Popular Unity government could not remedy the shortage of health professionals simply through academization and internationalization. The NHS workforce was still at a premium. Where nurses were concerned, policies sought to double their number up to 6000.[61] Even though this was a remarkable match with the prerogatives of the nurses' association,[62] it could not hide the strict pragmatic approach of the Popular Unity. Already since 1971, possibly even initiated during the Frei government, the nursing section of the NHS ran a program called "emergency plan." The emergency plan made it possible to choose a track of technical training during the fourth year of secondary education (*cuarto año de enseñanza media*) or sixth year of baccalaureate in the old system (*sexto año de humanidades*), leading to a nursing auxiliary diploma.[63] Other health professions designed similar tracks to make auxiliary staff more readily available in their respective areas.[64]

One could expect an aversion toward the increased value of nursing auxiliaries in health policy considering the elite self-image the *CECh* propagated. However, no reactions circulated in the print media, possibly relying on the board's earlier messages that framed auxiliaries as mere "hospital maids." That was different in the case of the health brigades. The claims of the health professionals during the 1972 strike suggest a severe confrontation with the volunteers. At the same time, nurses failed once again to persuade the government to allow them to enter the tariff scale of Law No. 15.076, and proposals for the restructuring of *Medicina Curativa* remained unheard. One might expect that nurses' negotiations with the Popular Unity ended at this time, but surprisingly, even in times of severe confrontation, they continued.[65] However, the events of 1973 would show that the unrest was growing constantly and the discussion about healthcare, and welfare more broadly, would make ideologies collide.

5 The New Opposition in the Healthcare Sector

In December 1971, Chile witnessed the first hint of a wider movement against the Popular Unity. Mostly women, the protesters gathered in an attention-catching demonstration known as the "March of the Empty Pots" (*marcha de las cacerolas vacías*).[66] Beating on pots, they reminded the shortages of basic groceries and foodstuffs.[67] Carmen Saenz, one of the leaders of what was later called the Feminine Power movement (*Poder Femenino*), was also the vice president of the most influential right-wing party, the National Party (*Partido Nacional, PN*). Another *PN* member was the Red Cross volunteer Silvia Alessandri Montes, niece of the former president Arturo Alessandri Palma (1920–1925/1932–1938).[68] It is very likely that she was just one of many other women of the upper class, and

US-trained nurses more specifically, to join the movement. This echoes the account by Margaret Power, who situates the marchers in the right-wing conservative spectrum of well-off Chileans.[69] Nevertheless, this movement mobilized women across social classes, as rightist women campaigned outside their own immediate circles.

The Women's March of the Empty Pots ended in a confusing confrontation. During the following months, demonstrations and counter-demonstrations led to clashes in the streets which broke the relative stability that had existed since the elections of 1970. Protests and military/police interventions, common for Latin American politics during the Cold War,[70] also became a feature of political and social life in the large urban areas.

The march was also a decisive moment in Allende's term of office. On the one hand, right-wing women used their organizing tactics, mobilization, and networking. On the other hand, this event also uncovered that the Popular Unity did not have a strong base within the united feminine movement.[71] Both of these traits implied a significant threat to the coalition's claims of a more egalitarian society, even though the March of the Empty Pots remained the largest occurrence in a public setting.[72] Women would further make important public appearances during the strikes of 1972 and 1973.

Until today, it has been mistakenly propagated that the healthcare professionals and workers joined the 1972 strike only when truck drivers cut the supply chain, in October. But, in fact, the strike in the healthcare sector started six months earlier. The trigger being a conflict which caused a violent clash in the hospital of Fresia, a small town in the region of Los Lagos (1000 km south of Santiago). Three newspapers, *El Mercurio*, *La Prensa*, and *El Clarín*, would widely document the backdrop and the events which followed in the next months. By then, *El Mercurio* was the most prominent voice of the conservative political spectrum, and the most credible among the lay readership, and had the third highest circulation figures in Chile.[73] The press of the Christian Democratic Party, *La Prensa*, represented the opinion of the most important opposition group in parliament, while the pro-government *El Clarín* was the second highest selling daily newspaper in Chile.[74]

Fresia counted in the early 1970s as few as 10,000 inhabitants.[75] *El Mercurio*[76] and *La Prensa*[77] reported that on April 14, 1972, radicalized inhabitants of the periphery occupied the local hospital to force physicians and nurses to hand them some medical certificates. Both newspapers focused on the angry protesters' threats against health professionals. But the circumstances in which these events took place remained unexplained. Nevertheless, the incidents in Fresia were also registered in the minutes of the Parliament; they read that a violent conflict between *pobladores* and *Carabineros* (Chilean police) had begun a few days earlier. The staff had refused to issue certificates for the emergency services provided, because these would confirm the use of force by the police in previous confrontations.[78] Following the argument of *El Mercurio*, the aggression of the *pobladores* was initially addressed to hospital physicians, but acts of violence quickly targeted, as confirmed by *La Prensa*, other health workers as well. Nurses of the hospital, for example, were threatened with rape. From our search there is no evidence that *El Clarín* reported this incident.

A few days after the Fresia incident, the president of the medical association Emilio Villaroel and the general secretary Edgardo Cruz criticized the communication strategy of the government during this episode.[79] Villarroel and Cruz used the opportunity to circulate broader criticisms against the government's health policies and called on their colleagues to stop working. With similar statements in newspapers and pamphlets, from then onward the physicians' association became the most salient voice among professionals against the Popular Unity.

At first, a number of physicians in Santiago and Valparaíso went on strike. By the beginning of May 1972, the mobilization extended to the southern areas of Osorno, Llanquihue (therein Fresia), Chiloé, and Aysén.[80] The northern regions remained quiet, or at least the three major papers did not report on them. One would thus say that initially this was not a nationwide movement, though discussions in the private sphere remain unknown. But the tone was caustic enough to uncover for the first time the widespread discontent among physicians throughout the country.

There is no clear sign about the participation of nurses and other health professionals in industrial action until July 1972. However, the confrontation affected various hospitals and healthcare centers, although nurses at least became witnesses of the disputes within healthcare. It is likely that in times of staff shortage the strike meant for them overtime hours. In various cases nurses and other health professionals and workers must have felt the obligation to express their sympathy for the cause of the medical association or their rejection of the strike movement.

El Mercurio stated that the Popular Unity attempted to dissuade strikers by dismissing hospital directors and replacing them with pro-government individuals. Replacements stirred up the unrest further.[81]

This happened against the background of a growing popular discontent. Parallel to the conflict in the healthcare sector, there were violent confrontations between the police and *pobladores*, which continued to escalate on the grounds of illegal land occupation.

The Popular Unity responded to the growing resistance among the physicians by declaring cities, and even entire regions, as areas of sanitary emergency (*zonas de emergencia sanitaria*). From May 9th, this was the case in Santiago, Linares, and Talca (300 and 250km south of Santiago, respectively). Other health professionals were caught in the crossfire. This was clear when the NHS director and the health minister were granted temporarily greatly enhanced powers to relocate not only physicians but all professional groups to different municipalities, towns, or regions, or to dismiss them at once.[82] As in the case of Fresia, this relocation policy was not reported in *El Clarín* either.

Groups from the conflicting poles accused each other of using propaganda. However, the sheer magnitude of oppositional press releases imbued the memory of this event with the striking health professionals' version of the occurrences. The then health minister Concha stressed during an interview in 2017 that the opposition overestimated the strikes, which obscured other voices. In an interview he told us that most of the workers and employees did not actually go on strike.[83]

Like in 1970, the most powerful federation of health workers, professionals, and auxiliaries, *FENATS*, came into action.[84] However, as their members belonged to the opposite ends of the political spectrum the federation failed to effectively intervene in the conflict.[85] A gradual fragmentation indeed debilitated the once powerful union. The physicians' association, on the other hand, took advantage of the power gap that the situation exposed and built its own set of alliances.

Already in April 1972, the dentists and the pharmacists appeared signing one of physicians' statements in *El Mercurio,* in which they reproached the government for not wanting to clarify the events in Fresia.[86] No later than July of that same year, the three associations formed a new union, namely the Confederation of Professional Associations (*Confederación de Colegios Profesionales*). The first association to join soon after this broader conglomerate, and whose wages were not under the umbrella regulation of Law No. 15.076, was the *CECh*.[87] On September 27th, the four professions formed the National Front of Professionals (*Frente Nacional de Profesionales*), and just a month later the midwives and the psychologists joined them as well.[88] By the eve of the big nationwide strike, those two conglomerates had become powerful competitors of *FENATS*, though different in their demands. Rather than speaking on behalf of all health workers, Confederation and Front were the battle force of an elite network of professionals.[89]

Only three days had passed since the creation of the National Front of Professionals when, on September 30th, the 1100 health workers of *Hospital San Borja*, one of the largest NHS facilities in Santiago downtown, were involved in a major work stoppage. This action was in response to the dismissal of the director Dr. Agustín Denegri by minister Concha. *El Mercurio*[90] and *La Prensa*[91] claimed that everybody, even the auxiliary personnel, joined the strike. *El Clarín*, however, remained silent on the matter.

While there were some instances of successful mediation, those never really effaced the fact that Popular Unity was continuously losing momentum, while the idea of multiple local strikes began to spread like a wildfire.[92] Still in 1972, an agreement between the NHS and the medical association, signed on October 6th, remained futile.[93] It rather showed the disagreement within the government. Concha did not even attend the negotiations.

After one and a half years in office, the Popular Unity seemed to struggle. The entire governmental coalition was unstable and grew vulnerable in different areas. Allende's cabinet reshuffles were ineffective as well.[94] He and Concha were not to amalgamate with one another against the closing ranks of the opposition or, even less, against the health crowd.

6 End of Negotiations: The 1972 Strike

In the existing historiography, the 1972 strike started in Aysén and extended within a few days over the entire country. It lasted almost four weeks and provoked restrictions in all aspects of public and private life. Lawyers and notaries stopped working, air traffic was paralyzed, freight and food transportation shrank to a minimum, mining halted, and so forth.

On October 11th, the healthcare workers announced a nationwide strike, which in practice meant that what was initially planned as focal seizures in hospitals and healthcare centers extended quickly throughout the country and across areas.[85] As the analytical emphasis tends to be placed on the conflict between the private sector and the government, the health sector protest is often seen as a mere backdrop of the truck drivers' strike and thus of much lesser importance. Yet, unlike closed mines and canceled flights, the health professionals and auxiliaries refused to provide emergency procedures and the important medical cares. This was a parallel strike with its own dynamics and conditions to exert political pressure.

While in the preceding months nurses made headlines every now and then, since October 1972 they merged gradually into the strike movement. The members of this interest grouping no longer distinguished themselves from physicians, midwives, nurses, dentists and pharmacists, socialists, Communists, Radicals, and so on. The becoming of a bogeyman, that this movement was, reached its first peak. From then on, the Popular Unity period was felt very much like "health professionals" versus "Allende and his supporters."

Constant negotiations between the health minister, the NHS director, the president himself, and the professional associations did not lead to any satisfactory solution. On November 2nd, the strike reached its peak when the professional associations together with the unions and federations dropped out of negotiations with the government. On the same day, the associations of physicians, dentists, pharmacists, and, as the only organization of female health professionals, nurses, issued the following public release in *La Prensa*, naming the underlying reasons of the industrial action:

1. Fragmentary and mistaken information [from the government] about the state of medical supplies in healthcare centers
2. The physical, moral, and administrative oppression [on the health staff] with inappropriate goals leading but to toughening the positions at the negotiation table
3. The brigades of collision [referring to the health brigades], created illegally with the aim of intimidating employees and creating a climate of hate
4. The use of physician mediators [*médicos interventores*] in areas and hospitals which the National Audit Office rejected.[95]

The content of the accusations would not change until the coup d'état, in September 1973. The professional associations criticized that Popular Unity was using unlawful measures in both administration and delivery of healthcare. Beneath such claims lay the idea that, among other things, engaging volunteers was a threat for their own bargaining power. An equally strong view developed against employing foreign professionals.

The claims became openly nationalist and anti-Communist, while *El Mercurio* and *La Prensa* fueled fears about Cuban physicians.[96]

The second peak of the opposition was reached when the health professionals announced their solidarity with lawyers, agricultural engineers, schoolteachers and journalists, as well as the unions of *Lan Chile* airline employees, and the professionals and auxiliary staff hired through municipal administration.[97] Once again, the specific type of a joint endeavor led to adapting claims which did not pertain to health politics at all, like nationalizing the paper-producing industry or reframing contents of school education, often referred to as socialist "political indoctrination" through public schools.[98]

As the country faced the nationwide spread of the strike, in early October, *El Clarín* finally started to touch upon the healthcare situation. On October 30th, it published a statement which clarified the position of the Popular Unity. In the second part of the article, *El Clarín* editors published an announcement of the government:

> "We state that this country will not come to a standstill. Most of the factories keep on producing, transport via railways and roads continues as per usual, the hospitals are operating, patients are being treated. We congratulate our comrades, patriotic physicians, nurses, dentists and pharmacists, who have doubled their efforts to ensure the health care provision."[99]

After this introduction, an author in *El Clarín* applauded the work of the trade union confederation *Central Única de Trabajadores de Chile* but did not mention the volunteers of the health councils and brigades, not even the health workers affiliated with *FENATS*.[100] Along with the silence about local strikes like the one in *Hospital San Borja*, this omission suggests a rather weak connection between the healthcare workers and the Popular Unity, much as *FENATS* affiliates represented its power base and may have identified themselves with its ideals.

Afterward, *El Clarín* made an allegation against the health professionals, one that would be repeated several times in the following months, about a very sensitive issue, the refusal to give patients care. The allegation read that the strikers "led the country to sickness and death."[101] Such an accusation had a high impact on the public opinion, considering that it seemed to contradict professionals' assurances of medical care for emergencies, constantly reiterated by the health professionals themselves in articles that appeared in *La Prensa* and *El Mercurio*.

Collier and Sater (2004) stated that some 600,000 to 700,000 people took part in the strike.[102] Though it is not clear how many out of the 80,000 professionals joined,[103] as the votes per each professional association were incompletely reported.[104] However, the information in the newspapers does provide more detailed information. The most precise piece referred to the medical association where it was reported that within the two largest sections, in Santiago and Valparaíso, the vast majority voted for the strike (75 and 80 percent, respectively).[105] These figures confirm the assertion by Chanfreau (1979), who talked about 30 percent of strike breakers.[106] *El Clarín* only gave details when it stated that "most of the physicians' association affiliates" in Antofagasta (1330 km north of Santiago) voted against the strike.[107]

The same holds for the participation rate of nurses in the strike. Just one result was properly documented in the public archives. It covers a regional section in Punta Arenas (far south) where 56.5 percent of the members voted for the strike.[108] Nevertheless, it can be inferred that most of the nurses, at least in Santiago, followed the directions of the *CECh* board to stop working.

It would seem that overthrowing the government was the only issue the nursing association board cared about by November 1972. What, then, happened to equal participation in political decisions, resistance to patriarchal institutions and their self-perception as a social force, and the improvement of nursing policies? Did Peake and Garrido really believe that replacing Allende and appointing another man as head of the state would improve their position dramatically in future negotiations about healthcare? It is understood that they had a powerful voice in the strike movement, and probably the most powerful of all participating women. But this movement did not precisely stand for healthcare issues properly. By then nationalist ideas had somewhat slowed down the movement, and this backward-looking policy became more powerful with each new vote for the strike.

The transparency of the voting in the general and regional councils of the professional associations can be seriously doubted. Following from Chanfreau (1979), already in 1960 the physicians' association had established in its statutes that members who refused to follow the majority's decision to go on strike would lose their license to practice.[109] Belmar and Sidel (1975), on the other hand, explained that such level of pressure of the national board was exerted only immediately before the 1972 strike.[110] But even under pro-government boards, conflict between breakers and supporters arose, as suggested by a statement of the physicians, dentists, pharmacists, and, once again as the only female health professionals, nurses from November 1st in *La Prensa*. This included a threat against those not conforming to the board's guidelines, as follows:

> "Any member who refuses to put this order [to go on strike] into practice shall face preliminary proceedings on the grounds of violation of professional ethics."[111]

Nurses who adhered to Popular Unity affirmed that most of their colleagues supported the strike, and strikers secretly reported against those who continued to work. This information would become crucial later as to justify the dismissal or relocation of left-wing nurses after the coup d'état.[112] However, the supporters of the government either represented a minority or their absence from newspaper headlines was another sign of socialist newspapers like *El Clarín* underestimating their support among health professionals. As a consequence, we rely on information about Garrido, who enthusiastically supported the claims of the Confederation of Professional Associations in her capacity as the president of the nursing association. She was the only woman to give a speech in a general assembly of the striking professionals in October.[113] As the general secretary, she promoted the politicization of the nursing workforce. Therefore, she strengthened the image of nurses as alibi women within a male-dominated movement.

Surprisingly, written as well as oral sources ignored the participation of the auxiliaries in the strikes altogether. The few traces which exist are not enough to fix class-blindness in the health historiography. Belmar and Sidel (1975) not only claimed that the biggest part of the health team did not support the strike; they also ensured that "hospitals and health centers" kept running with the help of the health councils and medical students. They also stated that pro-government workers supported healthcare and thereby the Popular Unity.[114] Contemporary researchers, like public health physician Hadjez-Berrios (2014), confirm this observation.[115] It is worth noting, however, that nursing auxiliaries represented by far the largest stand-alone group of healthcare workers (about 20,000). The shortages in healthcare provision further suggests that most of them also stopped working and marched in the streets.[116] This decision may, indeed, sound contradictory. Nevertheless, refusing to join the protests could have meant administrative sanctions at the workplace, which was controlled by those from the professional ranks.

Beginning in November, the merger of the health professionals, voluntary or enforced, took effect. The conflict between the opposition and the government, most prominently represented by Concha and the NHS director, became entrenched. The state's fundamental institutions, like the ministries and the parliament, were losing momentum as well. In the meanwhile, the streets became more and more the locus of the conflict. Several new umbrella organizations appeared (see Chart 2.1); some of them lasted for mere days, like the Command of Professionals (*Comando de Profesionales*)[117] or the Unified Confederation of Professionals (*Confederación Única de Profesionales*).[118] In all those mergers of professionals (i.e., health, finance, economy, agriculture), the lawyers moved quickly to the leading roles.[119]

Well into 1972, the Popular Unity was under overwhelming international pressure. The US, secretly acting through the CIA, actively

Chart 2.1 Organisations of health care workers

Name	*Members*	*1972–1973*	*After September 1973*
FENATS—Federación Nacional de Trabajadores de la Salud	professionals and auxiliaries	1972/1973 divided in political camps	first documented strike in 1985
FEPROTEC—Federación de Profesionales y Técnicos	professionals and auxiliaries	1972 supporting the Popular Unity, 1973 divided in political camps	no sign of operation since October 1973
(Con)federación de Colegios Profesionales (Universitarios) de Chile	professionals	1972/1973 opposition against the Popular Unity	negotiations with the Health Ministry in 1980, protest against governmental measures in 1984 and 1985
Frente Nacional de Profesionales	professionals	1972 opposition against the Popular Unity	no sign of operation since October 1973
CUPROCH—Confederación de Profesionales de Chile	professionals	1972/1973 opposition against the Popular Unity	no sign of operation since October 1973
CUT—Central Única de Trabajadores de Chile	professionals and auxiliaries	1972/1973 divided in political camps	reactivated in 1987

supported the opposition.[120] The strike catalyzed the economic slump of the country and further reduced the margin of the Popular Unity to respond to economic constraints, as evidenced by the increasing inflation and the shortage of consumer goods.[121] The shutdown of nearly entire hospitals, like *San Borja*, affected thousands of care-seeking individuals. Politically, this damaged the trust in the government's ability to solve the healthcare problems, trust that many genuinely had.

At Popular Unity some attempted to compensate for the decline of political influence by cooperating with the Armed Forces. That was not the first time. During the previous state of emergency episodes, like in May 1972 in Valparaíso, the heads of the military had the chance to seize control and expand their influence on the executive.[122] Considering this, the restriction of civil rights, such as freedom of expression and freedom of assembly, proved to be a useful governing measure which young Chileans had a taste of for the first time during Allende's government.

On November 2nd, Allende appointed Gen. Augusto Pinochet as the Supreme Command of the Armed Forces,[123] replacing Gen. Carlos Prats González (1915–1974) who became Minister of Home Affairs. Two days later, Prats summoned all the striking leads to his office. As he announced, he sought to end the strike, though his main tactic was threatening the leads. Some 48 hours later, the strike ended.[124] According to the document, signed in Prats' presence, nobody would be put on a trial, either instigators or participants of the strike, and further negotiations would not be possible.[125]

The conflict would no longer be managed by the government, the Catholic Church, the parliament, the health minister Concha, or even Allende.[126] From then onward, the Commander-in-Chief of the Military would take part in national politics, being granted large discretion to mediate and intervene.[127]

However, nothing and no-one seemed able to reverse the social schism, not even the Armed Forces. The use of force by both sides was particularly gruesome. Over a period of six months, violent clashes, misinformation, and disappointments shaped public life,[128] and mutual distrust would determine the further course of events. By way of example, just two weeks after the agreement between the government and the strike leaders, the medical association reported the Ministry of Health for violating the *Medicina Curativa* provisions contained in the regulations.[129]

Interestingly, Garrido, president of the nursing board, was the only female health professional summoned by Prats on November 2nd. No information is available about her actual influence on the outcome. But her presence alone underlined nurses' self-image as an equal stakeholder in negotiations that concerned national politics. They had become the apprentices of other negotiators as far as the linkage between professional associations and politics is concerned.

7 The Hardened Fronts

By early 1973, Garrido and Peake had lost hope to involve nurses in the *Medicina Curativa* Act through negotiations with the Popular Unity. But without changes in the agenda-setting it became difficult for them to find support among fellow associates, or convince them to go on strike, even if congresses did not seem conceivable under a state of emergency. And yet, the nurses' board was already committed to the opposition movement of the other professional associations.

The Popular Unity had to face the oppositional front of both the professionals and right-wing conservative congressmen, company owners, and unions. Allende hoped for a favorable sign in the parliamentary elections of March 4, 1973. The outcome was viewed by both sides as an appraisal of the president who would remain in power until 1976. The Popular Unity obtained a significant number of votes (44.03 percent), which implied that impeachment proceedings, only possible with a high quorum, could be averted. But the government still lacked a parliamentary majority.[130]

Allende continued to rule with decrees, which only hardened the fronts. Then, only six months after Prats' intervention, the confrontation went back to the streets. The first setting was copper mining, vital for Chilean economy. On April 19th, most workers of the largest mine, *El Teniente*, stopped working,[131] but pro-government forces of the *CUT* managed to avoid a full standstill.[132] Nonetheless, this strike, which would last 74 long days, slowed down productivity and provoked a disastrous impact on the state budget.[133]

To avoid a complete halt of a large industrial complex, the clinical staff on the site intervened. The work of physicians, nurses, and nursing auxiliaries was an important prerequisite for the continued employment of strike-breaking miners.[134] Nurse Patricia Talloni was appointed as the new nursing coordinator at *El Teniente*, right at the pinnacle of the conflict, toward the end of June. In an interview, she stated that she had sufficient staff to assure medical care along with other pro-government professionals.[135] Quite possibly, the strike eventually affected Talloni's crew at the mine's nursing station.

In June 1973, the strike in *El Teniente* spilled over into other medical facilities. The decisive factor was the stoppage at the *Hospital del Salvador* in Santiago. As in the case of *Hospital San Borja* in 1972, the strike cut off medical care for an entire urban district. From June 20th, the staff only accepted emergency patients.[136] Again, the physicians took the lead in a conjoint movement of dentists, pharmacists, and nurses. A week later, their local leads rejected an agreement negotiated between the NHS, the national board of medical association, the new health minister Jirón, and Allende.[137] This showed not only the president's loss of standing as a mediator but also, for the first time, the differences in interests between the national and the regional boards of the physicians' association.

One day before the negotiation deadlock in the *Hospital del Salvador*, the strike extended to one of the grandest facilities in Santiago downtown, the *Hospital San Juan de Dios*. The headline of *El Clarín* showed how the fronts had hardened by then:

> "Evil plan of the patient-killing rightists: fascists will occupy the hospitals to take care of their victims during civil war."

Insulting words, such as "parrot" (*perico*), were used to refer to the medical director of *San Juan de Dios*, García Nuño, or the term "fascists" for the physicians who refused to treat patients. This made it clear that, from one year to another, the dispute acquired a personal and more aggressive connotation.[138]

The most aggressive insults from the opposition were published in the newspaper *La Tribuna*, the outlet of the right wing. Authors there referred pejoratively to Allende as the "moustache of La Moneda" and his supporters in public facilities as "Marxist elements."[139] The newspaper also stated that Chileans had to prevent an upcoming "dictatorship" from happening.[140]

On June 27th, the negotiations with the staff of the *Hospital Del Salvador* failed to achieve any results. The situation in the *Hospital San Juan de Dio*s and at *El Teniente* also got bogged down in the political issues. Two days later, a regiment of the Armed Forces attempted a coup d'état in Santiago.[141] Prats, wanting to back democracy, hindered the assault and once again saved the Popular Unity.[142] More than ever, Allende depended on his loyalty, but this time he decided against putting any government responsibility on him. The president still believed in solving the crises without permanently involving the Armed Forces.

8 The End of the Socialist Experiment: The 1973 Strike

The coup attempt of June 29th, even if failed, weakened the Popular Unity. As a direct consequence, Jirón had to make concessions to the professional associations. But the agreement, reached on July 9th, came too late. The professionals and workers led by physicians and nurses at the hospitals *Del Salvador* and *San Juan de Dios* did not appreciate the instructions of the association's national boards. Two weeks later, the rebel hospitalists forced them to cancel the agreement.[143] On July 25th, the second national strike started.

Aware of their might, the union of truck drivers blocked virtually all the supply chains. But unlike the previous year, there was no collaboration between the health professionals and the other professions who joined the truck drivers, except a few statements made jointly in *La Prensa* and *El Mercurio*. They acted like an independent unified movement albeit led by the medical association,[144] while the only stable linkage with the other opposition members was their determination to overthrow the government.[145]

As is often the case, there is a dearth of evidence about female leadership during the hospital strikes. However, it is safe to affirm that at *San Juan de Dios* hospital at least two figures gained salience. One was Margarita Soza, who would later become a board member of the *CECh*,[146] sitting by the time of the strike as the deputy secretary of the nurses (*subjefe de enfermeras*) in her hospital.[147] The other was Zunilda Pizarro Ramirez, permanent contributor of *Enfermería* magazine, working in a pediatric unit.[148] As both these nurses remained appointed in their posts, the backing from the opposition is evident. This also leads us to the view that, although undocumented, women did take part in the strike, with nurses mobilizing the trained female workforce.

On August 9th, Allende called Prats into the cabinet again. But this time the general failed to put an end to the strike. On the contrary, he came under enormous political pressure. Finally, on August 21st, he resigned all civil and military missions and duties. Gen. Pinochet, until then serving as Commander-in-Chief, was then appointed as Prats' successor in the Armed Forces.[149]

On August 23rd, the opposition in the parliament led by the Christian Democrats contested the legitimacy of the government on the basis of an alleged violation of the constitution.[150] On such a critical moment, Popular Unity supporters still intended to back the government. The left wing of *CUT* organized a demonstration against the blockades.[151] A broad alliance of parties and movements marched on September 4th through the streets of Santiago. Margaret Power (2002) suggested "hundreds of thousands" of participants.[152] However, those figures raised some controversy,[153] a controversy that extends to the question of how many health workers actually broke the strike.[154] Beyond these differences, however, it is important to bear in mind that any estimate is expected to be questioned so long as the political orientation of the female auxiliary personnel, the very bottom of the pyramid, remains unknown.[155]

On September 7th, Allende made his last, though unsuccessful, attempt to mediate with the representatives of health professionals.[156] Physicians, nurses, and other allies extended work stoppage indefinitely.

The last radio speech of Allende, on September 11th, was aired by *Radio Magallenes*, the only station not yet shut down or turned inoperative during that morning. After mentioning some general accusations and saying words of thanks, the president became very precise as he addressed the women and the professionals as if wanting to highlight the pains of the ones contrasted to the privilege of the others:

> "I am talking specifically to the modest women of our country, to the female peasants who believed in us, to the grandmothers who worked harder, to the mothers who knew our concern about the children."
>
> [speech goes on]
>
> "I am addressing the professionals of our fatherland, the patriotic professionals who continued to work against the complot planned by the professional associations, associations of a class society that defended the capitalist system which benefits a small group."[157]

Allende mentioned the health professionals only once, but what is remarkable is that he addressed them right after addressing the women of the country. Of course, the life-threatening atmosphere must have made it difficult for him and his advisors to structure and summarize the speech. Nevertheless, as it was more of a spontaneous product, it shows what came to his mind first when he rethought the experiences he had lived for two convoluted years between ardent opponents and fierce supporters. Specifically, Allende treated women and professionals as distinct groups. Then, he associated women with agriculture and motherhood. And afterward, he did not differentiate between physicians, nurses, dentists, or midwives. For him, all those who had joined the strikes and the broader movement did not pertain to the solidary society he sought and were part of a small separate class. This demonstrates that Allende, just like his opponents and close friends, was situated within the patriarchal *Zeitgeist*—he, too, embedded the spirit of his era. On September 11th there came the end of a fight between two groups of powerful men. Some of them certainly had good intentions and may have acted in good faith, but because of the ideological and nationalist delusion they either neglected nurses and nursing more broadly or used them as a means for their movement.

Nurse Talloni recalls soldiers entering the medical facility of *El Teniente* on September 11. They called the staff together. The Commander-in-Chief opened his speech on a high note with the words: "We won!" Then, everybody had to go home, keep an ear to the radio, and wait for instructions.[158]

9 Conclusion

Assessments of the Popular Unity health policy have traditionally been overlaid with ideologically motivated arguments. The most striking example is the criticism of the use of volunteers to support healthcare staff.[159]

The Allende administration may have reached some positive outcomes. The increase in staff and supplies for the *materno-infantil* sector and the trouble-free cooperation with PAHO and the UN reduced major problems like child mortality. Nevertheless, much as his policies aimed for universal coverage, those encountered strong resistance. The creation of the health councils and brigades or attention-catching actions like the health train, which one might label as populist, were not supported by a broad consensus in the parliament and, most importantly, not backed by the majority of healthcare professionals. Probably not even by the auxiliaries. In the case of nurses, pro-government groupings with as much power and visibility as the women sitting on the board of the nursing association were rare. Nurses being an important element in any attempt to policy implementation.

Only the health projects planned and subsidized with international funding and education agreements proved to have a constant expansion. However, they depended on the cooperation with the NHS, the universities, and the professional associations. As already seen during the Frei administration, the main focus of health policy was ultimately narrowed down to *materno-infantil*. While doing so, PAHO was *the* major actor in Chile to collaborate in the preparation and implementation of a health policy.

The 1972 strike was the turning point during the Popular Unity government, which began with an almost unnoticed incident in a small township. Unlike common beliefs, nurses, midwives, and nursing auxiliaries played a key role in this social and political conflict. They may not have appeared in Chile's historiography yet, but were still devoted to the care of thousands of individuals and raised awareness about Allende's halo slip. Their action preceded a national strike that was going to take place five months thereafter. What is more, the organizations of the healthcare professionals on different levels became a blueprint for future mergers against the Popular Unity.

Apart from the continuation of measures undertaken by previous governments, the politization of healthcare also remained an important heritage of the 1000 days of the left-wing government in Chile. The most vivid example being the small but powerful group of university-trained nurses. For the first time since its foundation, the board of the nursing association positioned itself openly in a political camp.

All signs of progress in reaching poorer sectors suffering from malnutrition and epidemics were overshadowed by the ideological confrontation. By the time the coup d'état took place, confrontation made it difficult to follow up any evidence of improved healthcare. And, eventually, confrontation threatened the physical and psychological well-being of the entire Chilean society.

Chilean nursing did benefit from the increasing investment in healthcare. Through this development, the academization of training continued and strengthened the political representation of the *CECh*. The reforms initiated in the previous years had established a framework which was evidentially firm enough to guarantee the ongoing progress in *materno-infantil*. Though this, the cooperation (or rather confrontation) with the health brigades and councils, perhaps the only new concept in healthcare between 1970 and 1973, remained a passing occurrence.

Interestingly though, the socialist regime did not generate a new sort of "socialist nursing." The *CECh* board first tried to show political neutrality. Then, it cooperated with the government or, rather, tolerated some measures in healthcare. However, this was a fragile peace. Once the opposition gained more power, disagreement of the *CECh* board toward the involvement of volunteers and foreign professionals resurfaced. This fueled dissatisfaction with the continuing exclusion of nurses from the *Medicina Curativa* plan and Law No. 15.076.

Nursing auxiliaries only appeared in a few sources. The changes introduced by the Popular Unity to improve their training remained a short spotlight on work life, as did the indirect mentions when media tried to convince readers that either "everybody" or only "a small group" of healthcare workers joined the strikes.

And yet, we must entertain the view that the nursing association was the most powerful formal body of professional women during Allende's presidency. Despite its elite character, the *CECh*, a strong voice among the female health professionals, played a leading role in this context. They had representation in high politics holding speeches and signing treaties with the new civil-military government. Even though all decisions were taken by men, at least one woman validated them. And who but a nurse, the mother of the nation, would be a better match among health professionals to craft this image of "gender solidarity"?

Intriguingly, nurses did not appear in the press as women, but as nurses. Yet, their involvement in the 1970s strikes marked a very high point in political participation alongside the right to vote, in 1949. But can those achievements in organization and participation be seen as the first step on the way to destabilize the healthcare patriarchy?

In September 1973, for some there reigned a spirit of stabilization and reconstruction, the annulment of reforms, and new ideas. However, nurses' story of "success" beneath the strikes and the political crises is much more difficult to visualize. Nevertheless, it raises the question of whether the Popular Unity established a new set of rules or a new atmosphere, and whether nurses' participation in the strikes increased or diminished their bargaining power.

One may argue that nurses did expand their power as they were on the winning side. But they did so by exerting non-transformative agency, which is to say they did as much as they could within male-dominated institutions, frames, and arrangements. As a consequence, they were not able to turn their specific prerogatives as nurses into an actual gain.

Notes

1. The political diversity of the Popular Unity ranged from Soviet Communists and Socialists to Social Democrats, represented by the Radical Party (*Partido Radical*), in: Duffner, Georg: Partner im Kalten Krieg. Die politischen Beziehungen zwischen der Bundesrepublik Deutschland und Chile, Frankfurt am Main [Campus Verlag] 2014, p. 206;

   On October 24, 1970, the Chilean congress ratified Allende as president of the Republic. On September 4th, 1973, his coalition had won only 36.6 percent of the seats in the Congress.
2. Belmar et al. (1975), p. 53, 56–64.

   In 1988, gender researcher Carmen del Pilar Campaña also described a working plan for healthcare in rural areas. See: Del Pilar Campaña, Carmen: Participación comunitaria y salud rural en Chile, in: Salud rural [Ed. grupo de investigaciones agrarias, Academia de Humanismo Cristiano], Santiago 1988, p. 44.
3. Waitzkin, Howard; Modell, Hillary: Medicina, Socialismo y Totalitarismo: Lecciones de Chile, in: Participación Popular en la salud en América Latina—Experiencias de Chile, Cuba y Nicaragua, Colección "PRAXIS," Vol. I, Santo Domingo (República Dominicana) [Ed. Guarocuya Batista, Santiago Gómez M.] 1982;

   In its election program from 1964, the Popular Unity aimed to build a unified public healthcare system on a "national structure," in: Candidatura presidencial del Dr. Salvador Allende [Oficina Central de Planificación Grupo de Salud]: Plan de Salud, atención médica y medicina social, in: Cuadernos médico sociales, Vol. 46, Suplemento 1 [Colegio Médico de Chile], Santiago 1964, p. 20;

   Nevertheless, in public announcements Allende did not emphasize this plan. According to sources of *El Mercurio*, sometimes he even denied it, in: Así lo señaló el presidente Salvador Allende al presidente del Colegio Médico, Dr. Emilio Villaroel," in: *El Mercurio*, 01.-07.05.1972, p. 5.
4. Ley No. 17416, 09.03.1971, Fija sueldos y salarios que indica. Modifica las leyes que señala. Otras materias.
5. Belmar et al. (1975), p. 58.
6. Morales (1981), p. 55.
7. Decreto 602, 21.09.1971, Crea Consejos Locales de Salud";

   The Ministry of Health published flyers with guidelines for the health brigades, in: Consejaría Nacional de Desarrollo Social (Chile): Brigadas de Salud [Ed. Editora Nacional de Quimantú], Santiago 1972 [National Libary of Chile, No. 000430100].
8. Interview with Concha, Santiago, March 2017.

9. Müller-Plantenberg quoted an article of Alfonso González for the newspaper *El Siglo* with the title "Increasing the Participation" (*A Impulsar la Participación*) from June 1972; then she stated that "a huge part of the councils existed only formally and showed no activity," in: Müller-Plantenberg (1983), p. 105;

   In 1972 and 1973, Müller-Plantenberg visited Chile for several months. By request of the Popular Unity and UNESCO, she paved the way for a Ministry of the Family. As far as we know, those plans were never put into effect.
10. Ministerio de Salud Pública: Oficio No. 0799, Solicita colaboración para constitución de los Consejos Locales y Paritarios de Salud, 0799-1817-1972, 12.05.1972, p. 1–2.
11. Müller-Plantenberg described that most of the participants refused to accomplish the training hours because it was too time-consuming for voluntary work. They had expected to learn a "real job." Once they noticed that they would not get paid, they quit the training. That is why in some cases, the participation requirements had been loosened: In order to employ the volunteers as soon as possible, the training was reduced to an intensive course of some weeks, in: Ibid., p. 107-109.
12. Interview with Concha, Santiago, March 2017.
13. The authors of *La Prensa* mentioned the employment of volunteers on one occasion, in November 1972, when the professional associations protested against the Popular Unity, in: Inserción: Colegio Médico, Colegio de Enfermeras——Colegio de Químico-Farmacéuticos——Colegio de Dentistas de Chile. "A la opinión pública," in: *La Prensa*, 02.11.1972.
14. One example was the failed implementation of measures to control the work hours. The Frei administration had failed in a similar attempt, in: Interviews with Concha and Jiménez, Santiago, February 2017;

   The plan to raise the work hours was discussed since January 1972, in: Ministerio de Salud Pública: Oficio No. 0018, Situación que afecta a trabajadores del Servicio Nacional de Salud, 0018-1816-1972, 05.01.1972, p. 1;

   The first attempt to implement the control measures dates back to August 1973, in: Ministerio de Salud Pública: Oficio No. 1467, Indicación a proyecto de ley que beneficia a funcionarios afectos al DFL. 338/60, del Servicio Nacional de Salud, 1467-1844-1973, 17.08.1973, p. 1
15. The resistance of the medical association forced Concha to stop the implementation, in: Proyecto para modificar la Medicina Curativa, in: *El Mercurio*, 28.06.-02.07.1972, 27.06.1972, p. 5.
16. Salud. Nuevos ataques, in: *El Mercurio*, 22.-28.05.1972, p. 8.

17. It seems that the hiring of physicians increased constantly until the coup d'état, in: Ministerio de Salud Pública, Oficina de Asuntos Internacionales: Oficio No. 1549, Contratación de médicos extranjeros, 1549-1844-1973, 16.08.1973, p. 1-2 [8/21].
18. The first Cuban physicians arrived in 1960 after the earthquake of Valdivia, in: Gómez Dantés, Octavio: The Dark Side of Cuba's Health System: Free Speech, Rights of Patients and Labor Rights of Physicians, in: *Health Systems and Reform*, Vol. 4, No. 3, 2018, p. 175-178, 178.
19. Two articles in which the physicians expressed their disagreement with the employment of Cuban physicians:
    1. Salud. Contrataciones, in: *El Mercurio*, 25.-30.09.1972, p. 8;
    2. Anuncian, in: *La Prensa*, 04.11.1972, p. 9.
20. Waitzkin et al. (1982), p. 12.
21. Ministerio de Salud Pública, Oficina de Asuntos Internacionales: Oficio No. 0443, Informe primer trimestre 1972, proyecto Chile-3105, 0443-1816-1972, 20.03.1972, p. 1.
22. Again, the positive effects were inherited by the Frei administration. The construction of 24 new healthcare posts in rural areas started in August 4,1970, in: Dr. Concha G., Juan Carlos: Oficio No. 0358, Propuestas [estatales] al PMA-584, 0358-1816-1972, 07.03.1972;

    19 NHS facilities (institutes, hospitals, and children's homes) in Santiago already existed when the Popular Unity came to power.
23. Ministerio de Salud Pública, Subsecretaría: Oficio No. 0191, Sobre Petición de matronas y practicante para posta de Puerto Ibañez, 0191-1816-1972, 01.02.1972, p. 1.
24. In June 1972, the governor of the Region of Maule warned the general director of the NHS that the shortage of physicians and midwives in the hospitals of Cauquenes and Chanco (350 to 400 km south of Santiago) would "cause a real unrest among citizens," in: Ministerio de Salud Pública: Oficio No. 1111, Transcribe Oficio No. 295 del Intendente de Maule, 1111-1818-1972, 04.06.1972, p. 1.
25. Ministerio de Salud Pública: Oficio No. 1568, Sobre Atención Médica en la Ciudad de Talca, 1568-1844-1973, 20.08.1973, p. 1.
26. Waitzkin praised the measures to distribute milk as successful, in: Waitzkin et al. (1982), p. 10.

    A study of PAHO from 1980 suggests that the distribution of milk and basic foods like rice reached its highest peak during the government of the Popular Unity and declined during dictatorship, in: González Toro, Nicolás; Infante Barros, Antonio: Programas de alimentación complementaria del Sector Salud en Chile, in: *Boletín de la Oficina Sanitaria Panamericana*, No. 89, 1980 [PAHO/WHO Institutional Repository for Information Sharing], p. 563-571, 565.

Nevertheless, the program could never reach full supply. An example for the shortage of milk was found for the Maule region. Especially in public health areas, the delivery of milk was insufficient, in: Ministerio de Salud Pública: Oficio No. 1379, Entrega de leche Maule y Constitución, 1379-1819-1972, 09.08.1972, p. 1.

27. Modell et al. (1982), p. 14.
28. Waitzkin et al. (1982), p. 12.
29. The only related source found in the documentation center of the Ministry of Health tells us about the start of the project, on December 9, 1972, and the end of the project on February 28, 1973. Some 65 health volunteers were involved, in Ministerio de Salud Pública: Oficio No. 2152, Sobre gastos Tren de Salud, 2152-1821-1972, 29.12.1972, p. 1-1 [9/12].
30. Low, Brian: The hand that rocked the cradle: A critical analysis of Rockefeller philanthropic funding, 1920—1960, in: *Historical studies in education*, 2004, p. 33-62;

    O'Connor, Alice: Contradictions de la philanthropie libérale face aux mouvements sociaux, in: *Lien social et Politiques*, No. 65, 2011, p. 19–42.
31. The conference took place from October 2 to 9, 1972, in: Ministerio de Salud Pública, Oficina de Asuntos Internacionales: Oficio No. 0519, Sobre Reunión de Ministros de Salud de la Américas, Santiago, 2 al 14 de octubre de 1972, 0519-1816-1972, 03.04.1972, p. 1–2;

    The health ministers formulated the Ten-Year Health Plan for the Americas, in: Regional strategies of health for all by the year 2000. Evaluation of the ten-year health plan for the Americas, Washington 1980.
32. Ministerio de Salud Pública: Programas del Sector Salud de Chile con las Naciones Unidas y sus agencias especializadas año 1972, 1817-1972, 06.1972, p. 1–2.
33. Lavados, Iván: Evolución de las políticas sociales en Chile 1964-1980, in: Estudios ILPES UNICEF sobre Políticas Sociales, Inscripción No. 57.318, Santiago 1983, p. 104.
34. In the case of the PAHO, 86.29 percent (799.690 USD) of the joined resources were spent for *materno-infantil* projects, in: Ibid., p. 1-2;

    Chilean attributions for UNICEF, in: UNICEF: Report 1972, p. 16, https://sites.unicef.org/about/history/files/unicef_annual_report_1972.pdf [2021-10-15].
35. Ministerio de Salud, Oficina de Asuntos Internacionales: Oficio No. 0137, Proyectos temporales, 0137-1816-1972, 25.01.1972, p. 1–2;

    In two of the 30 projects, the University of Chile was involved. The projects with the numbers 4103 and 4201 relied on a cooperation with the Medical Faculty, in: Ministerio de Salud, Oficina de Asuntos

Internacionales: Ref. No. 0137, Proyectos temporales, 0137-1815-1972, 25.01.1972, p. 1–2.

36. In 1972, Chile owed the PAHO the amount of 524,559 *Escudos*. In June 1972, the organization waived 127,300 *Escudos*, in: Ministerio de Salud Pública: Oficio No. 0923, Aportes del Gobierno a la Reunión de Ministros de Salud de la Américas y del Consejo Directivo de OPS. Deudas pendientes, 0923-1817-1972, 12.06.1972, p. 1–2.
37. In the case of the WFP, Chile contributed with 1.015.400 USD in three years, about 335.133 USD yearly, in: Ministerio de Salud Pública: Programas del Sector Salud de Chile con las Naciones Unidas y sus agencias especializadas año 1972, 1817-1972, 06.1972, p. 1–2.
38. Convenio para el desarollo de los servicios de salud materno-infantil, in: *El Mercurio*, 05.-11-06.1972.
39. Since 1968, there existed the program Family Planing Actions of the NHS (*Acciones de Planificación Familiar del SNS*), in: Ministerio de Salud Pública, Oficina de Asuntos Internacionales: Oficio No. 0530, Incluye Informaciones relacionadas con planificación familiar, 0530-1816-1972, 03.04.1972, p. 1;

    A summary of the UN projects in Chile and South America for 1973, in: Agency for International Development: The Population Program Assistance. United States Aid to Developing Countries, Annual Report, Fiscal Year 1973, Washington 1974, p. 100-101.
40. The Ministry of Health listed the professionals as officials (*funcionarios*). For a survey, it analyzed all seminars and scholarships health professionals attended abroad. It counted only activities from eight days to nine months, in: Ministerio de Salud Pública: Oficio No. 1047, Decretos de permiso para viajar al exterior de becarios del sector salud, 1047-1818-1972, 26.06.1972, p. 1–2.
41. Ministerio de Salud Pública: Oficio No. 0297, Sobre misión para adquirir materias primas y productos terminados farmacéuticos, 0297-1815-1972, 16.02.2972, p. 1–2.
42. In July 1973, health undersecretary Molina stated that a joined venture of UN and WHO (*Plan Cuadripartito de Operaciones de un Programa de Extensión de Servicios Materno Infantil y Bienestar Familiar*) from December 1972 had not been implemented yet, in: Ministerio de Salud Pública: Oficio No. 1340, Solicita la aprobación de los acuerdos que señala, suscritos por el Gobierno de Chile, 1340-1844-1973, 23.07.1973, p. 1;

    UNICEF, which in 1972 had opened a regional office in Santiago to manage the cooperation with the Chilean government, also had to adapt to the growing difficulties: In March 1972, it shrank the food delivery for children in 23 hospitals located in two regions (since August 1970) to 20 hospitals in only one region, in: Ministerio de Salud Pública: Oficio No.

0358, Propuestas [Estatales] al PMA-584, 0358-1816-1972, 07.03.1972, p. 1–6.

43. Jerez, Directora Depto de Enfermería Sede Santiago Norte, U. de Chile: Discurso de la Profesora Sra. Idilia Jerez, in: *Enfermería*, No. 40, 04-05-06-1974, p. 7–9, 7.
44. The cooperation with the NHS did not end with the transition of its nursing schools to the universities: nurses who worked in the NHS administration also participated in PAHO seminars in Peru, Mexico, and Argentina, in: Ministerio de Salud Pública: Oficio No. 768, Cursos Básicos de Planificación para 4 enfermeras en Perú, Argentina y México, 768-1843-1973, 25.04.1973, p. 1-1 [9/17].
45. Ministerio de Salud Pública, Oficina de Asuntos Internacionales: Oficio No. 0342, Sobre solicitud de lista de maestros y materias que imparten Escuelas del S.N.S., 28.02.1972, p. 1.
46. Ministerio de Salud Pública, Oficina de Asuntos Internacionales: Oficio No. 0431, Curso materno-infantil para enfermeras en U. del Valle, Cali, Colombia, 0431-1816-1972, 17.03.1972, p. 1;

    First Evaluation Level of a Master's Program in Community Health with a concentration in Nursing in Mental Health and Psychiatry (*Curso de Magister en Salud de la Comunidad con mención en Enfermería de Salud Mental y Psiquiatría*), in: Ministerio de Salud Pública, Oficina de Asuntos Internacionales: Oficio No. 0620, Consultoría de Dra. Claire Pagin a la Escuela de Enfermería de la U. Católica, 0620-1843-1973, 29.03.1973, p. 1-1 [5/17].
47. The Ministry of Health listed Monardez as the director of the University of Chile's nursing department, in: Ministerio de Salud Pública, Oficina de Asuntos Internacionales: Oficio No. 0379, OPS-beca para Nidia Nuñez Alvarado - Puerto Rico, 0379-1816-1972, 10.03.1972, p. 1;

    The Ministry of Health listed Krebs as the director of the nursing school of the Medical Faculty, in: Ministerio de Salud Pública, Oficina de Asuntos Internacionales: Oficio No. 0442, OPS asesoría Dra. Marion Murphy para Escuela de Enfermería, U. de Chile, 0442-1816-1972, 20.03.1972, p. 1;

    At least until 1971, Krebs worked in a leading position in the Catholic University of Santiago, in: Krebs, Vicerrectoría Académica de Institutos y Escuelas, U. Católica de Chile, in: *Enfermería*, No 28, 04-05-06-1971, p. 20–22.
48. The last time the opening of a new nursing school was discussed dated back to July 1972, in: Ministerio de Salud Pública: Oficio No. 1091, Posibilidad de crear Escuela de Enfermería en Arica, 1091-1818-1972, 03.07.1972, p. 1.

49. Letter of Jirón to the NHS, in: Ministerio de Salud Pública: Oficio No. 1526 Solicita opinión sobre incorporación de Enfermeras a Ley 15.076, 1526-1844-1973, 14.08.1973, p. 1.
50. Memoria de la Contabilidad e Informe del Balance General al 30 de Junio de 1982, in: Enfermería, No. 72, 04-05-06-1982, p. 47–56.
51. The 7th national congress of Chilean nurses took place from October 8 to 14, 1972. In May, Concha confirmed his participation, in: Ministerio de Salud Pública: Oficio No. 0885, Celebración del VII Congreso Nacional de Enfermeras, 0885-1817-1972, 06.06.1972, p. 1.
52. Interview with Concha, Santiago, March 2017.
53. The so-called Compensatory Fees of Midwives (*Arancel Único Compensado de Matronas*), in: Ministerio de Salud Pública: Oficio No. 2014, Sobre Reajuste Arancel Único Compensado de Matronas, 2014-1821-1972, 05.12.1972, p. 1-1 [3/12].
54. Programa de Educación de Enfermería en Chile, in: Ministerio de Salud Pública, Oficina de Asuntos Internacionales: Oficio No. 1759, Sobre integrantes de la Comisión de Educación de Enfermería, 1759-1820-1972, 19.10.1972, p. 1;

    The Program for the Development of Nursing Education was meant to "give and regulate post-graduate education in nursing," in: Ministerio de Salud, Oficina de Asuntos Internacionales: Oficio No. 0147, Reitera Oficio No. 1213-A del 13 julio 1971, Acuerdo para Programa de Desarrollo de la Educación en Enfermería, 0147-1816-1972, 25.01.1972, p. 1;

    The Program of Progressive Patient Care (*Programa De Atención Progresiva De Pacientes*) of the nursing school in Valparaíso was rejected by the Foreign Affairs Institute of the Ministry of Health. The reason for this decision was the lack of a similar research area in Chile, in: Ministerio de Salud Pública, Oficina de Asuntos Internacionales: Oficio No. 1270, Solicitud asesoría Escuela Enfermería Universidad de Valparaíso, 1270-1818-1972, 27.07.1972, p. 1.
55. Statement of costs of the program, in: Ministerio de Salud Pública, Oficina de Asuntos Internacionales: Oficio No. 1104, Programa de Provisión de Textos de Enfermería, Chile-6310, 1104-1818-1972, 04.06.1972, p. 1–2;

    Garrido for the *CECh* and Lía Santibáñez R. for the NHS led the commission, in: Ministerio de Salud Pública, Oficina de Asuntos Internacionales: Oficio No. 1759, Sobre integrantes de la Comisión de Educación de Enfermería, 1759-1820-1972, 19.10.1972, p. 1.
56. Even the documentation of the Ministry of Health shows that the PAHO, among all female health professionals, mostly subsidized nursing pro-

grams, but, also offered scholarships for other professionals such as midwives. Afterwards, scholarships for midwives of the Universidad Austral were rejected, but the document also refers to positive responses in similar cases, in: Ministerio de Salud Pública, Oficina de Asuntos Internacionales: Oficio No. 1040, Becas para tres matronas rechazadas por OPS - voluntad del MdS apoyar a la creación de la profesión de enfermería obstétrica, 1040-1818-1972, 22.06.1972, p. 1.

57. Zunilda Pizarro Ramírez and Margarita Soza Aranda, nurses from the hospital *San Juan Dios* in Santiago received PAHO scholarships for studies in Mexico, Cuba, and Puerto Rico, in: Ministerio de Salud Pública, Oficina de Asuntos Internacionales: Oficio No. 0303, Zunila Pizarro y Margarita Soza (San Juan de Dios) becas a México, Puerto Rico y Cuba, 0303-1816-1972, 17.02.1972, p. 1;

    Six nurses received scholarships for seminars in methodology and planning. The seminars took place in Lima, Buenos Aires, and Medellín, in: Ministerio de Salud Pública, Oficina de Asuntos Internacionales: Oficio No. 0328, Sobre cursos destinados a preparar a enfermeras en metodología de la planificación, 0328-1816-1972, 25.02.1972, p. 1;

    In 1972, Mirella Ortega Carvallo, investigator and active member of the *CECh*, applied for a one-year scholarship in Cali and Medellín, in: Ministerio de Salud Pública, Oficina de Asuntos Internacionales: Oficio No. 0659, Solicitud de beca de la Srta. Mirella Ortega, 0659-1817-1972, 24.04.1972, p. 1;

    Lilian Viveros, president of the Chilean Society of Nursing Education, chose three nurses (from Valdivia, Antofagasta, and Temuco) for short-term intensive seminars (*cursos cortos intensivos*) in *materno-infantil* nursing, funded by the PAHO and executed by the University of Valle, Colombia, in: Ministerio de Salud Pública, Oficina de Asuntos Internacionales: Oficio No. 1760, Becas para cuurso intensivo materno-infantil en la U. de Valle, Colombia para tres enfermeras [working title], 1760-1820-1972, 19.10.1972, p. 1-1 [3/10].

58. Williams in her capacity as a WHO consultant, in: Stanhope, Marcia; Lancaster, Jeanette: Public-Health Nursing. Population-Centered Health Care in the Community, St. Louis [Elsevier] 92016, p. 172;

    One example of Williams' work in Chile, in: Ministerio de Salud Pública, Oficina de Asuntos Internacionales: Oficio No. 1309, Acciones financiadas por Convenio Chile-6300, 1309-1844-1973, 17.07.1973, p. 1;

    Cammaert in her capacity as a WHO consultant, in: Saskatoon Star Phoenix: Margaret Cammaert, 09.04.2016, https://thestarphoenix.remembering.ca/obituary/margaret-cammaert-1065300755 [2021-10-15];

One example of Cammaert's work in Chile, in: Ministerio de Salud Pública, Oficina de Asuntos Internacionales: Oficio No. 1339, Srtas. Irma Acevedo, Rosa Chiang y María Ramírez, 1339-1819-1972, 03.08.1972, p. 1.

59. No sign of the hiring of Cuban nurses in Chile between 1970 and 1973 was found. The only clue in this direction is the participation of nurses (in cooperation with the *CECh*) in a delegation of Chilean health professionals in September 1971 to Cuba, in: Boletín Informativo No. 8, quoted in: Memoria de la Contabilidad e Informe del Balance General al 30 de Junio de 1982, in: *Enfermería*, No. 72, 04-05-06-1982, p. 47–56, 48.
60. A foreign nurse had to present the following documents: Request of revalidation from the dean of a medical faculty, title or diploma awarded by a professional school, summary of the studied subjects, certificate or bachelor certificate in humanities (i.e., secondary school) or equivalent, birth certificate, certificate of earlier employments, PAHO validation of the nursing exam, letter of application, membership in a professional organization, and certificate of religion, in: Ministerio de Salud Pública, Subsecretaría: Oficio No. 0181, Informa acerca requisitos para ingresar como Enfermera al S.N.S., 0181-1816-1972, 1972, p. 1.
61. *El Mercurio*, 22.-28.05.1972, p. 8.
62. Raising the number of nurses scientifically trained was a long-term claim of the *CECh* and several times demanded by Pincheira in the *Enfermería*. For example, in the edition published in the same month the Popular Unity came to power, in: Editorial, in: *Enfermería*, No. 26, 10-11-12-1970, p. 3–4.
63. The only sign of this project was found because of its disastrous outcome acknowledged in 1973. Of 1000 participants, only 55 percent finished the training. Out of the 450 graduates, only 226 worked later for the NHS, in: Ministerio de Salud Pública: Oficio No. 875, Sobre convenio formación auxiliares de enfermería, 875-1843-1973, 04.05.1973, p. 1-2 [10-11/17].
64. In November 1972, the dentists' association refused to train dental technicians in the University of Concepción. After only two years of training, instead of five, the trainees would receive the title of dentist, in: *La Prensa*, 06.11.1972, p. 8.
65. In August 1973, the Christian Democratic Senator Ricardo Valenzuela Sáez introduced a bill in the Congress in order to intensify the control measures for nursing schools, in: Moción del honorable Senador Señor Valenzuela, con la que inicia un proyecto de ley que define lo que se entiende por atención de enfermería y dicta normas acerca de la profesión de enfermería, in: República de Chile: Diario de sesiones del Senado, Sesión 63a, 28.08.1973 [Biblioteca del Congreso Nacional], p. 2791-2792.

66. The food shortage had been the subject of a controversial debate. Toledo explains that the criticism against the governmental politics that prominently appeared in oppositional newspapers like *El Mercurio* or *La Prensa* did not reflect the reality, in: Toledo, Ana Corina: Partizipation von Frauen während der Militärdiktatur in Chile (1973-1990), Berlin [Ergon Verlag] 2000, p. 124;

    Power also does not confirm a general popular discontent. Nevertheless, she states that the supply of food became difficult since the beginning of 1972, in: Power (2002), p. 143.
67. Silvia Alessandri was a Red Cross nursing volunteer. Therefore, she had no *CECh* membership, in: Silvia Alessandri Montes. Reseñas Biográficas [Biblioteca Nacional];

    Alessandri arranged the permission for the march, in: Power: Mujer de Derecha. El poder femenino y la lucha contra Salvador Allende, 1964-1973, Santiago [Centro de Investigaciones Diego Barros Arana] 2008, p. 195.
68. Power (2002), p. 65;

    Power also interviewed Lisa Baldez in the early 1990s, in: Women Lead the Opposition to Allende: Interview with Carmen Saenz, in: The Chile Reader. History, Culture, Politics [Ed. Quay Hutchison, Elizabeth; Miller Klubock, Thomas; Milanich, Nara B.; Winn, Peter], Durham and London 2014, p. 406-409, 407.
69. Palermo, Vicente: March of the Empty Pots, in: *Encyclopaedia of Latin American History and Culture*, Vol. 4, 2008, p. 368-369, 368.
70. For example, political repression under Isabel Martínez de Perón, in: The Faces of Human Rights [Ed. McCall Smith; Wouters, Jan] 2019, p. 270;

    Political repression in Chile, in: Power (2002), p. 156;

    Also described in: Collier, Simon; Sater, William F.: A History of Chile, 1808-2002, Cambridge [Cambridge University Press] 2004, p. 349.
71. Only a few hours after the march started, female supporters of the Popular Unity requested permission for a counterdemonstration. Allende rejected the request because he feared an escalation of violence, in: Baldez, Lisa: Why women protest. Women's movements in Chile, Cambridge [Cambridge University Press] 2002, p. 82.
72. Toledo states that it was men who normally organized the demonstrations. She states that the women repeated the march of empty pots every 14 days, in: Toledo (2000), p. 120, 130;

    Even if marches were repeated, they did not appear in the print press anymore.
73. In 1972, *El Mercurio* was the newspaper with the third highest circulation, in: Uribe, Hernán: La Prensa y el periodismo político en los años 1960/70, in: Carmona, Ernesto: Morir es la noticia, los periodistas relatan la historia de sus compañeros asesinados y/o desaparecidos, Santiago [E. Carmona] 1997.

74. *La Prensa* had a print run under a million copies, in: Ibid., p. 7.
75. The number of inhabitants was estimated due to the census of 2017, in: Instituto Nacional de Estadísticas: Censo de Población y Vivienda 2017.
76. Declaración del Colegio Médico frente a asalto contra un facultativo, in: *El Mercurio*, 10.-16.04.1972, p. 6, [1/1].
77. In *El Mercurio*, the attack on the hospital in Fresia is dated to April 14th. *La Prensa* did not give an exact date, in: Ministro en visita para los asaltantes del hospital de Fresia, in: *La Prensa*, 13.04.1972.
78. Documentos proporcionados por el Presidente del Colegio Médico de Chile sobre los hechos ocurridos en el Hospital de Fresia, in: Informe de la comisión de acusación deducida en contra del Señor Ministro del Interior, Don Hernán del Canto Riquelme, in: República de Chile, Cámara de Diputados, 26.04.1972, https://www.bcn.cl/laborparlamentaria/wsgi/consulta/verDiarioDeSesion.py?id=591383 [2021-10-15].
79. In May 1972, Cruz was mentioned for the first time as the undersecretary of the medical association, in: Se mantiene el paro de los médicos, in: *El Mercurio*, 01.-07.05.1972, p. 5 [2/7];

    In April, the critics of Cruz and Villaroel against the Popular Unity were published for the first time, in: *El Mercurio*, 24.-30.04.1972, p. 6, [7/9].
80. Se mantiene el paro de los médicos, in: *El Mercurio*, 8.-14.05.1972, p. 8, [1/1].
81. In July 1972, *El Mercurio* announced the resignation of 19 physicians from the medical section of the mine *El Teniente*, one of the most important state-owned companies, in: Renuncia de 19 médicos en el hospital de la mina El Teniente, in: *El Mercurio*, 03.-09.07.1972, p. 5 [1/1].
82. *El Mercurio*, 15.-21.05.1972, p. 3.
83. Ensalaco (2000), p. 18; Interview with Concha, Santiago, March 2017.
84. Molina Bustos states that health professionals joined one another as *FENATS* members, but also cooperated with the largest union, the Workers Central (*Central Única De Trabajadores*, *CUT*), in: Molina Bustos, Carlos Antonio: Una mirada historiográfica acerca del desarollo de la institucionalidad sanitaria chilena: 1889-1989, Santiago 2007, p. 7-19.
85. Director del SNS hace fracasar arreglo del Hospital de Curicó, *El Mercurio*, 06.-12.11.1972, p. 4.
86. Paro médico en Santiago, in: *El Mercurio*, 24.-30.04.1972, p. 6 [7/9].
87. Casals Araya, Marcelo: Estado, contrarrevolución y autoritarismo en la trayectoria política de la clase media profesional chilena. De la oposición a la Unidad Popular al fin de los Colegios Profesionales (1970-1981), in: *Izquierdas*, No. 44, 2018, p. 91-113, 100.
88. *El Mercurio*, 25.-30.09.1972, p.7 [1/4-3/4].

89. The professional associations started consultancy departments (*asesorías jurídicas*) in order to protect the professionals against possible attacks of the government. It is unclear whether they offered legal protection to the auxiliary personnel, in: *El Mercurio*, 17.-23.07.1972, p. 7 [4/5].
90. Se mantiene el paro de los médicos, in: *El Mercurio*, 25.-30.09.1972, p. 7.
91. Se mantiene el paro de los médicos, in: *La Prensa*, 30.09.1972.
92. Talloni stated that she and her colleagues compensated for the absence of staff, in: Interview with Talloni, Santiago, February 2015.
93. Convenio entre el Colegio Médico y el SNS el 06.10.1972, in: *El Mercurio*, 12-18.02.1972, p. 7 [1/2].
94. Nuevo Gabinete del gobierno el 13.06.1972, in: *El Mercurio*, 12.-18.06.1972, p. 1 [1/1].
95. "Inserción: Colegio Médico, Colegio de Enfermeras—Colegio de Químico-Farmacéuticos—Colegio de Dentistas de Chile. A la opinión pública," in: Se mantiene el paro de los médicos, in: *La Prensa*, 02.11.1972;

    Announcements like this did not appear in *El Mercurio*, which rather published summaries of such actions in articles with titles like "Professionals of the Country claim to return to a constitutional State," in: *El Mercurio*, 25.-30.09.1972, p. 7;

    The National Audit Office (*Contralaría General de la República*) following a description of Ensalaco had power possessions like a High Court. It was initiated due to the constitution of 1925, in: Ensalaco (2000), p. 51-52.
96. One example, in: Se mantiene el paro de los médicos, in: *El Mercurio*, 25.-30.09.1972, p. 8;

    Second example, in: Anuncian, in: *La Prensa*, 04.11.1972, p. 9.
97. List of participants: "carriers, traders, professional associations and," as the author of *La Prensa* called it "other gremios," in: Continúa indefinido paro gremial: Suspendidas las conversaciones entre los gremios y el Gobierno, in: *La Prensa*, 02.11.1972;

    LAN Chile and municipalities' employees also stopped to work, in: *El Mercurio*, 16.-22.10.1972, p. 1.
98. About the planned nationalization of the paper industry, in: Se mantiene el paro de los médicos, in: *El Mercurio*, 25.-30.09.1972, p. 7;

    About criticism against reforms of the education, in: La instrucción proselitista y concientizadora en la Educación, in: *El Mercurio*, 25.-30.09.1972, p. 7.
99. "Paro médico es un atentado contra Chile," dice la CUT, in: *El Clarín*, 31.10.1972, p. 7.

100. Flyers or handouts were distributed by both movements and political parties. For example, in November 1972 the Central Committee of the Socialist Party thanked (in this particular order) the *CUT*, the so-called Patriotic and Professional Fronts (*Frentes Patrióticos y Profesionales*) and the women and the health councils for their efforts to keep the country running during the strike, in: Partido Socialista (Pleno del Comité Central): Resolución política, in: Haria, Victor: La Izquierda Chilena (1969-1973), 2002, Vol. 5, p. 3322.
101. *El Clarín*, 31.07.1972, p. 7.
102. Collier et al. (2004), p. 349;
    There are no exact numbers in *El Mercurio*. Its authors listed 400,000 farmers, 120,000 small- and large-scale manufacturers and 30,000 students. But they did not provide similar information about the other groups, in: Decisión del Comando de Defensa Gremial——Negociaciones en una sola mano, in: *El Mercurio*, 23.-29.10.1972, 27.10.1972, p. 1.
103. Valentín Robles, leader of the National Front of Professionals, counted 80,000 professionals in 1972, in: *El Mercurio*, 25.-30.09.1972, p.7 [3/3];
    According to Lavados, 68,188 professionals worked in 1972 in Chile, in: Lavados (1983), p. 105.
104. Casals (2018) stated that a large majority of professionals voted for the strike. For this, he analyzed the reporting in the *Vida Médica* and *El Mercurio*, in: Casals (2018), p. 102.
105. The regional council of Santiago also represented the region of O'Higgins, 140 km south of Santiago, where about 75 percent of the physicians had voted for the strike, in: *El Mercurio*, 16.-22.10.1972, p. 1.
106. Chanfreau (1979), p. 99.
107. Colegio Médico de Antofagasta ordenó volver a trabajo, in: *El Clarín*, 30.10.1972, p. 4;
    Also documented in *El Mercurio*. There, it is described as "medical meeting convoked by the left-wing professionals" (*una reunión médica solicitada por los profesionales de izquierda*), in: *El Mercurio*, 30.10.-05.11.1972, p. 2 [4/10].
108. En Antofagasta sigue el paro médico y bancario, in: *El Mercurio*, 30.10.-05.11.1972, p. 2.
109. Chanfreau (1979), p. 99.
110. Belmar et al. (1975), p. 59.
111. A cualquier colegiado que contravenga esta orden, se le instruirá un sumario por falta grave a la ética profesional, in: *La Prensa*, 01.11.1972.
112. Interviews with Patricia Talloni, Patricia Grau, and Margarita Reusch, Santiago, March 2016.
113. Profesionales de la salud reafirman defensa gremial, in: *El Mercurio*, 30.10.-05.11.1972, p. 4 [7/10].

114. Belmar et al. (1975), p. 59.
115. Hadjez-Berrios, Esteban: A socio-psychological perspective on community participation in health during the Unidad Popular government: Santiago de Chile, from 1970 to 1973, in: *Journal of Health Psychology*, Vol. 19, No. 1, 2014, p. 90-96, 94.
116. But nursing auxiliaries were only mentioned in September 1972, as the strike began in the Hospital San Borja. The following groups appeared in *La Prensa* article: physicians, nurses, dentists, medical-technical assistants, social workers, midwives, inspectors, nursing auxiliaries, and cleaning staff (*médicos, enfermeras, dentistas, tecnólogos, asistentes sociales, matronas, inspectores de saneamiento, auxiliares de enfermería y personales de servicio*), in: *La Prensa*, 30.09.1972.
117. A los médicos, dentistas, químico-farmaceúticos y enfermeras, in: *La Prensa*, 02.11.1972.
118. *El Mercurio*, 16.-22.10.1972, p.1.
119. Politicians and professionals like the president of the lawyers Valentín Robles or the lawyer Julio Durán played important roles both backing and opposing human resources policy in the public sector during the 1970s. In 1979, Durán eventually led the professional associations in a heated debate about the transformation into private associations (Chap. 4).
120. The US government indirectly announced the severance of the diplomatic relations; it introduced trade restrictions and blocked credits to avoid the recovery of the Chilean copper exportation after its nationalization, in: Barrios, Harald: Chile im internationalen System, in: Chile heute. Politik, Wirtschaft, Kultur [Ed. Imbusch, Messner, Nolte], Frankfurt am Main [Vervuert] 2004, p. 457-478, 459.
121. The boards of the revolting professional associations blamed the Popular Unity for the high inflation rate, in: Profesionales del país piden retorno al estado de derecho, in: *El Mercurio*, 25.-30.09.1972, 28.09.1972, p. 7.

    Especially the shortage of consumer goods was constantly criticized by the opposition, For example in *La Tribuna*, the extended arm of the Chilean right-wing parties and movements, in: A los profesionales y al país, in: *La Tribuna*, 16.10.1972, No. 494, p. 9.
122. The first incident took place in May 1972 in Valparaíso. As the government had enforced state of emergency, a member of the Navy Command became the new governor, in: Vicealmirante asumió Intendencia de Valparaíso, in: *El Mercurio*, 15.-21.05.1972 [2/3].
123. En calidad de subrogante, General A. Pinochet U. asumió comandancia del ejército, in: *El Mercurio*, 30.10.-05.11.1972, p. 1.

124. Decisión del Gobierno entregó Ministro del Interior: "Solución del paro dentro de las próximas 48 horas, in: *El Mercurio*, 30.10-05.11.1972, 04.11.1972, p. 1.
125. Conferencia de *La Prensa*—General Prats analizó situación nacional, in: *El Mercurio*, 06.-12.02.1972, 07.11.1972, [10/10].
126. Seven bishops attempted to mediate between the two political sides, in: Allende analiza la situación, in: *El Mercurio*, 15.-22.10.1972, 21.10.1972, p. 1.
127. Molina (2007), p. 90.
128. Profesionales de la Salud reafirman defensa gremial, in: *El Mercurio*, 30.10.-05.11.1972, p. 4 [9/10].
129. The accusation was documented by *El Mercurio* in 1972, in: *El Mercurio*, 11.-17.12.1972, p. 5 [3/5];
    And in 1973, in: *El Mercurio*, 16.-22.04.1973, p. 5 [2/3].
130. Collier et al. (2004), p. 351.
131. On June 23, an undefined number of women took part in the march from Rancagua to Santiago. Power states that especially because of their participation, right-wing groups within the Armed Forces found themselves constrained to act, in: Power (2002), p. 214.
132. Bitar, Sergio: Chile: 1970–1973: Asumir la historia para construir el futuro, Santiago [Pehuén Editores Ltd.] 1996, p. 380.
133. For example, the copper mine *El Teniente* counted in 1973 about 11,000 workers and employees. They generated almost a third of the whole outcome of Chilean mining, in: Bitar (1996), p. 242.
134. The first time health workers went to strike in *El Teniente* was in July 1972, in: Profesionales de la Salud reafirman defensa gremial, in: *El Mercurio*, 03.-09.07.1972, p. 5 [1/1].
135. Talloni knew a physician who worked for the Ministry of Health. He advised her to the join the Popular Unity, in: Interview with Talloni, Santiago, March 2017.
136. Médicos de Santiago prolongan su huelga, in: *El Mercurio*, 18.-24.06.1973, p. 5 [1/1].
137. Sigue Paro en hospital Salvador, in: *El Mercurio*, 25.06.-01.07.1973, p. 5 [6/11].
138. "Siniestro plan de los matasanos momios. Fascistas se tomarán los hospitales para curar sus heridos de la guerra civil," in: *El Clarín*, 26.06.1973, p. 4.
139. *La Tribuna*, 496, 18.10.1972, p. 10.
140. *La Tribuna*, 494, 16.10.1972, p. 9.
141. Bürgerkrieg in Chile? in: *Der Spiegel*, 20.08.1973.

142. Chile: A Chronology. Report prepared by the staff of the Congressional Research Service, Library of Congress, in: Hearing before the Subcommittee on Interamerican Affairs of the Committee on Foreign Affairs, House of Representatives: United States and Chile during the Allende years, 1970–1973, Washington [U.S. Government Printing Office] 1975, p. 390.

    The tight cooperation with the Armed Forces was criticized not only by the opposition but also by members of the Popular Unity, in: Power (2002), p. 222.
143. Most important subject of discussion was the case for flat fee system for physicians, dentists, and pharmacists, in: *El Mercurio*, 16.-22.07.1973, p. 8 [3/3].
144. *El Mercurio* reported about a healthcare strike like it was a parallel movement to that of the truck drivers, in: Salud. Paro médico, in: *El Mercurio*, 03.-09.09.1973, p. 8;

    Already in June, health professionals had declared their solidarity with employees of *Canal 6*, a TV broadcaster of the University of Chile, which had been investigated by the police, in: *El Mercurio*, 18.-24.06.1973, p. 5 [1/1].
145. Power (2002), p. 226.
146. Collier et al. (2004), p. 356; Espinoza Ciudad et al.: Proceso de atención de enfermería en el ejercicio profesional región metropolitana urbana, in: *Enfermería*, No. 76, 04-05-06-1983, p. 31–35.
147. Espinoza Ciudad et al.: Estudio de necesidades del perfeccionamiento post grado de la Enfermeras del área Occidente año 1976, in: *Enfermería*, No. 50, 10-11-12-1976, p. 27–37.
148. Pizarro worked in the pediatric unit of the *San Juan de Dios* hospital in 1971, in: Comisión de Enfermería Pediátrica: Exposición del Colegio de Enfermeras sobre la Atención de Enfermería del Recién Nacido, in: *Enfermería*, No. 27, 01-02-03-1971, p. 24-45;

    Pizarro was working in the pharmacy of the same hospital in 1979, in: Dra. Pinto C., Enfermera Jefe Pabellón Quirúrgico, Hospital San Juan de Dios et al.: Esterilización, Desinfección y Antisepsia, in: *Enfermería*, No. 59, 01-02-03-1979, p. 24–32.
149. Collier et al. (2004), p. 356.
150. Paro total de actividades, in: *El Mercurio*, 06.-12.08.1973, p. 1 [1/2].
151. Cámara de Diputados: Acuerdo adoptado por la N. Cámara de Diputados, 23.08.1973, https://obtienearchivo.bcn.cl/obtienearchivo?id=documentos/10221.1/13377/1/mj_00061.pdf [2021-10-15];

    El Mercurio, Ed. Extraordinario, 08.1973, p. 2 [12/17].
152. Power (2002), p. 235.

153. The US government (1975) counted 100,000, in: Chile: A Chronology. Report prepared by the staff of the Congressional Research Service, Library of Congress (1975), p. 394.
154. According to reports used in a hearing before a commission of the US Senate from July 1974, under the label "escapees and refugees," strike breakers had been arrested after September 1973 all over the country. An unknown number were tortured and murdered. According to Amnesty International, the report states 65 murdered physicians and various health professionals including some arrested nurses, in: Refugee and humanitarian problems in Chile [microform]: hearing, Ninety-third Congress, first session, 23.07.1974, p. 235.

    The written sources from nurses did not draw a clear picture, but mention, without giving a number, nurses who were "questioned" after the coup d'état, which means they had supported the Popular Unity, in: Colegio de Enfermeras de Chile: Posición del Colegio de Enfermeras frente a las colegiadas funcionarias cuestionadas, in: *Boletín Informativo*, Nos. 34, 35,36, 1973, p. 9.
155. Quote: "los gremios de profesionales, técnicos, trabajadores independientes y campesinos demuestran su disciplina y su eficacia," in: *El Mercurio*, 16.-22.10.1973, p. 3;

    The nursing auxiliary Yvette Cap de Ville (*Hospital San Borja*) and the technical auxiliary (*auxiliar en tecnología médica*) Teresa Aburto (*Hospital J.J. Aguirre*), both interviewed for this research, told us that there were auxiliary workers who continued to work in order to support the government of the Popular Unity, in: Interview with Teresa Aburto and Ivette Cap de Ville, Santiago, March 2017.
156. Involucrados en las negociaciones: médicos, dentistas, químico-farmacéuticos y enfermeras, in: *El Mercurio*, 03.-09.09.1973, p. 8 [3/4];

    After the coup d'état, the board of the medical association called itself the War Board (*Directiva de Guerra*), in: *El Mercurio*, 03.-09.12.1973, p. 5.
157. Last speech of Allende, September 11th, in: Discurso del presidente Salvador Allende en la Radio Magallanes, 11 de septiembre de 1973.
158. Interview with Patricia Talloni, Santiago, March 2017.
159. Belmar et al. claimed it had significantly reduced the impact of the October 1972 strike, in: Belmar et al. (1975), p. 59.

CHAPTER 3

Nursing Under the Civilian-Military Cooperation (1973–1979)

1 Introduction

The constant search for a nursing policy, and the necessary political alliances, shifts the spotlight on the nurse not just as a professional but also as an important social actor. Principles from the previous chapters, like the concept and implementation of public health, continued. Especially their closer bond with the state, beginning in the 1920s, reached a pinnacle during the Pinochet dictatorship.

Analyzing the years from 1975 to 1979 shows how an organization of female professionals worked under and experienced the control of the military. Based on sources from the Ministry of Health, daily newspapers, and nursing organizations, this chapter provides the first study devoted more purposefully to auxiliary nurses. In doing so, this story expands the knowledge about women during the dictatorial regime, especially those who worked outside of the home.

Until 1979, the *military junta* and civil collaborators laid the foundations for extensive healthcare reform. As nurses and auxiliaries represent a large portion of the healthcare workforce, they communicated and implemented the state policy, becoming both agents and victims of those policies. And because of the intersection of gender and social class, it is important to look at how the reform process mirrored the dynamics of exclusion.

© The Author(s), under exclusive license to Springer Nature Switzerland AG 2023

M. Thulin, R. A. Ayala, *Nursing, Policy and Politics in Twentieth-century Chile*,
https://doi.org/10.1007/978-3-030-90835-5_3

2 The Establishment of the Civilian-Military Cooperation

On September 11, 1973, a military board (*junta militar*) took power and declared state of siege.[1] They suppressed the parliament, took over the media, censored the press, and forbade unions, political parties, and all kinds of gatherings. The press and the education system came under their control.[2] For the next 16 years, an Army general and an Air Force general, both of whom had no healthcare training, would have the last say when it came to deciding about nursing. Air Force Commander Gen. Gustavo Leigh (1920–1999) was in charge of the healthcare ministry[3] and Gen. Pinochet of the Ministry of the Interior and the universities. To govern, they mostly ruled by decree (*decreto ley*), in other words issuing de facto laws without the need for debate among the ruling group and simply imposing them. Such an approach gave their measures a near-democratic veneer while in reality deciding laws by a small circle of men who derived their power not from popular but from armed sovereignty.

For nurses, the new rulers had no reason to use coercion, as the nursing association simply obeyed. But they did so not only because of mortal danger. In September 1973, Garrido and Peake as well as the other board members moved from submission to civilian male power to subordination to military male power, and it would seem that nursing auxiliaries, *practicantes*, and Red Cross nurses acted likewise. As a consequence, while state powers were transformed, the social ladder remained unchanged. What changed was the political frame and the consequences nurses had to face when they criticized the rulers.

The generals issued an endless amount of decree laws. The underlying idea being to disguise the military administration as legal rule, although the basis of rule enforcement was repression, which redistributed powers and gave a new organization to the state.[4] In 1991, an independent commission reported about 2930 cases of human rights violation due to direct political repression.[5] This number was updated in 2010, when another commission counted 40,018 victims, of which some 3065 were either killed or reported as missing.[6]

By mid-1974, the military junta had established and secured control, and one might think that this would have been the right moment to hand the direction of the country back over the state's three power branches. But although arguing the opposite, the generals had no intention to return to the regime that the army and the rightists interrupted in September 1973.[7] They remained in power, with Pinochet becoming the de facto successor of Allende.[8]

From October 1973, a wave of criticisms washed over the junta.[9] The Conservative paper *El Mercurio*, however, labeled this criticism an "international campaign against Chile."[10] Though stable domestic affairs may have seemed, they could not dissimulate the problem of legitimacy the military junta had to face when it came to negotiations with the center-left governments of Western Europe and the US Democratic Party.

The professional associations' boards used this opportunity to voice their views. Several of them wrote letters justifying the coup d'état before American and European governments or took part in what they called "information tours" across Europe and North America.[11] Nurses responded to a letter of the Nicaraguan Nurses Association explaining there was "false information [accusations against the military] being spread by certain individuals and organs of the foreign press." They also wrote to the United Nations defending what they considered to be the truth behind the charges.[12] The pharmacists' association contacted partner entities in various countries.[13] The medical association sent correspondence to Pope Paul VI about "the real situation."[14] The Confederation of Professional Associations sent about 15,000 letters written in five different languages to partner organizations in Europe and the Americas.[15]

For the military junta, the most reliable partner among professional organizations was the association of lawyers (*Colegio de Abogados*). In 1974, its president, Julio Durán, accompanied the minister of finance in a journey to Europe. The goal of their "crusade" was to "explain to government officials the reasons for the military uprising."[16] Only a few reports talked about how the Chilean delegations were received or the reactions to their explanatory letters, and those which survived the passing of time seem generally positive.[17]

To run the public sector institutions, the military junta relied not only on a stable bureaucratic apparatus, mostly assured by professionals. Its administration also benefitted from the expertise and networks of economists, advisors of the former president Jorge Alessandri (1958–1964), and members of the former National Party. The ideology for the new society was shaped by the rightist leadership movement (*gremialismo*).[18]

The *gremialismo* movement, as mentioned in Chap. 1, appeared for the first time during the 1960s in the Catholic University in Santiago. During the 1970s, its influence spread over various state and civil institutions. Finally, at the turn of the 1980s, its institutionalization concluded. For the leader, the influential jurist and statesman Jaime Guzmán, the professional associations played an important role in his vision of a restructured society:

> "The ones who participate are only those who can choose from a variety of consume options within an open competitive economy. The ones who participate are only those who feel free to enroll in or disenroll from corporations, labor unions and professional associations, in the spirit of true freedom of association and work."[19]

Foreign affairs, internal administration, and political ideology; the generals could not operate without the professionals and their associations. And they had to quickly find a way to communicate and collaborate with them. After a three-year period of economic downturn, strikes, and clashes, the population would not remain quiet if there was no solution for hyperinflation (up to 376 percent in 1974), unemployment, and impoverishment.[20]

The economy did not come to a complete breakdown principally because the coup d'état did not bring about a complete rupture with the past. International relations, established by the Frei government and strengthened by Popular Unity, remained stable, and foreign money continued to flow into Chile, even though the most important donor countries had been criticizing the human rights violations since 1973. Regarding healthcare, PAHO alone financed at least one-third of the Chilean system. The UN continued to cooperate with civilian professionals based in Chile, and through the back door of development policy it legitimized the military junta.[21] Except for the Kellogg Foundation, which ended its involvement right after the coup d'état,[22] it would appear that no international organization relevant to healthcare changed its strategy regarding Chile.[23]

Despite the civilian-military cooperation and international aid, it took internal affairs a good three years before the military government stabilized. From then until 1983, however, no external factor could jeopardize the new leaders. It was a personal conflict within the junta members that became the most dangerous threat to the new order. One of the conflicting scenes was the healthcare sector, controlled by Leigh's Air Force.[24] By the beginning of 1976, Pinochet had given the go-ahead to a package of state reforms, including changes to the health legislature and the way to finance it. Leigh opposed it vehemently,[25] this being one of the most important reasons why he was dismissed from the ministry.[26]

During the following years, civilians regained more power in the ministries of health and labor (i.e., undersecretary and minister, respectively). However, the Ministry of the Interior, supervising all conferences of the health professionals and controlling the cast of the professional associations' boards, remained under the control of the Army.[27] In this way, the civilian-military cooperation became a cornerstone of the Pinochet regime of the 1980s.

Nurses, as we will see in the next section, joined the civilian-military cooperation. One might think that this was strategic to settling their claims. Female professionals thought that, perhaps, they could put aside ideological constraints and work toward achieving the target goals for their professions. This was not the case. Up until September 1973, they could lead strikes, publish position statements, and protest in the streets. After, fearful silence fell like a curtain on their associations. And as they waited and obeyed, the generals consolidated their power. For nurses this meant new working conditions and relationships. In the following we shall take a closer look at the dictatorial frame within which nursing policy developed over the next 16 years.

3 The Labor Policy

Since the foundation of the NHS, nurses had fought for better pay schemes and an equal treatment in healthcare institutionality. However, very soon they found out that the military policymakers had no intention whatsoever of looking at the specific needs of specific populations. To stabilize the state budget, the generals imposed drastic cuts on public spending.[28] They emphasized informal employment, reduced pensions, implemented programs of precarious employment, and did little to correct the high redundancy rate, on average 20 percent during the 1970s.[29] As seen in other recovery or adjustment programs then and now, the people with the lowest income often have to bear the brunt.

Between 1972 and 1975, the number of the unemployed in the social services quadrupled (11,500 to 75,800).[30] At least three waves of redundancy, in 1973, 1975, and 1977, took place in the healthcare sector.[31] During the first wave, people were laid off on the grounds of suspected or confirmed political involvement.[32] This "political adjustment" of the early months was followed by economic redundancies in 1975 and 1977. This staffing policy also hit the education sector. In the University of Chile, the most iconic and geographically extended academic center for health professionals, around 20 percent of the professors were laid off.[33]

The junta extended the low-wage sector by implementing a plan called Program of Minimal Employment (*Programa de Empleo Mínimo, PEM*) in 1975. The participants were mostly professional individuals working in exchange for a subsidy in areas as diverse as agriculture, education, craftsmanship, and healthcare.[34] The beneficiaries did not belong to the public administration and received only a daily payment. Severely criticized for legitimizing cheap labor, changes in working hours and redundancies could be set out unilaterally at any time. The nurses who would stand up to *PEM* in the 1980s recall that the program never offered year-long contracts.[35] Once again, the pressure was too high to keep an eye on the lower social strata. Even though *PEM* grew as ubiquitous as to affect 200,000 people nationwide,[36] the nurses we interviewed could not tell for sure whether nursing auxiliaries were also affected.

On December 31, 1973, the junta implemented payment guidelines for professionals and workers, the Unified Salary Scale (*Escala Única de Sueldos, EUS*). It listed 48 professions, 18 of them in the health sector, and sorted them across 32 wage categories or *grados*. The four highest grades were only accessible to professionals working in the ministries' bureaucracy. Physicians, pharmacists, lawyers, architects, and engineers usually started their career in the administration on the 15th grade and could be promoted up to the 5th. Nurses, midwives, and social workers, however, started on 18th grade and could reach up to the 12th. Nursing auxiliaries, in turn, ranked between the 29th and the 20th grades.[37] Health authorities praised the *EUS* as a harmonization of criteria and simplification of pre-existing wage systems. The medical association, however, did not agree, but as they were not allowed to strike, they only published their criticisms in the press.[38]

Another target of the labor policy was unionism. The labor unions were suppressed, but physicians, nurses, lawyers, architects, engineers, and the like could keep their associations functioning. A decree law from March 1974 shows the rationale behind that decision:

> "The government recognizes the valuable contribution of community organizations, professional associations and other similar organizations as supporting structures which help to solve the nation's problems."[39]

Yet the outcome for the professional associations was altogether unanticipated. Neither those warm words in the introduction of the decree law nor the propagandistic solidarity of the associations' boards toward the junta could prevent them from coming under direct state control and intervention. In fact, the Ministry of the Interior controlled all aspects of political affairs related to professional matters.[40]

The only labor union of professionals, the Common Union of Workers in Education (*Sindicato Unico de Trabajadores de Educación*, *SUTE*), gathered the majority of all professionals working in schools.[41] Unlike the boards of the professional associations, which became visible in the strikes of 1972 and 1973, the educationalists did not actively support the movements against the Popular Unity. In return, the junta backed the creation of the Association of the School Teachers of Chile (*Colegio de Profesores de Chile*) in 1974 and banned their union the following year.[42] Such level of oppression explains why from among the schoolteachers there emerged the most radical movement of professionals against the dictatorship, which would become an inspiration for left-wing nurses in the decade to follow.

In June 1978, the military junta implemented another labor policy. A new guideline for white- and blue-collar workers was enacted in the decree law 2.200. This regulation became one of the most decisive labor policies of the dictatorship, because it paved the way for the 48-hour week, also shortening the notice period when laying off employees and lowering the legal working age to 14 years.[43] University-trained nurses lost their most important argumentative basis for their salary raise claims. For nursing auxiliaries, the law simply confirmed the precarious conditions in which they worked.

The implementation process of the labor reform was important for a reason the military junta did not anticipate. Due to the growing international pressure led by the Carter administration, the military decided to lift press censorship in 1976, and for the first time since the coup d'état critical voices accompanied the implementation of a decree law. They mostly contested the enhanced decisional power of employers as the new legislation enabled state and private companies to modify or end contracts unilaterally without having to give any reasons.[44] They also condemned the reduction in payment arising from the extension of the work time.[45] Female professionals and workers remained silent about such drastic changes. However, their wait and see attitude began to deteriorate when the military junta interfered in and used elections to introduce submissive board members in the associations.

Four months after decree law 2.200, the Ministry of the Interior conducted a concerted action to fully reform the organization of workers and professionals. On October 31, 1978, it ordered the replacement of the board members (i.e., president, general secretary, treasurer) of all labor unions throughout the country and the election of new ones within three days.[46] Candidates deemed suitable were those who had not had any active political involvement during the previous 10 years.[47] This was the intent of the Pinochet regime to disempower left-wing individuals who were already active in political unionism.[48]

The labor policy of the 1970s implemented significant changes. At first glance, there was no difference between female and male professionals and workers; only those who counted on a strong lobby group, like physicians and dentists, were able to block severe implications. The claims of nurses and auxiliary nurses appeared in neither *El Mercurio* nor *Hoy.* They had to accept the terms of the *EUS*, of the *PEM*, and of decree law 2.200. Labor policy remained a male business.

4 The Healthcare Policy

From the very first day in power, the military junta made it clear that the structures of the health sector were obsolete. The necessary investments were too high and the healthcare coverage too low.[49] But economic crises inhibited any major changes during the first five years. The expansion and strengthening of the private sector and the reorganization of the health insurance scheme were put on hold.[50] The only measure the generals could introduce was a setting for the centralized state agencies like those which managed healthcare and universities.

The basis for the health system had been settled six months before, with a restructuring of the country by regions (*regionalización*). They redistributed the 25 regions into 13,[51] each having a regional ministerial secretary (*secretario regional ministerial*), appointed by the junta and entrusted healthcare coverage together with the NHS authorities.[52] The University of Chile was "regionalized" as well. Administration, financing, and study plans on offer came under the responsibility of its regional branches, with the biggest campuses in Santiago and Valparaíso.[53]

The other important change introduced by the military was an austerity approach in the budget for healthcare. Until 1982, the expenses fell by 15 percent compared to 1973.[54] The decrease was disastrous regarding the urgent needs in the rural areas and the slums of the suburbs. In the periphery of the cities, demographics aggravated the problem, especially in

Santiago where the population, already the largest in a single city, grew by 40 percent between 1970 and 1980.[55]

The condition of healthcare provision was so inadequate that even *El Mercurio* mentioned it several times between 1975 and 1979. The system lacked medicines, staff, and infrastructure.[56] In several cases, health personnel charged patients additional payments illegally or simply denied care because of the lack of stock.[57] The archives at the Ministry of Health confirm cases of refusal to see patients, critical infrastructure, and lack of medical instruments, although without quantifying the issue.[58] Only the slight relaxation of the press censorship at the end of the 1970s brought the long-term consequences of the austerity measures out of obscurity, notably the spread of infectious diseases.[59] Regionalization seemed more of an additional burden rather than a helpful reorganizing. Still in 1978, four years after its launch, understaffing threatened stable healthcare coverage in all 13 regional health services.[60]

5 The Origins of Resistance in the Healthcare System

The spring of 1973 was a major point of divergence for the opposition movement within healthcare. More than that, it was the highlight and the collapse of the health professionals' political involvement. By the beginning of September, they had brought the government to its knees. By the end of the year, they had become one of the many civilian co-operators of the military junta. From this point on, the only way for them to shape policy was to organize themselves outside of the Ministry of Health and NHS structures. Professionals who did not agree with the new rulers had to develop a new network and find an alternative communication medium and a place to meet.

From the coup d'état, the most important meeting places for the victims of the dictatorship were the facilities owned by the church.[61] In January 1976, several of them merged into the newly founded *Viacría de la Solidaridad* forming a powerful social network in Santiago.[62] *Vicaría* offered legal advice, food for the poor (children in particular), handcraft workshops and basic healthcare services.[63] By 1980, *Vicaría* housed 74 healthcare centers, which served some 2200 patients yearly.[64] That was certainly not enough to fix the deficiencies that the state policy produced, but at least it gave a clearer picture of a gap in the system. Furthermore, hundreds of health professionals had found a place outside the healthcare sector. There, they did not only exchange work methods. Alternative political ideas spread and the *Vicaría* became much more than just a provider of basic care for the community.

Vicaría became the meeting place for those who wanted to work for an alternative social model.[65] It encouraged reform-minded Chileans by publishing the magazine *Solidaridad*. For the first time, a constant critical medium protected by an institution, generally away from the Armed Forces and the police, reported openly on the failures of the social system and informed about the work of opposition groups.[66] *Vicaría* authors helped to speed up the development of the human rights movements in the country. *Solidaridad* set an exemplary standard for the founding of new print media and channeled the views of think tanks opposing the government and its policy.[67]

Higher international pressure followed the murder of a former member of the Popular Unity in Washington, alongisde Carter's human rights policy, further catalyzed activism on the part of oppositional journalists. After the loosening of censorship, there appeared the first edition of the weekly magazine *Hoy*. In just a few years, it was regarded as one of the most important sources for alternative information about the Chilean healthcare system.[68]

Another pioneer of alternative information about the healthcare system was the magazine *APSI*, published fortnightly. It was founded in July 1976 and, as with *Hoy*, their authors gravitated toward the left wing of the Christian Democratic party.[69] *Análisis*, another magazine, also spoke critically about the situation in the healthcare system.[70] Conversely, authors writing for *El Mercurio* did not seem to blame the military for the deficits in healthcare. They rather pointed fingers at civilians.[71]

Except for one incident at the medical association, which was commented on in *Ercilla,* in 1975,[72] it would seem that oppositional ideas encountered strong resistance at the professional associations' boards. Even though oppositional members regained their voice, the power remained in the hands of the right-wing elite,[73] which served actively in the civilian-military cooperation, as we will see in the case of the nursing association.

The first sign of resistance among health professionals, not political in its origin but very political in its consequences, took place in March 1979. Reported only in *El Mercurio*, a group of recently graduated physicians occupied the national headquarters of the medical association. They wanted to call attention to the very few job offers there were. A unit of *Carabineros* brought them out of the premises and arrested all of them.[74]

However minor an event, and even if media coverage was brief, the occupation of the headquarters of the medical association proved once again that no professional group received as much attention from *El Mercurio* as the physicians.[75] *Qué Pasa* and *La Tercera*, also among the most important pro-government outlets, followed this trend.

The most prominent conflict in healthcare continued to be the medical association's struggle for law reform of *Medicina Curativa*. And even if their tone became more aggressive by the end of the 1970s, they never moved beyond symbolic acts.[76] That was a general problem of all sorts of oppositional work. The regime suppressed even the tiniest of signs of confrontation, during the 1970s and 1980s, this time using the military forces to do so. Authors of the alternative magazines found themselves in the same trap. Furthermore, except for *Solidaridad*, they could not refer to healthcare organizations or movements of health professionals as members of a new democratic society and, as a result, the rebelling physicians failed to suggest suitable solutions to the urgent problems, the basis for shaping policy.

By the beginning of the 1980s, the first steps toward a new opposition movement were being taken. Undoubtedly, *El Mercurio* remained the key source for the formation of political opinion, while *Vicaría*'s influence was minor compared to the shaping power of the official health institutions. On top of that, the first rebellion of the physicians had crashed. But it also became clear that the junta had to tolerate at least a small opposition. Nurses did not appear in this picture. This is surprising as they continued to be the most powerful voice of female health professionals. To understand their silence, we have to analyze their working conditions and their status after the coup.

6 Nursing in Times of Dictatorship

6.1 *Privileged and Subordinated*

The history of nursing in previous years has shown that throughout the modernization of the system some caregivers were privileged, but most of them were actually subordinated. While nurses who trained academically had to follow the orders of privileged men, nursing auxiliaries had to obey the same men *and* the academically trained nurses, while trained nurses themselves were controlled by elite nurses. In fact, the biographies of *CECh* board members seem to be the only ones that were worth being written down. A number of them held leading positions in universities, NHS facilities, or hospitals. Moreover, the biographies of six privileged nurses contain marginal notes on their subordinates, likely a trait arising from class relations between them.

During the Pinochet era, Gladys Peake was still the most powerful nurse in the NHS—head of the nursing section and the *CECh*'s general secretary.[77] As she was also the editor-in-chief of the traditional nursing magazine *Enfermería*, she defined the tone of the discourse in nursing politics. Furthermore, Peake was one of the most influential nurses in South America. From 1974 to 1976, she held the position of general secretary in the Pan American Nursing Federation (*Federación Panamericana de Enfermeras*).[78] In addition to that, she had the support of the military junta, as in 1978 she was designated a Chilean delegate for the ILO conference in Geneva.[79]

Conversely, Pincheira continued to maintain her seemingly apolitical position.[80] As in the 1970s, she never sat for a long time at the top management of the *CECh* board. Her still prominent figure in the nursing affairs resulted from her work as a counselor in nursing congresses[81] and the writing she did for *Enfermería*, especially editorials.

Another important role was played by Rosalba Flores. At least from September 1973 onward, she edited the Informative Bulletin (*Boletín Informativo*). In this capacity, in November 1973 Flores decided to write about the political involvement of the *CECh*.[82] In her writing she documented the most important events in nursing politics. It was her who reported on the correspondence with Pinochet, communicated with international partners, and organized the political involvement of the nursing association.[83]

Lidia Díaz, on the other hand, did not appear in nursing journals. Unlike Peake, Pincheira, or Flores, her role in the Ministry of Health only became visible when the junta came to power. From 1975, she was, after Peake, the most quoted name in nursing policies in the ministerial papers.[84] While she was the editor-in-chief, Díaz coordinated the most extensive study on nursing employment during the dictatorship (1979). However, she made certain to avoid any reference to state politics. Her study focused on nursing in three regions and had the goal to persuade the authorities to hire more university-trained nurses. Hence the fact that she avoided mentioning nursing auxiliaries when referring to nursing staff.[85]

Special consideration merits the biography of Elisabeth Gudelhoefer, advisor to the first undersecretary of the health minister in 1973. Her résumé was the most prominent among the nurses who benefited from personal relations. It may be the case that Gudelhoefer arranged the first and most decisive meeting of the *CECh* board with the health minister (to be explained hereinafter) only a few days after the coup.[86]

The archives of the Ministry of Health and the few surviving copies of *Enfermería* also shed light on nursing professors' biographies, most importantly that of Idilia Jerez Klopfer, president of the regional council in Santiago. In 1974, she became the director of the school affiliated with the Medical Faculty of the University of Chile in North Santiago.[87] As will be shown, until 1979 she would transform this institution into a distinguished study center for nursing on national (NHS) and international levels (PAHO). Her work on *materno-infantil* shaped the perception of her profession in this area (Chap. 6). Jerez's legacy materialized in 1977 in the relaunching of the Chilean Society for Paediatric Nursing (*Sociedad Chilena de Enfermería Pediátrica*).[88]

Oral narratives about the director of the nursing school of the University of Concepción, Irene Bocaz, are remarkable. It would seem that her institution had not only a deep impact on a conflict with the midwives' association about the new nurse-midwife degree program. She also managed to impose a different, prima facie more liberal regime. All this was possible, at least partly, because of her close relationship with the highest military authorities of the region which she knew how to manipulate to their full advantage.[89]

Peake, Pincheira, Flores, Díaz, Gudelhoefer, Jerez, and even the more autonomously acting Bocaz depended on the will of the men who led the civilian-military cooperation. They had to follow the orders of generals, hospital directors, and NHS authorities. Nevertheless, they still published a magazine and a bulletin, traveled abroad, presided over international organizations, and could contact the press. These women, especially Peake, were among the most influential women of their time in the country, and this is probably why the subordination they experienced was not comparable with the power they themselves exerted over the nursing auxiliaries and other fellow nurses.

By 1978, some 24,087 nursing staff worked in the public healthcare system. Only 3000 of them were university-trained nurses, while the remaining 21,087 had not attained a university education. They were cast in the subordinate group of nursing auxiliaries,[90] which overall represented the female working class. In an article in *Enfermería* (1978), Peake and Pincheira saw them "under supervision of a professional nurse."[91] But the lack of professional nurses, ever more severe since the 1920s, showed that this idea of supervision did not really hold true for the suburbs and rural areas. Even Peake admitted that the auxiliary staff there performed most of the nursing tasks.[92]

Officially, nurses also oversaw both classroom contents and practical training of the nursing auxiliaries in vocational schools (*institutos profesionales*), hospitals, and healthcare centers.[93] But the reality was altogether different. In 1975, in four of the 13 regions the NHS did not have any nursing professionals.[94] And, as the case of Ivette Cap de Ville showed (Chap. 1), part of nursing auxiliary training relied on apprenticeship and self-learning.

Nursing auxiliaries continued to be absent from official records. However, they were organized as well. An unknown number of them registered in the National Association of Nursing Auxiliaries (*Asociación Nacional de Auxiliares de Enfermería, ANAECH*), but unlike the *CECh*, it had no co-determination rights in national health policies. This means that its board could not sign contracts with national or international organizations[95] and that only the Ministry of Health was allowed to represent them. For example, in 1975 the Ministry rejected the request of *ANAECH* to raise the educational requirements for students to enroll in a vocational institute. An eight-year school certificate remained the only condition for the nine-month training,[96] while professional nurses had to complete 12 years in school before entering nursing training.[97]

The directory of *ANAECH* did not only try to raise the educational requirements. In 1977, its president, Francisco Jara, also sought to reduce the control of the professional nurses over *ANAECH* members. Peake, responsible at the NHS for their curriculum, interfered at the Ministry of Health to secure nurses' domination.[98] She was always right, as far as the board was concerned. And so Jara's proposition was turned down,[99] and another law by decree in 1978 confirmed the administrative and clinical dependence of the auxiliary staff on university nurses.[100]

The international relations of *ANAECH* remained poor and the little contacts they could establish were blocked by the Ministry.[101] In a bill which followed the coup, they were only referred to as "extensions" of the nurses. This view contrasts to the increasing number of nursing auxiliaries appointed by the NHS, especially to work in rural areas,[102] where they usually worked rather autonomously. In doing so, the military junta continued on the path drawn by previous governments, paying less attention and granting less privilege to the stratum most needed for expanding healthcare coverage.

Nurses and nursing auxiliaries were socio-politically connected through their importance to the health policies, especially in public health and *materno-infantil*. However, the example of *ANAECH* shows that they were only allowed to address the Ministry of Health when they communicated through a male spokesperson. It would seem that health authorities did listen to Francisco Jara, but despite his gender privilege, his job title of *auxiliar de enfermería* discredited him in a way that the minister and his spokesmen did not concede to his demands, even though Jara tried to defend a cause of the majority. Hence, *materno-infantil*, the showcase of national and international cooperation, was the project of a health elite built on dominance. In fact, auxiliary staff also engaged actively in *materno-infantil*, notably in subsections such as midwifery, social work, and clinical laboratory, much as information about their study plan remains in obscurity, if any ever existed. Conversely, for nurses who trained in university there was continuity in national policy.

Despite the status quo remaining between nurses, the state, and the physicians since 1973, the figure of women forging their aspirations but within a symbolic cage did not disappear. If nurses were systematically denied participation in decisions about nursing policy, such dynamics were reflected in auxiliary workers being excluded from decisions that affected them. The continuity in both biographical trajectories and state nursing divisions rather mirrored the privileges of (a group of) university-trained nurses.

6.2 Donors and Cooperators

How did the change of state ideology and the oppression by the Armed Forces alter the work life of nurses and auxiliary nurses? Was it even possible not to interact with the military administration by professing an "apolitical" type of nursing? And if so, what did this imply for women?

At the beginning of the dictatorship, the *CECh* still represented a collective of women led by strong female figures. By 1973, about 2700 women made up the trained nurses registry.[103] It would seem that most of them had strongly opposed the socialist government and manipulated both desire and behavior. Naturally, they expected gratitude from the military junta.

Only 20 days after the coup d'état, Garrido, president of the *CECh* (1971–1976), and general secretary Peake visited the health minister Col. Alberto Spoerer (1973–1974).[104] There are no records of the topics they discussed. But as two other delegations of professional associations visited the minister on the same day, the meeting may have been a regular appointment, perhaps even an obligation.[105] Only four days after, on October 5th, the ministry received from the *CECh* a donation amounting to 3,000,000 *Escudos*, the currency at the time, to be made effective through nurses' additional five hours of work per week to "support the noble intention of national reconstruction."[106] A donation in kind was not unusual back then.[106]

Unusual, though, was the attempt of Spoerer to facilitate something that could be called a small consideration for the nurses' efforts. In that same month, Spoerer proposed to the minister of finance a salary upgrade for the NHS nurses, meaning a wage equating the scale of the medical Law No. 15.076.[107] For the nurses, it appeared that the claims raised during the Frei and the Allende presidencies were finally heard. After eight years hearing governments repeatedly use the word "revolution" in political programs, Peake and Garrido hoped to exert political leverage within the junta. They were willing to bet everything by proceeding strategically as they did with earlier governments—exchanging political support for better wages. Unexpectedly though, the Ministry of the Interior, already under army control, rejected Spoerer's suggestion.[108]

The offer of additional work hours did nothing on the fixed plan of the military junta, much as the initiative was well received. Moreover, from October 14th all workers in all professions and all sectors were requested to work overtime—four additional hours per week for the sake of the so-called "reconstruction" of the nation. What began as an innocent offer of the nurses was transformed into a legal obligation for everyone.[109]

On top of that, in October 1973 the *CECh* board saw their enduring vindication crash. The privileges associated with *Medicina Curativa*, just like the wages granted by Law No. 15.07, were confirmed not to be applicable to any professions other than physicians, biochemists, and pharmacists.[110] Hurriedly, Peake and Garrido called on Pinochet himself.[111] However, he did not engage with or approve the claims and, in fact, refused any further discussion about wages until a new salary scale was designed.[112] As if regretting their unconditional support, Peake and Garrido informed their associates across the country of this outcome and did not seek to address the salary issue anymore.

In 1975, on the occasion of the 155th anniversary of Florence Nightingale's birth, several homages to nurses illustrated the importance of the profession in public life. Even *Vida Médica*, which barely mentioned professionals other than physicians, dedicated two pages to nurses. The *CECh* sent invites to a celebration to be held in the banqueting hall of the University of Chile. Expectedly, no nursing auxiliary was invited. Of course, Gen. Pinochet was, but he excused himself and Gen. Leigh attended on behalf of the junta. In his speech, Leigh quoted a study of PAHO which recommended an average of 4.5 nurses for every 1000 inhabitants, but he admitted that Chile could only provide 2.6. Leigh promised to increase the number of nurses,[113] but once the ceremony was over nursing disappeared from the headlines for some seven years.

Behind the scenes of the national press, the nurses did not sit back in resignation. Until 1979, the board shared with the Ministry of Health four studies about the shortages of nurses.[114] None of the studies were mentioned in the upcoming nursing policy papers of the government, which again showed just how poorly grounded nursing policies were during the regime, and the little say nurses had, even as the main stakeholders.

The donation of work hours in 1973, and the ceremony in 1975, made no impact on Chilean nursing. Both events left not even a slight contour in the profession. Or, at least, that is what was believed until the field research for this book, when three issues of the *Informative Bulletin* published by Flores were found in the National Library archives. In particular, the content of the December 1973 volume was part of the first social history article on nursing policy and politics in the country,[115] leading to the intriguing question of whether nurses individually, as women, and beyond their figurehead, the *CECh*, opposed or rather adapted to the dictatorial regime.

6.3 *Victims and Agents*

From September 1973, certain nurses became victims of political persecution. An anonymous piece in the *Informative Bulletin* (probably by Flores) admitted, even though indirectly, that a number of nurses lost their jobs when the military junta came to power. After an exchange with Pinochet about Law No. 15.076, she published a statement with the title: "Position of the Chilean Nurses Association to the members whose status has been questioned." Here, an author of the *CECh* magazine assured that every nurse dismissed since September 1973 had the right to reach out to the board for legal support. The author wrote about "failures" which had been committed by the government and about appeal committees (*comisiones de apelación*) the *CECh* had organized to examine those cases closely. Nurses accused of committing "direct political activity" were offered legal help to undo the dismissals or to propose displacements instead. But if political activism was proven, the *CECh* would simply withdraw its support.[116] On December 5th, 1973, the appeal committees ceased carrying out their functions. From then on, all nurses in need of further information or legal assistance had to reach the Ministry of Health, [117] which would inevitably make things worse for them, without any corporative representation or advocacy.

Patricia Talloni, a supporter of the Popular Unity, was one of the nurses being laid off on political grounds. She was the chief nurse in the healthcare center of the *El Teniente* mine.[118] Peake, who she knew personally and was also a member of the appeal committee she consulted, explained to Talloni that her solidarity with the strike breakers in 1972 and 1973 made her ineligible for legal support from *CECh*.[119]

In *Enfermería* magazine Peake provided no information about the dismissed nurses,[120] but for Flores the affair was worth receiving a minor note. On the occasion of the general council's yearly meeting, in September 1974, Flores' *Informative Bulletin* published brief summaries of the activity of the regional councils. It showed, for example, how "dysfunctional" the branches in Concepción, La Serena, Valdivia, Punta Arenas, and Santiago had become. Shortage of nurses was usually the reason, but only in the case of Concepción it was related to dismissals after the coup.[121]

Even if this information was more precise for regional branches, that would have remained but a rough indicator of the real extent of the issue, because not all cases were registered systematically by the *CECh*.[122] Least of all nursing auxiliaries, as they sat in a more fragile position—they did not receive any benefit from the nurses' association and could be fired without properly documenting it or legally negotiating it.

A dismissal was not the only penalty for nurses who supported the Popular Unity or felt identified with it, which applied to female activism too. The following cases give some insights about the way the regime dealt with those individuals: Patricia Talloni and Patricia Grau, both supporters of the Allende government, risked their lives while staying employed or looking for a new employer. They had to provide for their families. Grau was not dismissed on September 11th just because she was about to give birth to her first child, and decided not to go back to work after maternity leave,[123] whereas Talloni moved back to La Serena, a city where she had found her first job in the 1960s. Both these nurses hoped that the employers would not request their résumés from the NHS authorities—it did not work out for Talloni. She was rejected and had to leave La Serena immediately. To divert attention from her background, she temporarily stopped looking for a regular contract. For three months, the single mother made a living from sewing. At the beginning of 1974, she found a job in *Hospital Dr. Lucio Córdova,* in Santiago, which belonged to the NHS. As she accepted to work on an honorary basis, her résumé was never checked.[124] Grau was hired onto the German Clinic in Santiago. After six months working on the honorary system, too, the management offered her a permanent contract. They told Grau there would not be background checks on the condition that she would not take part in any kind of political movement.[125]

But not all nurses faced difficulties to the same extent. Until today, little has surfaced about the professionals who not only cooperated but even served as agents of the dictatorship. In 1984, the Danish journal *Sygeplejersken* (Nurses) quoted the reports of two physicians, Marianne Wallach and Ole Vedel Rasmussen, who had the chance to examine 19 Chilean individuals from that time period.[126] All of them were hunted by the police or Armed Forces, held in custody for up to 24 days in prisons before they could flee the country and find asylum in Europe. Some of them told that nurses in Chile took part in their interrogations, where they did a number of procedures, such as monitoring of vital signs, implementing life-sustaining measures, administering non-therapeutic substances (i.e., intravenous injections), hypnotizing the victims, examining before release or confirming death, and so on.

At the end of that article, the author asked readers to write letters to the Chilean secret police National Intelligence Center (*Dirección de Inteligencia Nacional, CNI*), to exert pressure to open an investigation which would force the *CNI* director to admit the crimes and stop the torture. The author also explained that a Spanish translation of the article was sent to Chile's medical association and to the *CECh*, as well as an English translation to the headquarters of the International Council of Nurses (ICN).[127] It is very likely that the ICN responded, but no evidence has surfaced.

In 1988, the UK-based journal *Nursing Times* published two articles referring to the situation of nurses and nursing practice in Chile. The first one, "Nurses in Danger—The Price of Protest," published in August, addressed the murder of nurse Jenny del Carmen Barra as an exemplary of other nurses who were victims of dictatorships worldwide.[128] In November, the article "Nurses in Danger—Agents of Repression" attempted to summarize the work of nurses in countries under political oppression or human rights violations.[129] The author drew on the report "Torture and the Medical Profession in Chile," published by the US human rights activist Eric Stover one year earlier. On several occasions, his interview partners also mentioned that nurses attended to the interrogations, normally in a team with a physician, but sometimes as the only health professional in the premises.[130] This information leads to the question of how authorities of the secret service recruited nurses, likely through families within the military environment.

As shown in Chap. 1, there were two groups of nursing effectives who were not recognized as nurses in the labor market and were not members of the *CECh*. Military nurses were one of those groups. According to magazine *Enfermería*, in 1978 some 125 nurses belonged to the Army.[131] They held ranks from second lieutenant (*subteniente*) to major (*mayor*)[132] and worked in the Military Hospital in Santiago, in military facilities throughout the country, or in premises of the secret services of the Armed Forces.[133] There were also close links between military staff and civilians working in the health division; for example, Nurse Elisabeth Guedelhoeffer was close to colonel Spoerer, first undersecretary of health during the dictatorship. However, a reality that often remains hidden but reminds the reader of nurses' potential participation in torture is the text of the oath (*juramento*) unusually published in the *Enfermería* magazine shortly after the coup. In March 1974, Peake recommended to use the oath in the graduation ceremonies of all nursing schools across the country. Nurses were expected to care for individuals from all walks of life, "regardless of their race, religion, political position and social standing."[134]

6.4 *Deceivers and Deceived*

Nurses' mandate was to "take care of children's health and nutrition," while the Armed Forces claimed to be "rebuilding the nation" and "destroying the wickedness." This is how Leigh saw division of labor in his speech to the *CECh* members in May 1975. On behalf of the military junta, he pledged to march on the "path of truth,"[135] words that seemed promising in an atmosphere that promoted a U-turn from socialism.

Leigh explained that five nursing schools had been inaugurated since the military junta was in power,[136] raising the number to 15. The civilian-military collaboration tolerated (and probably endorsed) the initiative of private universities to open nursing schools, but did not start or support the founding of any new public school; it just kept running the ones existing from before September 1973. The following years, the government would unveil its master plan for nursing policies.

Two weeks before Leigh's speech, the health minister Francisco Herrera (1974–1976) defined in an internal document his vision of a health assistant (*asistente de salud*) which would merge nursing and midwifery into a single profession.[137] Leigh went further, drafting how to implement a medical assistant (*asistente de salud*), a multipurpose professional (*profesional polivalente*) that mirrored at once the duties of nurses, midwives, and auxiliaries.[138] Busy at the NHS, Peake learned about those plans and hurried to call nurses' attention in *Enfermería*, albeit only in a brief note. She refused such plans but saw no need to take serious action on them. Peake still believed in the co-determination of the professional associations for such policy and waited for an invitation to a decision-making committee.[139]

However, the military junta preferred to accomplish facts. Until 1977, six of the 15 nursing schools were closed down, probably as a direct consequence of regionalization.[140] In his speech, in 1975, Leigh had promised to increase the graduate number of nursing students from 400 to 1000 within three years.[141] Yet the number of nursing students never fell as fast as it did during the dictatorship.

It would appear that the decreasing number of students was only one component in a broader process of care reform. As had happened to other female health professionals, jobs became scant in the course of the 1970s. The military limited new hires for the NHS,[142] increasing in the process the workload in hospitals and health centers. In addition to that, nurses were moved downward in the Unified Salary Scale, an overt depreciation of care work.[143]

Fearing a serious threat against the nursing profession, Peake and Pincheira wrote in *Enfermería* a statement of principles, which today would seem far away from reality. At the height of the shutdown of schools, in 1978, they wrote about "Basic facts of a Nursing Policy": First, they explained the respective guidelines of PAHO and WHO, which, as they stated, the military junta had ratified. Peake and Pincheira proposed a nursing policy applicable only to university-trained nurses, to be filed together with their "national partners" like other health professionals.[144] That seemed promising considering an active alliance with the most powerful group in healthcare, the physicians, which was in practice little more than a myth, albeit widely circulated in *Enfermería*.[145]

Peake and Pincheira praised their international allies (i.e., ICN, *FEPPEN*) but concealed the fact that none of them could interfere in Chile's politics. They misunderstood, or perhaps just ignored, the discrepancy between their goal to "respect every human being to reach maximum spiritual and material fulfillment" and day-to-day life in an inhuman regime. Peake and Pincheira even stated that the respect for every human being was at the core of the value system of the "honorable military junta." Their word choice is striking. In a moment of big losses for the profession it sounds almost ironic when they wrote about "convenient" payment and training, social security, and recognition of the nurses' efforts in the past few years.

The state of deep submission conveyed in Peake and Pincheira's writing almost rebutted the criticism, such as when they talked about low payment and long shifts combined with few recovery days. The "subsystem of nursing" they claimed for at the end of their article would get nurses involved in policy planning processes and assure them to have a say in wages and other important decisions.[146] Both probably ignored that this goal was virtually unattainable under military rule. Like the further advancement of career and promotion scheme (*carrera funcionaria*), a vindication appearing many times in *Enfermería*, or a plea for self-determination, Pincheira and Peake's dream of a united voice for nurses simply could not fit in a dictatorship.

The military junta, as far as records show, did not react to such publications. In the first years after the coup d'état, the generals justified their lack of dialogue on the grounds that the critical economic situation of the country needed their full attention.[147] But unlike Popular Unity, which did not address the nurses, the generals did talk with them. Nevertheless, it turned out that invitations to meet were pointless. In his speech from 1975, Leigh did not mention his plan to introduce a health assistant, the practitioner who would replace the nurse and other occupational categories. It would seem that this idea was hidden from the nurses, as even in the 1978 yearly plan of the ministry nurses still appeared as central as usual in the workforce.[148]

PAHO was still the most important financial supporter of nursing development and the only one to continuously keep advisers in Chile.[149] The *CECh* wanted to spend the foreign money in the career development project,[150] but the generals did not give them the chance to decide in the rather vertical policy-making approach. From a total of 12 PAHO projects run between 1973 and 1979, four mentioned cooperation with nurses. However, solely in one case could nurses decide for themselves about the use of the funding.[151] The rest of the financial, technical, and training support focused on medical care in rural areas. The same happened to other important aid organizations, like UNICEF, UNFPA, and the Inter-American Development Bank.[152] An additional problem here was that for most nursing students, a career outside of the cities or in the extending suburbs of the cities continued not to be attractive enough.[153]

The international ties of the *CECh* remained stable during the regime, sometimes they even grew stronger, and Garrido and Peake continued to cooperate with the ICN. Only six months after the coup, and being the strongest international lobby group of nurses, the ICN invited Garrido to speak in a seminar in Bogota, in 1974.[154] Their second important international partner was the Pan American Federation of Nursing Professionals, *FEPPEN*. In August of the same year, a delegation of the *CECh* joined the *FEPPEN*'s third congress, in Quito.[155]

Nevertheless, the *CECh* policy did not go totally unquestioned. Some nurses knew about the criticisms against the government they supported. This was one of the reasons why Peake used enthusiastic words when referring to the participation of Garrido in the ICN seminar in Bogota. She said that the *CECh* president was "received in a friendly manner" and that the hosts allowed them to "participate actively," which was a "nice gesture considering the background of the current circumstances."[156]

In the spring of 1974, the *Informative Bulletin* released its last issue.[157] Then, it was only Peake who reported on the activity of the nursing association and about nursing in general.[158] Except for some statements, as seen in an article co-authored with Pincheira in 1978, she maintained the apolitical tone of *Enfermería*.[159] Intriguingly, by doing so she continued to depict nurses in the way most male physicians regarded them: auxiliary staff essentially interested in technical matters.

In April 1979, Peake and Oye took part in the 5th Congress of *FEPPEN*, in Puerto Rico.[160] Critical voices against *CECh*'s close alliance with the military junta did not surface or remained unheard. Even though the chair of *FEPPEN* was assigned to another country, the interpretation of the human rights questioning was surprisingly dominated by the Chilean representatives. Indeed, since 1976 the *CECh* was in charge of the ethics commission of the *FEPPEN*.

Compared to its dominant position in the Latin American *FEPPEN*, the *CECh* board did not strengthen its ties with the ICN.[161] Peake did not even mention in her magazine that she was appointed by the junta in 1978 to join the Chilean delegation to the 64th Conference of ILO in Geneva.[162] An incident during the ICN congress 1977 in Tokyo may have well been the reason for that. Corrales, the then president, was unable to divert attention from national politics and the ugly *CECh*'s image associated with it, when the Spanish delegate criticized her for distributing political propaganda.[163]

Other international commitments remained minor when compared to the involvement of the *CECh* in *FEPPEN* and even the ICN.[164] Generally though, international events and seminars (i.e., scientific, academic, technical, or legal) were only possible when the military administration approved such gatherings and their ideas.[165] Cherry-picking was the order of the day, and this manipulated an image of nurses as members of an apolitical, loyal, conflictless, and unified collectivity.

The foreign policy of the *CECh* board shows just how easily deceivers could be deceived. This suggests that the board members were successful in persuading their colleagues in Bogota, Quito, and Tokyo about the good intentions of the "honorable military junta," a clear sign of a political strategy most likely prepared in meetings with other representatives of the civilian-military cooperation. Considering domestic issues, whereby the methods of propaganda and control used the same code, it is astonishing how blissful Garrido, Flores, Corrales, and Peake understood their loyalty to the military rulers. Information about the crimes of the military men were not unknown to anyone. Perhaps though, they hoped for a happier ending because the memory of bad experiences with the Popuar Unity was too fresh and the anti-Communist indoctrination of the 1940s and 1950s too solid. Ultimately, deceiving *CECh* members and international fellows may have been their best defense to not just accept with resignation more than a decade of a wicked policy process.

7 Conclusion

In this chapter, we have shown how civilian professionals worked closely with the representatives of the military. However, the caring professions, mostly female groups, appeared rarely in the print media, giving the impression that women had nearly no participation in social movements, and having a mere supporting role behind the active partakers.

Just as in the years before the coup d'état, the professional associations' debates and exchanges during nursing policy-making did not explicitly focus on the needs of their patients. And yet, nurses did use political transitions to voice their views. In doing so, they questioned social hierarchies, but also used them. Lobbyists were insistently concerned with their members' wages, work hours, and working conditions.

It would appear that the gradual lift of press censorship in the second half of the decade facilitated the possibilities for an alternate and non-governmental reporting, quoting most prominently male physicians. Since 1976, the military junta allowed the development of alternative care institutions, like the *Vicaría de la Solidaridad*. Under the protection of the church, lawyers and journalists criticized the devastating effects of state policy and a medical team offered services for those who had no access to public healthcare. But at the same time, this instance served as a place for nurses' networking and cross-pollination of ideas in non-health environments, where liberal priests, resisting professionals, and policy influencers met.

It is not clear how many of the 25,000 nursing staff were affected by political persecution, torture, and murder. For sure, everyone working as a nurse during the dictatorship heard about the military tactics. Peake and the *CECh* presidents negotiated with the junta or their civilian-military cooperation about dismissals, salary, statutes, political participation, and recognition. The board aligned itself with the military, although they set appeal committees for nurses being politically persecuted, which seems little more than a façade.

At the beginning of the dictatorship stands the cooperation of a group of nurses with the military junta in the form of worktime donation, participation in national and international propaganda and, arguably, in violence and inhumaneness. On the other hand, the regime planned to replace academically trained nurses altogether with a different type of professionals. The closing of almost half of all the nursing schools was the first step on the way to remove the achievements of a twenty-year haul. What happened since 1973 was perceived not just an attack against nurses. It was also the removal of one of the most important achievements of the 1940s feminine movement—the right to self-determination—and of the early 1900s—the modern scientifically informed professional system in nursing care. Nonetheless, such plans did not unfold.

Regardless of one's worldviews this part of history adds to the growing evidence of women as active agents in the defense of their collective interests. The expression "nursing under dictatorship" refers more purposefully to university-trained women navigating turbulent times and intending to gain control over the policies that affected them.

Notes

1. Decreto Ley No. 3, 18.09.1973, Declara estado de sitio;
   Decreto Ley No. 4, 18.09.1973, Declara en estado de emergencia las provincias y departamentos que indica.
2. Only *El Mercurio* and *La Tercera* were published in the first six months after the coup d'état, in: Ávila Dosal, Raquel: Memory struggles in Chile 45 years after the coup. A Critical Discourse Analysis on the role of the press, [Malmö University] 2019, p. 30;
   About the prohibition of unions, in: Decreto Ley No. 198, 29.12.1973, Establece normas transitorias relativas a la actividad sindical;
   About the temporary prohibition of universities, in: Reorganización total de las Universidades, in: *El Mercurio*, 01.-07.10.1973, p. 1;
   About the prohibition of political parties, in: Junta declara en receso a todos los partidos políticos, in: *El Mercurio*, 24.-30.09.1973, p. 1.
3. Castiglioni, Rossana: The politics of social policy change in Chile and Uruguay, London [Routledge] 2005, p. 27.
4. The decree laws were elaborated by advisory boards led by lawyers, in: Huneeus, Carlos: Pinochet - Institutionelle Faktoren, in: Chile heute. Politik, Wirtschaft, Kultur [Ed. Imbusch, Messner, Nolte], Frankfurt am Main [Vervuert] 2004, p. 227-251, 236.
5. Informe de la Comisión Nacional de Verdad y Reconcilación [also called Comisión Rettig], Vol. 1, Tomo II, Anexo VI, Santiago 1991, p. 944.
6. Comisión Nacional de Prisión Política y Tortura [also called Commisión Valech II], quoted in: The Pinochet Dictatorship: Military Rule and Neoliberal Economics, in: The Chile Reader (2014), p. 433-441, 436;
   In 2018, 1200 people were reported as missing, in: Cornejo, Marcela; Rocha, Carolina; Villaroel, Nicolás; Cácares, Enzo; Vivanco, Anastassia: Tell me your story about the Chilean dictatorship: When doing memory is taking positions, in: Memory Studies, 03-2018, p. 2.
7. For example, by the end of September 1973, during the visit of a Western German delegation, the military junta confirmed to limit the authoritarian rule to three years, in: Auf Menschenrecht gepocht, in: Süddeutsche Zeitung, 02.10.1973, quoted in: Chile Nachrichten, No. 7, Berlin 12.10.1973, p. 23-24, 24.

8. A decree law from June 1974 gave it the appearance of a legal act. The military junta had executive, legislative, and judiciary powers. Its president was also the head of state. The name "Pinochet" was not mentioned, but the new law implied that the president of the military junta was also the president of the state, in: Decreto Ley No. 527, 26.06.1974.
9. Ministerio de Salud Pública: M.S. Ord 0315, Solicita información sobre nuestro país para ser difundida en el exterior, 0315-1867-1974, 05.02.1974, p. 1-2 [4-5/12].
10. In June 1974, on the occasion of the WHO summit in Geneva, "verbal attacks of socialist countries" forced the Chilean health minister to defend the military junta, in: Salud. Acuerdo con OMS, in: *El Mercurio*, 06.1974, p. 8.
11. *El Mercurio* reported about a delegation (*Delegación Gremial*), which visited the US, Mexico, Spain, France, Italy, England, and West Germany, in: *El Mercurio*, 15.-21.10.1973, p. 4.
12. Garrido, Sonia: El Colegio de Enfermeras informa al mundo acerca de la situaación nacional, in: Colegio de Enfermeras de Chile: Boletín Informativo, No. 3, 1973.
13. Ministerio de Salud: M.S. Ord. 2630, Obj. Campaña defensa del país en el extranjero, 2630-1846-1973, 20.12.1973, p. 1-1 [30-43].
14. Salud—Rectificaciones, in: *El Mercurio*, 08.-14.10.1973, p. 8.
15. Casals Araya, Marcelo: Estado, contrarrevolución y autoritarismo en la trayectoria política de la clase media profesional chilena. De la oposición a la Unidad Popular al fin de los Colegios Profesionales (1970-1981), in: Izquierdas, No. 44, 2018, p. 91-113, 105.
16. "explicar las razones y fundamentos del golpe," in: Urquieta Ch. Claudia: El Acta Secreta que muestra la conivencia y colaboracionismo entre la Corte Suprema y el Gobierno Militar, in: El Mostrador, 13.09.2013, https://www.elmostrador.cl/noticias/pais/2013/09/13/el-acta-secreta-que-muestra-la-connivencia-y-colaboracionismo-entre-la-corte-suprema-y-el-gobierno-militar/ [20.05.2022]

    Casals Araya could verify the participation of lawyers in four other of these so-called information journeys, in: Casals (2018), p. 105.
17. Casals describes only two cases in which the delegations had been criticized, by a student protest in Madrid and by the president of the lawyer's association in Paris, in: ibid, p. 105-106.
18. Huneeus (2004), p. 243-244.
19. Quote: "Participa socialmente quien puede escoger entre diversas opciones de consumo, en una economía abierta y competitiva. Participa socialmente quien ejerce la libertad para afiliarse y desafiliarse a/o de gremios, sindicatos y asociaciones profesionales, en un cuadro de real libertad de asociación y de trabajo," in: Guzmán, Jaime: "Participación: ¿cuál es su expresión básica?," in: La Segunda, 04-1981, quoted in: Frontaura R.,

Carlos; Arqueros V., Claudio: Bases doctrinarias del gremialismo, in: 50 años del gremialismo [Ed. Arqueros], 2017, p. 103-126, 116.

20. Klein, Naomi: The Shock Doctrine: The Rise of Disaster Capitalism, New York [Metropolitan Books/Henry Holt] 2008, p. 115.
21. About the United Nation's support for Chilean public efforts in pediatrics, see Ministerio de Salud, Dirección PESMIB: M.S. Ord. No. 163-1721, Inversión de Fondos PESMIB por OPS/OMS, 1933-1721, 20.07.1976, p. 1–2;

    The WHO/PAHO also focused on projects in pediatrics, in: Ministerio de Salud, Unidad Normativa Salud de la Madre: M.S. Ord. No. 2015, Programa de detención del parto prematuro, 1934-2015, 18.08.1976.
22. In 1978, the Ministry of Health tried to re-establish relations with the Kellogg Foundation, in: Ministerio de Salud, Oficina de Asuntos Internacionales: M.S. Ord No. 604, Ref. Kellogg Foundation, institución privada norteamericana, 604-2025-1979, 02.02.1979, p. 1-2 [10/11-17].
23. In the course of the 1970s, the Inter-American Development Bank and USAID increased their support for Chile:

    1. Inter-American Development Bank, in: *El Mercurio*, 01.-07.10.1978, p. 8;

    2. USAID, in: Ministerio de Salud: M.S. Ord No. 0795, Mat. Agradece colaboración prestada a Jornada de Capacitación Nutricional, 0795-1991-1978, ¿03.1978, p. 1-1 [1-13];

    Private and semi-private organizations such as Peace Corps, the Latin American Society of Paediatric Research (*Sociedad Latino Americana de Investigaciones Pediátricas*, USA/Argentina), the Seventh Day Adventist Welfare Service, the Children's Television Workshop Foundation, the Kayser Foundation, and the Latin American Center for Educational Technology in Health followed their example:

    1. Peace Corps, in: Ministerio de Salud: No. 180, Aprueba convenio entre Ministerio de Salud y el cuerpo de Paz de los Estados Unidos de America, 180-1981-1978, 25.07.1978, p. 1-13 [1/13-22];

    2. Latin American Society of Pediatric Investigations, in: Ministerio de Salud: No. 312, Otorga Patrocinio Oficial y Ayuda Económica para la XVI Reunión anual de la Sociedad Latinoamericana de Investigaciones Pediátricas, 312-1984-1978, 27.11.1978, p. 1-4 [5/8-21];

    3. Children's Television W.F., in: Ministerio de Salud, Oficina de Asuntos Internacionales: No. 1110, Ref. Reunión de expertos en planificaciones, salud infantil y salud oral infantil a efectuarse en Buenos Aires, 1110-1993-1978, 29.06.1978, p. 1-1 [40-40];

    4. Kayser Foundation, in: Ministerio de Salud, Oficina de Asuntos Internacionales: Remite copias proyecto elaborado por ODEPLAN, 1990-1370, 02.06.1975, p. 1–6;

5. Latin American Center for Education Technology in Health, in: Ministerio de Salud, Oficina de Asuntos Internacionales: No. 724, Ref. Invitación para visitar sede universitaria y cooperación de la OPS en Seminario de Investigación sobre "Seguimiento de Graduados en Salud," 724-1960-1977, 19.04.1977, p. 1-2 [24/35-59];

Even the social-liberal Western German government rejected to cut relations with the Chilean dictatorship and facilitated in the following years two credits for healthcare programs:

1. In 1975, it was a credit of 21,000,000.00 German Marks for the NHS, precisely for "hospital installations," in: Crédito Alemán, in: *El Mercurio*, 01.-07.09.1975, p. 4;

2. In 1977, the *CORFO* received a credit of 50,000,000.00 German Marks of the Deutsche Bank for a nutrition program, in: Crédito Alemán por 50 millones de Deutsche Mark, in: *El Mercurio*, 07.04.1977, p. 8.

24. The sovereignty of the Air Force in the healthcare sector was confirmed in 1976, in: Ministerio de Salud, Asesoria Jurídica: Ord. No. 80 A.J./No. 1296, Acompaña copia de Oficio Circular No. 6353/122 del Sr. Presidente de la República, 1932-1296, 31.05.1976.
25. Castiglioni (2005), p. 25-34.
26. In order to destabilize his position, the president started to discredit Leigh. Pinochet knew that the austerity policy had caused or at least had not fixed serious deficits in the provision of healthcare. In 1976 and 1977, he visited several healthcare centers in different regions of the country. In interviews with *El Mercurio* he did not mention Leigh but complained about the public healthcare system.

    1. Pinochet's first journey, in: *El Mercurio*, 17.08.1976, p. 5;
    2. Pinochet's second journey, in: *El Mercurio*, 04.03.1977, p. 3.
27. In 1976, for the first time, a civilian physician became the undersecretary of the minister of health, in: *El Mercurio*, 19.03.1976, p. 7;

    Since 1976, the Ministry of Labor and of Social Welfare was led by a civilian. During the dictatorship, the Ministry of the Interior was only presided by military staff.
28. Between 1974 and 1984, the dictatorship reduced the average spending on healthcare for every citizen by 10 percent, in: López Cassou, Haydée: La municipalización en el contexto de la política de salud del régimen militar, documento de debate, No. 5, 1986, p. 2.
29. Ruiz-Tagle, Jaime; Urmeneta, Roberto: Los trabajadores del Programa de Empleo Mínimo en el Capitalismo Autoritario, Santiago [PISPAL, Programa de Investigaciones Sociales sobre Población en América Latina] 1984, p. 10.
30. Instituto Nacional de Estadísticas: Censos 1970-1982, Cifras comparativas, http://www.memoriachilena.gob.cl/archivos2/pdfs/MC0055468.pdf [15.03.2022].

31. Decreto Ley No. 1.056, 07.06.1975, Determina normas complementarias relativas a la reducción del gasto público y al mejor ordenamiento y control del personal;

    A high number of dismissals could be detected in 1977, in: Ministerio de Salud: No. 058, Renuncias no voluntarias de muchos jefes de unidades en el SNS, SERMENA y MdS, 058-1949-1973, 16.03.1977, p. 1-4 [14/17-27].
32. The dismissed employees could ask for legal assistance from appeal commissions, in: Ministerio de Salud Pública: M.S. Ord No. 23/AJ-0251, Remite reclamaciones que señala por las razones que indica, 0251-1867-1974, 28.01.1974, p. 1-2 [7-8/12].
33. Araya Espinoza, Alejandra: Declasificación de Archivos Universitarios en Dictadura, in: La dictadura de los sumarios, 1974-1985: Universidad de Chile intervenida, Santiago [Editorial Universitaria] 2016, p. 220.
34. Aspectos Relevantes de Política de Acción Social, in: *El Mercurio*, 15.03.1977, p. 5.
35. Interviews with Patricia Talloni, Patricia Grau (nurses) and Ivette Cap de Ville (auxiliary nurse), Santiago March 2017.
36. Sepúlveda Momberg, Matías: Del trabajo protegido al trabajo subsidario. Intervención, libre mercado y la situación de los trabajadores del PEM y POJH, 1974-1984, in: Seminario Simón Collier 2014, Santiago [RIL] 2015, p. 213-244, 217.
37. The Salary Scale was changed several times, most extensively in 1976, in: Decreto Ley No. 1.608, 07.12.1976, Dictar normas para implantar la segunda etapa de la carrera funcionaria y otras disposiciones.
38. From 1974, the medical association criticized continuously the Salary Scale, in: Sobre Base de Eficiencia y Medicina Privada - Sistema Mixto de Salud Propone Convención Médica a Autoridades, in: *El Mercurio*: 09.06.1974.
39. Quote: "Que el Gobierno ha reconocido en toda su extensión el valioso aporte que presentan las Organizaciones Comunitarias, Colegios Profesionales y demás organizaciones similares, como elementos cooperadores en la solución de los problemas nacionales," in: Decreto Ley No. 349, 13.03.1974, Prorroga mandato de directivas de Juntas de Vecinos y otras organizaciones.
40. For example the appointment of new members for the board of the kinesiologists' association in 1976, in: Ministerio del interior, Asesoría Jurídica: Of Ord. No. D-232-2598, Solicitud para proveer vacantes que indica, 232-2598-17880-1976, 1976, p. 1-1 [1/1].
41. In 1972, *El Mercurio* estimated the number of 80.000 professionals, in: *El Mercurio*, 25.-30.09.1972, p. 7 [3/3];

    Guzmán estimates that this number did not vary much, in: Guzmán Riquelme, Gabriel: Colegios Profesionales y Asociaciones Gremiales durante el proceso de la democracia en Chile, Santiago [Museo de la Memoria y los Derechos Humanos] 2012, p. 78;

The authors of *Solidaridad* counted 100,000 teachers in 1985, in: Colegio de Profesores. En busca del tiempo perdido Solidaridad, No. 215, 15.-27.12.1985, p. 17.

42. The historical review of the teachers' association stated that the professional association was forbidden directly after the Armed Forces came to power, in: Colegio de Profesoras y Profesores de Chile: Historia, https://www.colegiodeprofesores.cl/historia/ [17.10.2021];

    But the decree law dates back to 1975, in: Decreto Ley 1284, 19.12.1975, Cancela personalidad jurídica de los organismos que indica y crea comisión administradora de sus bienes.
43. Decreto Ley No. 2.200, 15.06.1978, Fija normas relativas al contrato de trabajo y a la protección de los trabajadores;

    The civilian-military cooperation called the new labor legislation "realistic," in: Elgueta Navarro, J. Bernardo: El realismo en el Decreto Ley 2200 de 1978, in: Revista de Derecho de la Pontificia Universidad Católica de Valparaíso, No. 4, 1980, p. 267-291, 278-279.
44. Tribunales del Trabajo, tres pasos atrás…, atrás…, atrás, in: *APSI*, No. 95, 24.03.-06.04.1981, p. 7;

    In 1977, *Solidaridad* reported about the dissolution of state institutions meant to protect labor rights, like the National Employment Service (*Servicio Nacional de Empleo, SENDE*), in: Desaparecen Servicios del Trabajo, in: *Solidaridad*, 12-1977, 01.-15.01.1977.
45. Economía y Sociedad. Inflación vs. Reajustes. ¿Se quebró el círculo vicioso?, in: *Hoy*, No. 9, 27.07.-02.08.1977, p. 25-26 [5/9-6/9].
46. *El Mercurio*, 28.10.1978, p. 1.
47. Quote: "No haber desempeñado actividad político partidista ni haber tenido militancia en partido político o haber postulado a cargo de representación popular o de otra índole, en representación de un partido político, en los últimos diez años contados desde que se adquiera la calidad de director sindical, ni incurrir en alguna de estas causales en el desempeño del cargo," in: Decreto Ley No. 2.376, 28.10.1978, Establece normas sobre organización y elección de las directivas sindicales.
48. Álvarez Vallejos, Rolando: ¿Represión o Integración? La política sindical del régimen militar. 1973-1980, in: Historia, Vol. II, No. 43, 2010, p. 325-355, 341;

    The Western German government supported the training of new union leaders, in: Colaboración alemana en la formación de dirigentes sindicales, in: *El Mercurio*, 15.11.1978, p. 7.
49. Miranda (1994), p. 5-66, 34.
50. Nueva Orientación a Servicios de Salud, in: *El Mercurio*, 31.02.1975, p. 5.
51. [68] Decreto Ley No. 575, 13.07.1974, Regionalización del país.

52. Ministerio de Salud: Delega Atribuciones en los Secreatrios Regionales Ministeriales de Salud, 1891-007, 19.11.1975.

    There exist different explanations as to why the reform slowed down after a fast start and ended only in 1976:

    1. Raczynski traced it back to the resistance of the medical association as the responsible, in: Raczynski (1982), p. 27;

    2. Castiglioni describes Gen. Leigh as the brakeman, in: Castiglioni (2005), p. 27;

    3. For Llambias-Wolff, both reasons led to the slow implementation, in: Llambias-Wolff (2013), p. 168-169.
53. Universidad y Regionalización, in: Revista de la Universidad de Chile, No. 60, 05-1977, p. [2/5-5/5].
54. Sherman estimates a reduction of 15 percent in public spending for healthcare between 1974 and 1982, in: Sherman, Jorge: Las políticas de salud y su impacto en los sectores populares. Chile 1974-1986, in: Salud rural, Santiago [Academia de Humanismo Cristiano] 1988, p. 57;

    Reichard states a reduction of 10 percent between 1974 and 1982, in: Reichard, Stephen: Ideology Drives Health Care Reforms in Chile, in: *Journal of Public Health Policy*, Vol. 17, No. 1, 1996, p. 80-98, 87.
55. Sperberg (2004), p. 142.
56. Some examples which demonstrate the resource problems:

    1. Shortage of insulin, in: Falta de Insulina en las farmacias, in: *El Mercurio*, 20.03.1976, p. 7;

    2. Labor staff shortage, in: Esfuerzos para mejorar atención en consultorios, in: *El Mercurio*, 23.-29.01.1977, 24.01.1977, p. 5;

    3. Shortage of physicians, in: Matronas pueden reemplazar médicos en caso de su escasez, in: *El Mercurio*, 17.12.1976, 17.12.1976, p. 7;

    4. Insufficient infrastructure, in: Esfuerzos para mejorar atención en consultorios, in: *El Mercurio*, 23.-29.01.1977, 24.01.1977, p. 5.
57. Three examples for the press reporting about illegal additional payments:

    1. Declaración Oficial: Postas: La atención no depende del pago, in: *El Mercurio*, 17.08.1976, p. 5;

    2. Beneficiarios del *SNS* exentos de todo pago en consultorios, in: *El Mercurio*, 25.02.1978, p. 1;

    3. Nacional. Gobierno. Reafirmación de principios, in: *Hoy*, 21.-24.03.1979, p. 7 [4/4];

    One example for the rejection of patients: No se construirán más hospitales gigantes, in: *El Mercurio*, 04.03.1977, p. 3.
58. Report about the rejection of patients as a national problem, in: Ministerio de Salud, Oficina de Planificación, Recursos Físicos: M.S. Ord No. 625, Mat. Anteproyecto de Centros de Desnutrición de Talca y Linares, Consultorio Externo Hospital San Javier y Constitución, y construcción Hospital Molina, 625-1960-1977, 06.04.1977, p. 1-5 [41-45];

Two reports, which describe the insufficient infrastructure:

1. Ministerio de Salud: M.S. Ord No. 1156, Programas Ministeriales [working title], 1156-1993-1978, 11.07.1978, No. 1-3 [19/21-40];

2. Ministerio de Salud, Depto. De planificación: M.S. Ord No. 1884, Mat. Preparación Programas Ministeriales 1979. Respuesta a cuestionario, 1884-1997-1978, 05.11.1978, No. 1-31 [40/70-81];

In a report from 1977, the Ministry of Health admitted that it failed to expand the public healthcare system in the VII Region (Maule), the fourth most populated of the country, in: Ministerio de Salud, Unidad de Planificación de Recursos Físicos: M.S. Ord No. 561, Mat. Remite Proyecto "Ampliación de la Cobertura de Servicios de Salud a las Áreas Rurales," 561-1960-1977, 29.03.1977, No. 1-1 [49-59].

59. More than that, there were significant problems in guaranteeing hygiene in other public facilities like sports venues and concert halls, in: Ciencia. Salubridad. Inspección a la carta, in: *Hoy*, No. 3, 15.-21.06.1977, p. [3/5-5/5].
60. Logros y Problemas de la Regionalización, in: *El Mercurio*, 17.07.1978, p. 6.
61. Ruderer described "acts in different speeds" at the hands of the Catholic Church. While aid for social ends was maintained from the early days of the dictatorship, reporting murders and disappearances began later on, in: Ruderer et al. (2015), p. 44-45.
62. Decreto Arzobispal No. 5-76, in: Memorias para construir la Paz, https://www.vicariadelasolidaridad.cl/cronologia [22.10.2021].
63. *Solidaridad*, 12-1977, 01.-15.01.1977, p. 18.
64. Ruderer et al. (2015), p. 47.
65. Guzmán (2012), p. 17.
66. The first opposition group presented by *Solidaridad* was the Ten Group (*Grupo de los Diez*), in: *Solidaridad*, 12-1977, 01.-15.01.1977, p. 15 [2/4].
67. De la Maza, Ocheniuss (2005), p. 19, quoted in: Guzmán (2012), p. 16-17;
68. Columna del director. La Verdad sin compromisos, in: *Hoy*, 01.-07.06.1977, p. [1/8-2/8].
69. Periodismo de la oposición (1973-1989): Hoy, http://www.memoriachilena.gob.cl/602/w3-article-96760.html [10.04.2022].

    About the prohibition of various *Hoy* editions, in: Hofmeister, Wilhelm: Die deutschen Christdemokraten und Chile, in: Auslandsinformationen, No, 7, Berlin [Konrad-Adenauer-Stiftug] 2004, p. 22-49.
70. It started to operate in December 1977. Like *Solidaridad*, many of the editors and authors had strong ties to the Catholic Church in Santiago.
71. Only one time, in 1977, an author of *El Mercurio* blamed the budget cuts for the public healthcare system as the reason for the shortages on medi-

cal supplies, in: Críticas a la Política de Salud, in: *El Mercurio*, 16.04.1977, p. 4.

72. In one of its fortnightly editions, in 1975, the *Ercilla* team had published a statement about acts of political repression against the medical association, in: Ministerio de Salud, Subsecretario de Salud: Artículo "Epidemia de censuras en el Colegio Médico" aparecido en Revista Ercilla, 1899-1175, 12.05.1975, p. 1–4.
73. Guzmán (2012), p. 27.
74. Even though the state of siege had ended, the state of emergency allowed authorities for 20 days to arrest people without giving any reason, in: Diferencias entre Estado de Sitio y Estado de Emergencia—Estado de Sitio y Estado de Emergencia—¿Simple Cambio de Denominación?, in: *El Mercurio*, 19.03.1978, p. 3.

    The association's board members vehemently argued against this procedure. However, they did not want to get too involved. This may explain their silence about the consequences the protesters had to face. It would seem that the students had reached a threshold of tolerance by making critical statements publically, in: Protest of the medical association: *El Mercurio*, 11.03.-17.03.1979, 13.03.1979, p. 7.
75. For the first time after the coup, in 1974 the medical association openly critized the governmental health policies. Above all, the Salary Scale, in: *El Mercurio*, 09.06.1974;

    In April 1977, the association protested against the budget cuts for the public healthcare system, in: *El Mercurio*, 16.04.1977, p. 4;

    In October 1978, the dispute about the *Medicina Curativa* came to the fore, in: *El Mercurio*, 26.10.1978, p. 6.
76. Raczynski was the first researcher to describe the conflict between the medical association and the Ministry of Health, in: Raczynski (1982), p. 27.
77. Peake, by then in her sixties, showed no intention to retire, in: Ayala, Ricardo; Thulin, Markus; Núñez, Rocío: Cold Interests, Hot Conflicts: How a Professional Association Responded to a Change in Political Regimes, in: *Nursing History Review*, No. 27, 2018, S. 56-87, 65.
78. Pincheira: Editorial, in: *Enfermería*, No. 41, 07-08-09-1974, p. 2.
79. Ministerio de Salud: No. 126, Designa en comisión de Servicios a la Sra. Gladys Peake Guevara, a Ginebra, Suiza, 126-1980-1978, 31.05.1978, p. 1-1 [6-40].
80. However, she did not oppose the military junta. For example, she participated in the (re)inaugural ceremony of the National Secretary for Women (*Secretaría Nacional de la Mujer*), one of the most important female organizations of the junta, in: Colegio de Enfermeras de Chile: *Boletín Informativo*, 10-11-12-1973, p. 15.

81. In 1974, for example, Pincheira was responsible for the *CECh* Department of Community Health (*Salud Comunitaria*), in: XXII Memoria Anual del Consejo General del Colegio de Enfermeras de Chile, in: Enfermería, No. 45, 07-08-09-1975, p. 24–37, 26.
82. *CECh*'s *Informative Bulletin* (*Boletín Informativo*).
83. Ibid., p. 55.
84. In 1975, Díaz made her first appearance in the documentation of the Ministry of Health, in: Ministerio de Salud, Oficina de Asuntos Internacionales: Asesoría Enfermera Srta. Lidia Díaz, 1896-0534, 12.03.1975;

    Her correspondence was controlled by the Ministry of Health. The WHO had to request the permission of the minister's office to talk to her, in: Ministerio de Salud, Oficina de Asuntos Internacionales: No. 0247, Ref. Asesoría D. Lidia Diaz, 0247-1959-1977, 17.02.1977, p. 1-1 [22-60].
85. Díaz, Lidia et al. (1979).
86. Ministerio de Salud: Envía nómina detallada del personal de esta Subsecretaría, 1845-1841, 04.10.1973, p. 1–2.
87. Jerez, Idilia: Discurso de la profesora Sra Idilia Jerez, in: *Enfermería*, No. 40, 04-05-06-1974, p. 7-9, 7.
88. Visión Actual de Enfermería, in: Enfermería No. 53, 07-08-09-1977, p. 32.
89. Ministerio de Salud, Oficina de Asuntos Internacionales: 2670, Beca para Irene Bocaz S., 2670-1846-1973, 28.12.1973, p. 1-1 [24-43];

    An interview with a former student of Bocaz's suggests that she had a special relationship with the military authorities and, in return, more autonomy to the nursing school, in: Interview with Luis Campus (nursing student in Concepción 1973-1977), Talca, March 2017;

    Midwife Anita Román Morra, who studied during the same period in Concepción, confirms this suggestion, in: Interview with Anita Román Morra, Santiago, February 2020.
90. Ministerio de Salud, Subsecretaría: Ord No. 1643, Mat. Conferencia Internacional sobre Atención Primaria en Salud, 1643-1995-1978, 27.09.1978, p. 1-32 [3-34];

    In 1978, Peake gave the exact number of 3000 nurses, in: Esfera de Acción de la Enfermera en Chile, in: *Enfermería*, No. 55, 01-02-03-1978, p. 7–11, 7;

    The state institutions and the *CECh* collected only data from affiliated nurses. As explained in Chap. 1, an unknown number of nurses worked with no registration in the informal sector and nursing auxiliaries did not need registration.
91. Quote: "Reafirmar la mantenición de las dos categorías de personal de enfermería existentes: Enfermera o Enfermero Profesional y Auxiliar de

Enfermería" [...] Las personas de esta categroría deben prestar asistencia preventiva, curativa y de rehabilitación en establecimientos asistenciales públicos y privados, bajo supervisión de la enfermera o enfermero profesional," in: Pincheira, Consejera General; Peake Guevara, Secretaria General CECh: Bases para una política de Enfermería, in: *Enfermería*, No. 54, 04-05-06-1978, p. 29–32, 29-30.

92. XXII Memoria Anual del Consejo General del Colegio de Enfermeras de Chile, in: *Enfermería*, No. 45, 07-08-09-1975, p. 24–37, 30;

    Peake even wanted to supervise the professional practice of other health professions, in: Memoria Anual del Consejo General del Colegio de Enfermeras de Chile, periodo Mayo 1976 y Abril 1977, in: *Enfermería*, No. 55, 01-02-03-1978, p. 33–44, 35.
93. Weitzel, Lidia: Rendimiento del Programa Nacional de Adiestramiento de Auxiliares de Enfermería, in: *Enfermería*, No. 35-36, 01-06-1973, p. 29-30.
94. Nursing professionals worked in the regions of Antofagasta, La Serena, Valparaíso, Santiago, Talca, Concepción, Temuco, Valdivia, and Punta Arenas, in: Sonia Garrido: En la paz y en la guerra siempre junto al dolor, in: *Vida Médica*, Vol. 27, 05-06-1975, p. 11;

    Nursing auxiliaries were missing, too. Especially in the slums of the suburbs, the lack of auxiliary nurses was alarming, in: Díaz, Lidia: Modelos de Atención de Enfermería, Santiago [Ministerio de Salud, Departamento de Apoyo a los Programas, Enfermería] 1979, p. 8.
95. Ministerio de Salud, Asesoría Jurídica: M.S. Ord No. 2037, Mat. Solicitud de personalidad jurídica presentada por la corporación denominada "Asociación Chilena de Terapeutas Ocupacionales," 2037-1997-1978, 21.11.1978, p. 1-2 [8/9-81].
96. Ministerio de Salud, Asesoría Jurídica: M.S. Ord. No. 2290, Obj. Envía Proyecto de Decreto Ley sobre Auxiliares de Enfermería, 2290-1846-1973, 19.11.1973, p. 1-4 [13-16/43].
97. Ministerio de Salud, Gabinete de Ministro: Modificación de requisitos para auxiliares de enfermería, 1898-0987, 24.04.1975.
98. In 1953, Peake participated in the commission which elaborated the national training program for nursing auxiliaries, in: Gladys Peake: Formación de la Enfermera y auxiliares de enfermería, in: Actas de las Segundas Jornadas de Salubridad, Organizadas por la Sociedad Chilena de Salubridad Santiago 1953, p. 84-116;

    Peake discredited the opinion of auxiliary workers. For her, surveys conducted by the *ANAECH* "lacked seriousness and validity," in: Memoria Anual del Consejo General del Colegio de Enfermeras de Chile, Periodo 18 de mayo de 1975 al 30 de Abril de 1976, in: *Enfermería*, No. 51, 01-02-03-1977, p. 34–43, 41.

99. Ministerio de Salud, Asesoría Jurídica: Ord No. 1930, Mat. Remite proyecto de Decreto Ley que autoriza a los auxiliares de enfermería el ejercicio libre de la profesión, 1930-1963-1977, 20.10.1977, p. 1-3 [3/5-92].
100. Quote: "Los auxiliares de enfermería podrán asistir en forma directa a pacientes y enfermos hospitalizados o ambulatorios [...] desempeñar sus funciones bajo la dependencia y supervisión de los profesionales universitarios correspondientes," in: Article No. 4 of the Decreto Ley No. 2.147, 31.03.1978.
101. In 1977, the health minister Matthei forbade the participation of *ANAECH* members in the Latin American congress of nursing auxiliaries in Chaclacayo (Peru), because of the "bad economic situation of Chile," in: Ministerio de Salud, Jefe de Gabinete: M.S. Ord No. 1305, Mat. 1. Congreso Latinoamericano de Auxiliares de Enfermería, 1305-1962-1977, 18.07.1977, p. 1-1 [42/43-54];

    Finally, Pinochet's head of office, Maturana Schulze, gave her permission. However, the participation could not be confirmed, in: Ministerio de Salud, Jefe de Gabinete: M.S. Ord No. 1909, Mat. Primer Congreso Latinoamericano de Auxiliares de Enfermería, 1909-1963-1977, 18.10.1977, p. 1-1 [6-92].
102. Ministerio de Salud, Asesoría Jurídica: M.S. Ord. No. 2290, Obj. Envía Proyecto de Decreto Ley sobre Auxiliares de Enfermería, 2290-1846-1973, 19.11.1973, p. 1-4 [13-16/43].
103. Ministerio de Salud: Envía nómina detallada del personal de esta Subsecretaría, 1845-1841, 04.10.1973, p. 1–2.
104. Ministerio de Salud: Actividades Ministerio de Salud día 1. de octubre de 1973, 1845-1798, 02.10.1973.
105. Ministerio de Salud: Actividades del Ministerio de Salud, día 5 de Octubre de 1973 [Contribución de horas extra de trabajo para el Gobierno], 1845-1855, 05.10.1973.
106. For example, the National Association of Magistrates (*Asociación Nacional de Magistrados*) donated five workdays, in: Vicaría de la Solidaridad: Memoria, https://www.vicariadelasolidaridad.cl/cronologia [22.05.2022];
107. Ministerio de Salud: Ord. No. 2645, Remite Proyecto de Ley que modifica la Ley No. 15.076 que benificia a personal dependiente del Colegio de Enfermeras de Chile, 1845-2645, 24.10.1973.
108. Colegio de Enfermeras de Chile: Boletín Informativo, No. 34, 35, 36 1973, p. 7.
109. Para la Reconstrucción—Jornada de Trabajo aumentó en 4 horas, in: *El Mercurio*, 14.10.1973, 15.-21.10.1973, p. 1.

110. Incorporación de las Enfermeras al Sistema de Medicina Curativa, in: *Boletín Informativo*, Nos. 34-35-36, 1973, p. 9-10.
111. Ibid., p. 7-8.
112. Ibid., p. 8.
113. Día Mundial de la Enfermera, in: *El Mercurio*, 13.05.1975, p. 6.
114. Two studies are described in *Enfermería*, in: XXII Memoria Anual del Consejo General del Colegio de Enfermeras de Chile, in: *Enfermería*, No. 45, 07-08-09-1975, p. 24–37, 30;

     The third study was published in 1977, in: Memoria Anual del Consejo General del Colegio de Enfermeras de Chile, Periodo 18 de mayo de 1975 al 30 de Abril de 1976, in: *Enfermería*, No. 51, 01-02-03-1977, p. 34–43, 42;

     In 1979, the most extensive study was published by Lidia Díaz. In 140 pages she and her co-operators described and evaluated the staffing structure in four different healthcare centers in three regions of the country, in: Díaz, Lidia et al. (1979).
115. Ayala A., Ricardo; Thulin, Markus; Nuñez, E. Rocío: Cold Interests, Hot Conflicts: How a Professional Association Responded to a Change in Political Regimes, in: *Nursing History Review*, Vol. 27, No. 1, 2019, p. 57-86.
116. Colegio de Enfermeras de Chile: *Boletín Informativo*, 10-11-12-1973, p. 9.
117. Colegio de Enfermeras de Chile: *Boletín Informativo*, 10-11-12-1973, p. 9.
118. Talloni reported that military units occupied the mine *El Teniente* on September 11, 1973. Workers and employees who had worked during the strikes were automatically dismissed, in: Interview with Patricia Talloni, Santiago, March 2016.
119. Interview with Patricia Grau, Santiago, February 2017.
120. In 1975, Peake reported in the *Enfermería* that 339 nurses had lost their jobs between May 1974 and April 1975. She gave no reasons, even though in no other moment did she provide such detailed information about dismissals, in: XXII Memoria Anual del Consejo General del Colegio de Enfermeras de Chile, in: *Enfermería*, No. 45, 07-08-09-1975, p. 24–37, 30.
121. Colegio de Enfermeras de Chile: *Boletín Informativo*, 10-11-12-1974, p. 6.
122. A study of the Ministry of Health from 1978 revealed that an unknown number of professionals were not registered in the lists of the *colegios profesionales*, in: Ministerio de Salud: Proyecto para el desarollo de los Registros de los Colegios Profesionales del Sector Salud, 1894, 1975.
123. Interview with Patricia Grau, Santiago, March 2017.
124. Ibid.
125. Ibid.
126. Interview with Nurse Patricia Grau, Santiago, March 2017.

127. Nielsen, L. B.; Hemmingsen, B. G.; Plougmann, S.: Nurses supporting torture in Chile [Translation from Danish to English by Lea Merz, University of Cologne, 07-2018], in: *Sygeplejersken*, 01-1984, Vol. 84, No. 4.
128. Nurses in danger: the price of protest, in: *Nursing Times*, Vol. 84, No. 33, 1988, p. 29-31.
129. Nurses in danger: agents of depression, in: *Nursing Times*, Vol. 84, No. 42, 1988, p. 45-47.
130. Stover, Eric: The open secret, torture and the medical profession in Chile, Washington [American Association for the Advancement of Science] 1987.
131. Esfera de Acción de la Enfermera en Chile, in: *Enfermería*, No. 55, 01-02-03-1978, p. 7–11, 7.
132. Article No. 173, Decreto No. 22, 03.05.1979, Aprueba reglamento complementario del Decreto Ley 2.306 de 1978, sobre reclutamiento y movilización de las Fuerzas Armadas.
133. The Valech Commission mentioned "military nurses" attending political prisoners, in: Ministerio del interior, Comisión Nacional sobre Prisión Política y Tortura: Informe de la comisión nacional sobre prision política y tortura, Santiago 2005, p. 243.
134. Ceremonias de Graduación en Escuelas de Enfermería, in: *Enfermería*, No. 39, 01-02-03-1974, p. 30.
135. Día Mundial de la Enfermera, in: *El Mercurio*, 13.05.1975, p. 6.
136. Ibid., p. 6;

    According to Peake, in 1975 14 nursing schools existed, in: XXII Memoria Anual del Consejo General del Colegio de Enfermeras de Chile, in: Enfermería, No. 45, 07-08-09-1975, p. 24–37, 29.
137. Ministerio de Salud: Las carreras de Enfermería y Obstetricia, 1898-983, 24.04.1975, p. 1–2.
138. Leigh was quoted by the Minister of Health in a letter to the *Colegio de Practicantes*, in: Ministerio de Salud: Colegio de Practicantes, 1895-0224, 31.01.1975, p. 1–3;

    Cruz Mena, undersecretary of health, had the vision of a more generalist professional (*profesional más generalista*), in: Ministerio de Salud, Depto. Recursos Humanos: M.S. Ord No. 086, Mat. Informe presentado en la XX Conferencia Sanitaria Panamericana, 086-2022-1979, 15.01.1979, p. 1-1 [40-53].
139. Memoria Anual del Consejo General del Colegio de Enfermeras de Chile, Periodo 18 de mayo de 1975 al 30 de Abril de 1976, in: *Enfermería*, No. 51, 01-02-03-1977, p. 34–43, 41.
140. Figueroa reported in 1991 that 14 nursing schools and nursing programs had been closed or ceased, in: Figueroa, María: Rol de la Enfermería Profesional, Concepción 1991 [Museo de la Memoria Santiago, 20/81, Fondo Patricia Grau], p. 9;

141. Día Mundial de la Enfermera, in: *El Mercurio*, 13.05.1975, p. 6.
142. Oye's request was rejected because the Ministry of Finance refused to pay for the additional costs, in: Memoria Anual del H. Consejo General del Colegio de Enfermeras correspondiente al periodo 31 de mayo de 1978 al 1 junio 1979, in: *Enfermería*, No. 61, 07-08-09-1979, p. 36–44, 40.
143. The Ministries of Health and Finance rejected the *CECh*'s complaints about a disadvantaged classification in the Unified Salary Scale, in: XXII Memoria Anual del Consejo General del Colegio de Enfermeras de Chile, in: *Enfermería*, No. 45, 07-08-09-1975, p. 24–37, 26-27;
144. Quote: "Enfermería fundamenta sus principios en el reconocimiento de los valores del hombre y de la familia, como núcleo fundamental de la sociedad, y en el derecho de cada uno de los integrantes de la comunidad de alcanzar su máxima realización espiritual y material dentro de sus capacidades, así como su participación en igualdad de oportunidades en la vida nacional para producir, contribuir al bien común y colaborar en la solución de sus problemas. Estos conceptos son coincidentes con los contenidos en la 'Declaración de Principios de la Honorable Junta de Gobierno del 11 de marzo de 1974,'" in: Pincheira, Consejera General and Peake Guevara, Secretaria General CECh: Bases para una política de Enfermería, in: *Enfermería*, No. 56, 04-05-06-1978, p. 29–32, 29.
145. Peake saw the cooperation with physicians, pharmacists, and biochemists as a step on the way toward a permanent union of professionals. She even had a name for it: The Four Associations (*Cuatro Colegios*) or "C-4," in: XXII Memoria Anual del Consejo General del Colegio de Enfermeras de Chile, in: Enfermería, No. 45, 07-08-09-1975, p. 24–37, 27.
146. Pincheira, Consejera General und Peake Guevara, Secretaria General CECh: Bases para una política de Enfermería, in: *Enfermería*, No. 56, 04-05-06-1978, p. 29–32, 30-31.
147. Memoria Anual del Consejo General del Colegio de Enfermeras de Chile, Periodo 18 de mayo de 1975 al 30 de Abril de 1976, in: *Enfermería*, No. 51, 01-02-03-1977, p. 34–43, 40;

     Between 1976 and 1977, several times the *CECh* board met with authorities of the Ministry of Health, but the nurses failed to reach an agreement, in: Memoria Anual del Consejo General del Colegio de Enfermeras de Chile Periodo Mayo 1976 y Abril 1977, in: *Enfermería*, No. 55, 01-02-03-1978, p. 33–44, 36.
148. Ministerio de Salud, Jefe de Gabinete: Ord No. 1868, Mat. Preparación Programa Ministerial 1978 - Sector Salud, 1868-1963-1977, 13.10.1977, p. 1-22 [39/60-92].
149. In 1976, the US-American nurse Patricia Ann Deiman (University of Minnesota) became the PAHO project manager for nursing programs in

South America, in: *Star Tribune*: Patricia Deiman, https://www.startribune.com/obituaries/detail/155825/?fullname=patricia-deiman,-csj [30.04.2020];

In 1977, Deiman participated in the *CECh* congress in Temuco, in: Ministerio de Salud, Oficina de Asuntos Internacionales, Juricic T., Jefe Oficina Asuntos Internacionales: No. 1987, Ref. Asesoría Srta Pat Deiman, 1987-1964-1977, 31.10.1977, p. 1-1 [41-41];

In 1979, another PAHO representative visited Chile for several months in order to advise the *CECh* board, in: Memoria Anual del H. Consejo General del Colegio de Enfermeras correspondiente al periodo 31 de mayo de 1978 al 1 junio 1979, in: *Enfermería*, No. 61, 07-08-09-1979, p. 36–44, 44.

150. XXII Memoria Anual del Consejo General del Colegio de Enfermeras de Chile, in: *Enfermería*, No. 45, 07-08-09-1975, p. 24–37, 30.

151. The *CECh* agreed with the University of Chile to use the money for the nursing school of the Medical Faculty in North Santiago, in: Ministerio de Salud, Oficina de Asuntos Internacionales: No. 1270, Integración Docente Asistencial en Enfermería, Sede Norte, Universidad de Chile, 1270-1962-1977, 12.07.1977, p. 1-1 [48-54];

The NHS used the rest of the budget for the following projects:

1. Investment in material, in: Ministerio de Salud, Oficina de Asuntos Internacionales: No. 0208, Ref. Material Encuesta de Nutrición, 0208-1959-1977, 02.02.1977, p. 1-1 [26-60];

2. Investment in information material, in: Ministerio de Salud, Oficina de Asuntos Internacionales: No. 0347, Mat. Publicación científica "El Papel de la enfermería en la atención primaria de salud," 0347-1989-1978, 15.03.1978, p. 1-1 [7-26];

3. Investment in scholarships for nurses in rural healthcare and *materno-infantil* projects, in: Ministerio de Salud, Oficina de Asuntos Internacionales: No. 1861, Ref. Becas viajeras PRUMIN (4). XI Región de Salud, 1861-1997-1978, 30.10.1978, p. 1-2 [73/74-81].

152. *CECh: Boletín Informativo*, 01-02-03-1974, p. 10-11.

153. Quote: "la política de contratación de las nuevas promociones se orientó a abrir contratos en provincias, con restricción en Santiago, Valparaíso y Concepción," in: XXII Memoria Anual del Consejo General del Colegio de Enfermeras de Chile, in: *Enfermería*, No. 45, 07-08-09-1975, p. 24–37, 30;

In 1978, from 2582 nurses registered in the *CECh*, 1386 worked in hospitals, 879 in health centers, 267 in private hospitals, and 50 in private health centers, in: Esfera de Acción de la Enfermera en Chile, in: *Enfermería*, No. 55, 01-02-03-1978, p. 7–11, 8.

154. Title of the seminar: Nursing Law in the 2nd Half of the 20th Century. The main topic was the collaboration of nurses with midwives and *practicantes*, in: XXII Memoria Anual del Consejo General del Colegio de Enfermeras de Chile, in: *Enfermería*, No. 45, 07-08-09-1975, p. 24–37, 31.
155. Peake described a conference of 2000 nurses from Latin America, who met in Quito, in: Campos S. et al.: Papel de la Enfermera en Servicios integrados de Atención Materno-Infantil, in: *Enfermería*, Nos. 43-44, 01-06-1975, p. 5–8;

   Ballerino held a speech about Chilean healthcare policies in *materno-infantil*, in: XXII Memoria Anual del Consejo General del Colegio de Enfermeras de Chile, in: *Enfermería*, No. 45, 07-08-09-1975, p. 24–37, 31;

   The *CECh* chaired the *FEPPEN* board between 1975 and 1976, in: Pincheira: Editorial, in: *Enfermería*, No. 41, 07-08-09-1974, p. 2;
156. XXII Memoria Anual del Consejo General del Colegio de Enfermeras de Chile, in: *Enfermería*, No. 45, 07-08-09-1975, p. 24–37, 31.
157. Memoria Anual del Consejo General del Colegio de Enfermeras de Chile, Periodo 18 de mayo de 1975 al 30 de Abril de 1976, in: *Enfermería*, No. 51, 01-02-03-1977, p. 34–43, 38.
158. As the *CECh* department of public relations was inactive since 1975, it seems that Peake was the only nurse with contacts in the media, in: XXII Memoria Anual del Consejo General del Colegio de Enfermeras de Chile, in: *Enfermería*, No. 45, 07-08-09-1975, p. 24–37, 27.
159. The articles with predominantly technical information were mostly written by the university professors. Regarding the content, psychiatry was the most important topic after *materno-infantil*, public health, and surgery.
160. Ministerio de Salud: M.S. Ord No. 568, Mat. Congreso Federación Panamericana de Enfermeras/os, 560-2024-1979, 29.03.1979, p. 1-1 [3-33].
161. In 1979, Peake criticized in her yearly report that the Latin American nursing associations had only a small margin in the ICN. It seems that the *CECh* organized then an initiative to act en bloc in the yearly meetings of the ICN, in: Memoria Anual del H. Consejo General del Colegio de Enfermeras correspondiente al periodo 31 de mayo de 1978 al 1 junio 1979, in: *Enfermería*, No. 61, 07-08-09-1979, p. 36–44, 43.
162. Ministerio de Salud: No. 126, Designa en comisión de Servicios a la Sra. Gladys Peake Guevara, a Ginebra, Suiza, 126-1980-1978, 31.05.1978, p. 1-1 [6-40].

163. The congress was mentioned in the *CECh* documentation, in: Memoria Anual del Consejo General del Colegio de Enfermeras de Chile Periodo Mayo 1976 y Abril 1977, in: *Enfermería*, No. 55, 01-02-03-1978, p. 33–44, 42;

    One of the Spanish delegates criticized Corrales. According to her, Corrales distributed political propaganda, in: Ma Eugenia Somalo, Congreso de Tokio. Tema del día 3 de Junio de (1977), in: *Boletín Cultural e Informativo del Consejo General de Ayudantes Técnicos Sanitarios*, 1978.

164. List of international congresses with the participation of Chilean nurses and Chilean nursing congresses with international participation:

    1. The participation of *CECh* board members in a nursing congress in 1976 in Buenos Aires, in: Ministerio de Salud: Decreto Comisión de Servicios a Congreso de Enfermeras a Realizarse en la Ciudad de Buenos Aires, de Funcionarias que se indican, 1922-284, 20.10.1976, p. 1–2;

    2. The participation of Elena Perich from the Argentinean Federation of Nurses (*Federación Argentina de Enfermeras*) in the Chilean Nursing Congress, 1977 in Temuco, in: Informe Final, in: *Enfermería*, No. 54, 10-11-12-1977, p. 44–46;

    3. No information about a cooperation with the National Association of Professional Nurses from Bolivia (*Asociación Nacional de Enfermeras Profesionales de Bolivia*, *ANEPB*), in: Memoria Anual del Consejo General del Colegio de Enfermeras de Chile Periodo Mayo 1976 y Abril 1977, in: *Enfermería*, No. 55, 01-02-03-1978, p. 33–44, 42;

    4. In 1977, two *CECh* nurses joined the Catholic Committee of Nurses and Social Workers (*Congreso del Comité Católico de Enfermeras y Asistentes Sociales*) in Rio de Janeiro, in: Memoria Anual del Consejo General del Colegio de Enfermeras de Chile Periodo Mayo 1976 y Abril 1977, in: *Enfermería*, No. 55, 01-02-03-1978, p. 33–44, 42.

165. For example, in 1976, the permission to take part in a *FEPPEN* congress, in: Ministerio de Salud: Decreto Comisión de Servicios a Congreso de Enfermeras a Realizarse en la Ciudad de Buenos Aires, de Funcionarias que se indican, 1922-284, 20.10.1976, p. 1–2;

CHAPTER 4

Nursing in Times of State Reforms (1980–1982)

1 Refounding the State[1]

The years from 1979 to 1982 became decisive for the relationship between professionals and the state. The military junta implemented quite an "avalanche" of decrees and laws meant to strengthen private initiatives and entrepreneurship. Another goal of Pinochet and his advisors was to suppress mergers of employees. For this, they facilitated concerted action against all workers and professionals, and only then they could resubmit the rules of employment relationship as well as the legal conditions for unions and associations' work. But the foundations for the reforms of the public and the private systems required a new constitution.

The 1980 constitution changed healthcare and nurses' living and working conditions. It meant a whole new social order, which informed healthcare reorganizing.[2] The most challenging policy arising out of the new constitution nurses retell was their shrinking political representation. And yet the empowerment of the auxiliaries as representatives of the workers is often consigned into oblivion, however threatening.

Up until 1982, the regime implemented a number of major state reforms. The state of emergency continued to be in force and restricted the possibilities for resistance among veto players. Since the fall of Gen. Leigh in 1978, opposition in the government was brought into line. By then, the junta became an executive board of Pinochet and his advisors. Here, the most prominent policy influencer was the engineer and

© The Author(s), under exclusive license to Springer Nature Switzerland AG 2023

M. Thulin, R. A. Ayala, *Nursing, Policy and Politics in Twentieth-century Chile*,
https://doi.org/10.1007/978-3-030-90835-5_4

economist Hernán Büchi (born 1949). Appointed as the undersecretary of the Ministry of Health (1981–1983) and then finance minister (1985–1990), he handled the execution of decrees and laws that, even today, define Chilean society.[3]

Men like Büchi were professionals who had decided to cooperate with the military junta. They ascended as the top group of civilians in the sixteen years of dictatorship, which granted them great decisional authority and political influence. Büchi and his colleagues were the heart of the civilian-military cooperation, because they advised the generals, assisted them to find political and economic solutions, and tried to build their personal careers within and throughout the political process. Most of the health professionals were obliged to negotiate with men like Büchi. But before we present the reaction of the healthcare sector, we will address the reforms of vocational institutes, the labor rights, the pension system, the public administration, and the private property political constitution.

1.1 Constitution: From the Façade of a Plebiscite to New Social Order

On August 11, 1980, a constitution with a disproportionate private property emphasis came into force.[4] It was one of the most significant legislation processes in Chilean history. But as the whole plebiscite process took place under the state of emergency law, the opposition was not allowed to campaign.[5] Moreover, the vote was a mere façade. The state of emergency itself, in force since 1978, was institutionalized and prolonged for five more years.[6] Pinochet stayed in power and continued to dispose of unlimited authority. The new de facto legislation backed imprisonment for up to 15 days with no investigation, expatriating citizens that opposed the regime and censoring the press.[7] By this legislation, the democratic appearance of state oppression was expanded and embedded in society; that is why such radical reforms in different areas, including healthcare and nursing, raised no systematic criticisms.

1.2 Pensions: From Public Cuts to Private Market

One of the legislation packages to introduce the new order was the reform of the retirement pensions in May 1981,[8] an outcome deriving from pressures from powerful groups. From then on, Chileans could either stay within the state-run welfare solidary system or move to one of the private fund savings plans, known as individual capitalization system (*capitalización individual*). Here, professionals were only categorized as employees.

While employers were waived from making contributions to the system,[9] those who entered work life after May 1st were obliged to enroll within the new pension funds. They had to hire one of the private investment companies called Administrators of Pension Funds (*Administradoras de Fondos de Pensiones, AFP*), which put the money on the capital market. By the time the insured reached the age of retirement, the interests on the savings but also the losses would be transferred. And yet, unlike in the previous system, a minimum pension was not enforced. Insufficient capitalization led to very low pension benefits.[10] Women were particularly disadvantaged by the new pension system. During family caregiving, most of them could not afford to pay contributions out of pocket for any length of time, and back then, caregiving was an overwhelmingly female task.[11] When nurses did work as such, be it as professional or auxiliary, their salary did not equate to that of males who, in turn, could enjoy a better-off retirement life. Taking a closer look, one will see that the new pension system only mirrored the principles of division of labor embedded in labor law.

1.3 Professionals: From Collective Bargaining to Collective Downgrading

Professional associations, unions, and other forms of organized social movements had proven to be central to both state planning and society more broadly. Since 1973, Pinochet and his advisors had successfully oppressed them, but threats and exclusion were not enough to part with their influence on national life. The leaders were tough. Within the framework of the upcoming constitution, the civilian-military cooperation looked for a way to restrict political mobilization once and for all.

In previous years, labor rights had been more of a vision than a reality, as the experience of nursing auxiliaries had shown. Nevertheless, three decree laws issued in July 1979 also put an end to the vision.[12] By the beginning of the new decade, hired employees were allowed to have only one union per company, had legally no chance to join federations across a single labor sector, and faced threat of dismissal when deciding to go on strike.[13]

Through this piece of legislation, the government deprived professionals and workers of their most powerful tool in negotiations with employers, which was the ability to halt production or deny services. For nurses, strikes like in 1972 and 1973 became impossible. The *CECh* was meant to deteriorate into a powerless discussion board.

1.4 Professions: From Public Law Bodies to Private Associations

As seen earlier in this book, Pinochet and his advisors sought to weaken professional groups, which by then had been an important force in public life and active policy shapers. In doing this, the junta board used an argument not many would have expected: democracy.

In 1979, all the professional associations were allocated the statutes of private associations (*asociaciones gremiales, A.G.*). At first glance, it was not evident that a new form of a professional organization was being founded because a wide range of organizations fell under this new umbrella legislation.[14] It defined an unusual status for the professions, as the term *gremio* did not mean just trade as in "professional association," but as in "private association." In fact, not only the leads of the professional associations but also company owners—and, by extension, rightist political leaders—were referred to as guildsmen (*gremialistas*). The principle of freedom of association thus translated into the choice whether to affiliate with a professional organization or not, which in practice meant a competition for members' votes.[15]

While the private association label triggered no particular resistance, the suppression of professional associations' right to co-decide upon wages raised the first complaints.[16] Most of the professional associations joined in an informal movement. Their dissent, expressed in public statements, was so vehement that Pinochet accepted for the first time since October 1973 to receive the representatives of seven boards. But that was only a symbolic action. For the law was eventually enacted without furnishing any consideration for professionals' claims and doing no further changes.[17]

Two years later, in February 1981, the professional associations would be formally stripped of their legal status as public law bodies.[18] They all were fated to become private associations, too. In a sense, the requirement of free and secret elections to form the boards of the reformed associations suggested Pinochet's will for some democracy on this level.[19] The boards had only one and half years to change their statutes, hold elections, and adapt their formal structure to the new charter.

Later on, nineteen out of the 30 professional associations, among them the *CECh*, opposed the reform.[20] The arguments of the government—individual freedom in choosing representatives, and preventing monopolization[21]—encountered criticisms for the four following issues:

- Loss of their overseeing authority in professional ethics
- Deregulation of wages, formerly controlled by the professional associations
- Fragmentation of professionals' representation
- Loss of an academic status for some professions[22]

Leading the protest were the journalists and the lawyers.[23] Not surprisingly, they focused on ethics and representation, but not on an academic status. As discussed below, only nurses, midwives, social workers, and other female professionals faced a status downgrade, among other disadvantages, like the wage debate not addressing gender equality. Like in October 1973, Julio Durán, president of the lawyers' association, became the spokesman of the professionals' resistance movement.[24] As per usual, it would seem that he appointed no woman to his circle of close advisors.

However, the professionals did not form federations or other alliances resembling the movements of the 1960s and early 1970s.[25] The opposition seemed something of a loose array of actors, organizations, and ideas, but as far as it was recorded in the press almost all professional groups formed a coalition of some sort.[26] Yet their methods seemed to have changed as they did not even try to organize strikes or demonstrations. The content they circulated differed from the harsh statements against Frei and Allende as well; for instance, Durán and his fellow campaigners were very careful not to make any criticism about Pinochet or any of his advisors, but about their policies.

The government did not react with repression, but still refused to negotiate.[27] It is 1981, and after two months of insistence Pinochet eventually receives the presidents of 24 professional associations.[28] He seemed open to discuss some minor issues, but the associations' legal basis as public corporations run and owned by the state was abolished regardless.[29]

One month later, the resistance collapsed. The first 19 associations agreed to become subjected to private law.[30] By 1982, all other professional associations saw the same fate befall them.[31] The critical voices became silent for some four long years. While print media generally ignored nurses, midwives, and other professions, exceptions were made for the physicians, the lawyers, and the journalists. In the following years, their associations continued to publicly target criticism to governmental measures, but in a much smaller scope compared to the years before.[32]

Ordinary people mostly ignored the movement of the professionals,[33] probably concerned by the never-ending barrage of laws and decrees, and so professionals' business simply dropped out of the spotlight. International voices, like the International Council of Nurses, failed to make any statement. One reason could have been the lack of knowledge, both in Chile and internationally, about the consequences the shift from public law to private law implied. By the beginning of the 1980s, the state was by far the biggest employer, when no nurse could be hired without holding a university title and *CECh* membership. The regime had thus arranged the social order for the long term.

1.5 Administration: From Regionalization to Municipalization

Until 1980, nursing, like midwifery or social work, had been centralized services. Even decisions on a local level, like hiring new staff, were forwarded to national authorities. This system was error-prone because it consumed time and did not respond to local requirements. The military junta wanted to transmit the responsibility for payment, administration, and staff issues to the mayors and city councils of *municipalidades*.

In June 1980, the ministries of internal affairs, education, and health started to transfer services to municipal ownership and responsibility. This was called *municipalización*[34] or reorganization of local administration.[35] Municipalities received a yearly budget, and from then on they had to provide education, retirement payments, and healthcare.[36]

In healthcare, a decree law from September 1980 specified that the municipalities had to guarantee primary care of their districts.[37] They, and not the NHS, would be the employers of the personnel,[38] and had to provide the facilities and equipment for them to function. To achieve those goals, it was allowed to cooperate with companies within the service sector (*corporaciones privadas*).[39]

In 1981 alone 17.4 percent (43 percent in rural areas) of the administrative units moved into municipal control. But in 1982, it fell to 3.4 percent and continued to shrink, while the process stopped altogether in 1983. The reasons for that were the economic crises of 1982 and the planned expansion of healthcare coverage. While the crises generally limited the financial scope of poorer municipalities,[40] the means for staff and material did not increase.[41] Money was at stake, and so the Ministry of Health urged the municipalities to expand their offer for private patients. Since 1979, the free choice system was supposed to be available for all Chileans who could afford it, no matter where they lived and to which social class they belonged. This implied further investment for additional staff and infrastructure[42] and the willingness of a number of health professionals to leave the cities to work in the country. But as in the decades before, public health remained unpopular for health professionals.

However, we found no trace of a substantial expansion of healthcare coverage in rural areas resulting from *municipalización*. The most important reason for the consistent undersupply was the economic crises—as discussed below—but external factors alone cannot explain the standstill from 1982 to 1986. Overcoming the urban-rural gap indeed consistently remained the main task of any government in Chile.

1.6 Students: From University to Non-university

At the beginning of the decade, eight universities offered study programs for health professions. The University of Chile had no fewer than 12 campuses throughout the country, and so most professionals trained there.

On January 3, 1981, a new decree law formally recognized academic freedom.[43] In practice, though, that was quite the opposite as public universities remained under the direct control of army commanders, and in all institutions professors and students had to conform to the socio-economic order embedded in the new constitution.[44]

During 1981, a number of decrees officialized the definitive detachment of the regional campuses of the University of Chile.[45] That meant that in the process 12 new public universities throughout the country started life, and the medical faculties of the universities were free to arrange collaborations with both the regional successors of the NHS and private companies.[46] The same aim had the reform of the accreditation procedure for private universities.[47] Between 1981 and 2015, some 35 private universities were founded, most of them after 1990, but their groundwork dates back to the overall reform process beginning in 1981.[48]

The number of job offers for health professionals in the public sector, already reduced because of the budget cuts in previous years, continued to shrink.[49] For example, in the medical faculties of the University of Chile in Santiago, the number of students fell from 4716 to 4073 (13.6 percent) between 1980 and 1982.[50] Our analysis of the nursing policies will demonstrate that this development affected mostly degree courses with predominantly female students.

As of 1980, only medicine, psychology, pharmacy, biochemistry, and veterinary medicine would have university training as the sole entry path to professional practice. As a result, training in nursing and other female professions could also be undertaken in non-university institutions[51] such as vocational institutes (*institutos profesionales*).[52] No later than a year afterward, *institutos* offered trainings in nursing, midwifery, social work, laboratory technology, dietetics, kinesiology, and occupational therapy. While the policy sought to enhance both the workforce and an educational market, it sent the message that there were first-class professions and second-class professions, which even today affects the way health professionals are perceived by the public. Within just months a large portion of the female workforce in health lost their status as graduate professions, whereas for most of that year references in the press were rather marginal, ignoring the social consequences this carried.[53]

1.7 *Auxiliaries: From Autodidact to Vocational*

Nowhere else in healthcare did entrepreneurship gain ground as fast as it did in nursing auxiliary education. By 1980, this was not anticipated because private companies played a small role in the financing and administration of training centers (*institutos profesionales*). By contrast, public and denominational institutes had been inherent to the higher education system. They have stood the test of time and, in fact, grown and diversified.[54] In 1978, universities counted 130,208 students, while in state-owned vocational institutes alone there were some 178,800 students.[55]

The spread of non-university institutes often led to conflicts. In May 1976, for the first time since the coup d'état, the Ministry of Health had to mediate between a professional association and a private vocational institute called the National Center of Paramedical and Agricultural Studies (*Centro Nacional de Estudios Paramédicos y Agropecuarios, PROPAM*). When *PROPAM* started to offer a training for laboratory technicians in Santiago, the president of the respective professional association decided this was unauthorized competition with study programs offered at universities, and asked the Ministry of Health to interfere to outlaw the courses.[56] Even though the decision was not documented, this incident would seem to be just the tip of the iceberg that, in reality, became a lengthy, abrasive dispute between the professional associations, the private vocational institutes, and the government.

A prominent figure in this conflict was the founder of *PROPAM*, Esteban Rocha Vera (1952–2008).[57] Between 1977 and 1979, he tried three times to get state accreditation for training programs in podiatry and nursing,[58] but the Ministry of Health was somewhat ambivalent. Undersecretary Edgardo Cruz Mena (1974–1981) rejected Rocha's requests. In an interview with *Hoy* magazine (1977) he criticized the "anomalies of the operating principle of those institutes," as well as their "weak standards of training."[59] In his decision, he was heavily influenced by the professional associations' arguments, as illustrated in the following excerpt:

> "This Ministry deems professional education in *institutos* inappropriate. Their pseudo-medical training only leads to much confusion with the already existing professions and their respective associations."[60]

Nevertheless, much as the minister publicly condemned health trainings in private institutes, he actually "tolerated" them.[61] Especially with *PROPAM*, it is unclear whether the institute eventually met the government's expectations or whether Cruz changed his mind for some other reason. Indeed, between 1977 and 1981 he increased the number of the institute's student intake from 400 to 3000 yearly.[62] By this, the post-coup policy to replace a part of the professional workforce with an auxiliary workforce entered its second phase.

There are three reasons why the government increased since 1978 the hiring of nursing auxiliaries.[63] Firstly, it was a necessity caused by the lack of academically trained nurses.[64] Secondly, as Chap. 3 has shown, the military junta gave quickly up to furnish university training in nursing. Finally, international engagement supported both types of caregivers, not only nurses who trained in university.[65] Businessmen like Rocha, but surely also students of auxiliary nursing, hoped that the expansion of institutes like *PROPAM* would improve auxiliaries' workplace situation and gain recognition for their work in society and by this a higher income.

The gradual educational reform accelerated with the healthcare reform (1979–1982). In 1981, Büchi became the new undersecretary. He allowed institutes to offer training for auxiliary workers, rebranded as technical staff, notably in such areas as nursing, midwifery, and social work. But then these were still the most sought-after areas among women who looked for a job in state healthcare.[66] Thus far, this policy of the Pinochet regime seemed successful.

And yet, at the turn of the decade Chile experienced a boom of higher education institutes, with diverse educational offers in different cities and aiming at different industries. Regulations of the ever-expanding auxiliary training sector fell short in regard to admission and supervision.[67] Soon after, misconduct became an alarming issue. Already in 1982, Büchi enforced a guideline for training conditions and certification, and from then on institutes, especially those where nursing staff trained, would undergo closer monitoring.[68] Nevertheless, as shown elsewhere in this book, institutes' procedural problems would never really be under state control. And although they became embedded in the higher education system, the quality of professional care was perceived to have lowered, despite that back then quality standards and assessment were still not integrated into the organizational culture.

But criticisms were rare—and when they came to light, they did not raise much debate. Several reasons can explain this silence. Firstly, the recent legislation for nursing training in private, non-university institutions was enacted as a quick passing mention within a wave of laws and decrees that rolled over the country by the turn of the decade. Secondly, the already weakened nursing association acted on several fronts, one of which was the dissolution of the professional associations' status within public law. The third reason for the lack of a strong criticism was the economic crisis, which since 1982 not only hit the wallets of Chileans but also created a disheartening atmosphere.

As it was for the university reform, the new set-up of the vocational institutes was decisive but had an effect only at the end of the 1980s. In fact, in 1981 some 3511 nursing auxiliaries graduated but only 653 studied outside public institutions (NHS).[69] Besides, the whole discussion neglected how the reform would deal with the tuition fees that private education implied. Former auxiliary workers, active in the 1970s and 1980s, recall that after eight years of mandatory schooling many of them could immediately start working in hospitals and healthcare centers. Not only was it unnecessary, but they could not really afford higher education. Many of them entered work life through the learning by doing approach[70] and then professionalized through NHS courses.

Moreover, education in private institutes did not really aid staff's mobility within the healthcare system. Their credentials led to wages so low that there was no actual leveling up in the salary ladder. This was probably an important strategy of Cruz and Büchi to increase the workforce and its usability as much as they could. [71]

As it states in the documents of the Ministry of Health, this unspecialized mass of auxiliary workers was employed in and moved across medicine,[72] pharmacology,[73] dentistry, clinical laboratory, and midwifery.[74] However, their training seemed carelessly planned, delivered, and assessed. Unlike for professionals, statistics about auxiliaries were imprecise and unreliable. They lacked a description of job profiles, workers' résumés, or even their names, which correlates with the high percentage of females in this sector, often from underprivileged backgrounds.

The way this training was handled suggests that a new generation of businessmen, like Rocha, took advantage of the state outsourcing training in the healthcare sector. The exemplary of *PROPAM* shows how the state nourished a neoliberal entrepreneurial self in areas as sensitive in social development as education and healthcare. The reform thus institutionalized an environment that was favorable to embracing capitalistic subjectivities, initially among managers and professionals, and then patients and citizens in general.

1.8 Healthcare: From Welfare to Business

The healthcare reform, which started in 1979, changed the administration and the workflow of health professionals and workers. Primarily responsible was the military junta, but also a group of economists and health professionals. With policies transposed from the Chicago School of Economics and the Columbia Business School, they fragmented the public providers, created a much larger private sector, and institutionalized political control. The reform became decisive for all following generations of health professionals.

Büchi was still the closest civilian advisor to Pinochet. He defined both policy and politics in the constitutionally altered healthcare system. Büchi was Pinochet's first and completely neoliberal chief executive, with large discretion to distribute the state's income and investment policy. Sitting on such high-ranking position, he established a system which fitted in the context of increasingly neoliberalizing reforms in other Latin American countries during the 1980s, and which consolidated over the following 40 years.[75]

Nevertheless, the reform was designed on the basis of previous arrangements under the old constitution. Achievements since 1973, like a newly implemented regional administration and a salary scale for public employees, had only been stepping stones for a much wider restructuring of the healthcare system under neoliberal rule, which demonstrates some continuity in such radical changes.

There are several reasons why Pinochet's close advisors recommended to abandon the Keynesian welfare of the post-war era. Not only they themselves but also the opposition perceived the inefficiency and the lack of flexibility of the NHS.[76] Even critical sociologist Diana Chanfreau stated that there had been no significant improvement in healthcare since its "grand opening," in 1952.[77] The military constantly blamed the NHS for the restricted access to healthcare. Gen. Fernando Matthei said during his office term as health minister (1976–1978) that NHS services fell somewhere "between bad and worse,"[78] while his successor Hernán Rivera (1980–1983) stated that most Chileans were dissatisfied with the NHS.[79] As dissatisfaction seemed to rise on different fronts, the reform was marked by the decree law No. 2.763 from August 3, 1979.[80] This being the biggest remodeling of the system since its foundation, in the 1920s, it comprised three main areas:

- The NHS and *SERMENA* merged into a single National System of Health Services, NSHS (*Sistema Nacional de Servicios de Salud)*, with each service covering a geographic district.
- The 27 constituents of the NSHS were requested to secure the constitutional guaranty of providing primary care for all Chileans.
- The financing, the supplies, and the staff of the NSHS were managed by a central state institution, the National Health Fund (*Fondo Nacional de Salud*, *FONASA*).[81]

In order to adapt the NSHS to the state' structure, budget, and expenses, the government implemented a nationwide registry of personal details and family status of all the insured of the public system. It was the first survey of this kind at a national scale in Chile's history, and it aimed at identifying cares (i.e., procedures or techniques) and codifying them within a master list of flat fee cases. The reason for this was the allocation of budget to the newly decentralized institutions on the basis of actual services being delivered.

From then on, beneficiaries of public healthcare contributed monthly to *FONASA* with a mandatory fee taken directly from the salary. The insured and their family could get care in a state-owned facility. Afterward, the respective district service would receive a refund from *FONASA*. And yet, the refund was calculated not on the basis of actual but predefined costs. Exceptionally the government could grant additional budget to *FONASA* in special circumstances, such as beneficiary's bankruptcy, or extreme economic hardship, or damage of health facilities.[82]

Interestingly, as the monetizing process unfolded, the regime seemed to put an end to a long-standing insurance system that set apart white-collar (*SERMENA*) from blue-collar workers (NHS) as it no longer offered separate services for each group. On the other hand, through private insurance or *ISAPRES*, what once was a hierarchy by type of work became more explicitly a hierarchy by wage. *ISAPRES* offered plans differentiated in accordance with the income level of the head of household and how much was available to "invest" in a health plan. Additional services, like free choice, were accessible for higher income groups or for larger co-payments.[83] This was not only a problem for individuals but also for municipalities. As explained, many of the rural and suburban communities could not afford the infrastructure or the staff to offer free choice medical care. Another problem for municipalities was providing free treatment for the unemployed or disabled.[84] Alongside coverage, regulated standards for the quality of the health service were missing, and all those circumstances together led to great disparities depending on the borough's financial endowment.

Aware of this gap, reformers presupposed that the deficits would be covered by the private sector and, in a smaller scale, the already existing religiously inspired initiatives. Owners of vocational institutes, like Rocha, picked the starting point out. His colleagues, who were also professionals, founded *ISAPREs* and private hospitals or healthcare centers. Private insurance functioned autonomously, except for some minor responsibilities from the state, such as auditing.[85] To ensure clientele differentiation, private clinics and health centers had to be built at least 300m away from any NSHS facility.[86]

One of the first corporations created within this frame was the Calvo Mackenna Medical Center Co. (*Sociedad Centro Médico Calvo Mackenna Ltda.*). In 1981, its board gave sponsorship not only for hospitals and health centers but also for the pharmacies of an entire urban district of the capital.[87] The number of partnerships with private companies rose fast between 1980 and 1981.[88] Nevertheless, as occurred with the reform of vocational institutes, privatization sped up only toward the late 1980s.[89] Chilean economists and politicians like Rocha and Büchi, representing private and state healthcare institutions, shaped the entire system because they counteracted the vision of a welfare state. Most of the professionals working in healthcare tolerated the realignment, irrespective of whether or not they rejected the changes. We are going to describe the disagreements, but before, we shall take a closer look at how the perception of the distinction between private and public changed in society.

During the course of the privatization wave throughout 1980 and 1981, the distinction between public hospitals and private clinics became more evident in everyday language as well as in the official documents of the Ministry of Health, journals, and newspapers. This does not mean that all clinics were entirely owned or funded by private companies, religious orders, or universities. The ministry subsidized with yearly payments both the private sector and religiously inspired institutions—and universities indirectly—to be able to ensure the constitutional right to basic care services. For example, in 1981 the hospital of *Colonia Dignidad* in Maule region was funded with 9.1 million pesos (roughly 233,000 USD), and the Archdiocese of Santiago some 45,924 million pesos (1,177,000 USD) for its *Hospital Parroquial de San Bernardo*.[90]

This same health reform also enabled the spread of private health insurance (*Instituciones de Salud Previsional*, *ISAPREs*), mentioned above. They provided not only insurance but also health staff and infrastructure. During the 1980s, an increasing number of *ISAPREs* managed hospitals and healthcare centers, as the law for municipalities and universities allowed cooperation with the public sector. For-profit business in healthcare was formally forbidden,[91] and yet constant criticisms, which have continued to rise until recently, have highlighted that this has never truly been effectively enforced. The private sector attracted mostly affluent clients, as cutting-edge technology, speedy access to care, and hyper-specialized professionals were prohibitively expensive for most Chileans. This is how stratification of health outcomes grew, too.

However, there is a sense in which the healthcare reform was groundbreaking. The fundamental principle being a shift from a Keynesian welfare state to a dual public/private system. Or, in neoliberal parlance, a public/private "partnership." However, with 70 to 80 percent of all policyholders, the public system continued to cover the majority of medical services.[92] Even nowadays, most Chileans contribute to *FONASA* and receive treatments in NSHS hospitals and public primary care centers.

As we have seen, the government converted the NHS into a system of local and regional healthcare providers. But it did not mean that they lifted the political control they exercised over the employees, as this still happened in the midst of the dictatorship. By the eve of its closing, the NHS was employing 5000 physicians, 2464 nurses, 1837 midwives, 690 nutritionists, 773 social workers, 500 untrained workers, and 21,286 nursing auxiliaries.[93] Before they could pass over to the employment relationship with the NSHS, they had to undergo a political check. In March 1979, Hector Concha Marambio, head of the Central Commission of Restructuring, asked to gather and file the résumés of all public employees[94] with the aim of facilitating a new method to assess the staff's technical and political performance (*encasillamiento*). This method eventually classified them into four distinct groups:

"A"—bad [and dismissed]
"B"—average [and dismissed]
"C"—politically active [and dismissed]
"D"—good [but dismissed]
"E"—good [contract extended][95]

The regional NSHS offices possibly returned questionnaire replies, but it can be assumed that the database was created and then erased from the archive after the staff assessment. Importantly though, this method shows that the reform became a powerful device of political control and was used at discretion to expel workers from the public sector. As being fired from an NSHS facility meant being unfitting for any of the other 26 branches, this measure carried with it fear and hardship among the health staff.[96]

If looking solely at the archives, it is difficult to estimate the magnitude of this part of the health reform. However, secondary sources help depict the situation. Authors like Labra speak of a general salary reduction and increasing redundancies in the public sector since 1979.[97] Greve also describes a shortage of jobs,[98] while Salazar and Pinto estimate 100,000 redundancies only in the public sector.[99] Archives from the Ministry of Health give further insights. Firstly, a 1980 directive granted a one-time payment to the staff who were categorized as "good" but had been dismissed because of institutional shrinkage.[100] For the year 1981, an increasing number of dismissals (*desahucios*) appear in the ministry's correspondence, and always on the grounds of being "unfit according to the appraisal method." Remarkable is also the increasing number of approved requests for retirement, compared to the previous years. Conversely, there is no evidence that such procedures were used in the private sector.[101]

The increasingly pressing question after the healthcare reform was whether or not there can be equal health insurance and medical treatment without a welfare state. The foundation of the NSHS, the easement for private companies, and the new employment relationship (as in the 1970s, politically controlled) showed that the government had no compunction about a full socio-political turn. However, this does not mean that the policy they opted for was a well-established pattern worldwide. By the beginning of the 1980s, many countries had small private sectors, while Chile constituted one of the first neoliberal "laboratories." Leaving aside the permanent problem of healthcare coverage and quality, one might think that the strategy worked out very well for the government. The problem was (and still is) that any private system—or a public system operating under private property rules—relies on investment. This may indeed be plausible in times of economic upturn and stability but not when economic crises hit.

1.9 Politics: From Cooperation to Resistance

The start of the reforms in 1979 did not encounter strong resistance. Not that nurses and other professionals were happy with reorganizing the whole institutionality. For, in fact, there were a few complaints about the dismissals during the implementation period.[102] The physicians' association criticized only the annual redoing of the typecasting (*encasillamientos*),[103] and even the response to such major changes as municipalization was marginal.[104] Likely because of the heavy-handed repression and the lack of information, up until 1986 the oppositional press criticized mainly the loosening of protection against dismissal and the flexibilization of the work time, rather than condemning the whole reform package.[105] Here, it is necessary to bear in mind that under the state of emergency strikes were banned. Nevertheless, associations and committees exerted opposition through, among other things, letters to the government and the print press.

In the beginning of the 1980s, there appeared new oppositional alliances, which also operated in this tight framework. Activists found a way to join and then raise a critical voice. They were pushed by the involvement of the Catholic Church in social affairs and politics. Founded in 1978, the Chilean Commission of Human Rights showed the activists how to adopt lawful means to counter state oppression. The most influential leaders of the opposition ranked among the Christian Democratic and ecclesiastic spectrum.[106]

The opposition needed a voice to spread their ideas and motivate others to join their movements. As customary, *El Mercurio* continued to publish public releases by the physicians but carefully avoided any critical view on the political system. Only the oppositional press welcomed some new voices. For instance, in April 1981 authors of *APSI* magazine interviewed Dr. Tegualda Monreal. She was a member of the medical associations' board, but was introduced as a "specialist in public health" and member of the Health Circle of the Academy of Christian Humanism (*Círculo de Salud de la Academia de Humanismo Cristiano*). She was indeed linked to the Catholic Church and sympathetic to left-wing groups. Unlike other doctors, Monreal referred to the catastrophic situation of *FONASA* insured in Santiago's hospitals in a more drastic tone.[107]

As per the records, Monreal was the first female professional to get her critical views of the healthcare policy published. For authors of the print press, women seemed like little more than background actors in the political scene, meaning they appeared incidentally in a nonspeaking capacity and exerting no agency by themselves, let alone making headlines in the way male professionals did. Article headings like "Women, go conquer dignity," published in 1980 in *Solidaridad*, underscored the astonishing revelation that the social workers referred to in the piece, who were females, had a voice.[108] In examining the written sources, we understood that female professionals often did not seem worth being named, quoted, interviewed, consulted, or lobbied for.

The fact that the press ignored women's voices became even more evident when reading about one of the most tragic events in healthcare during the military administration. Only two months after the junta announced the suppression of the NHS, four children died in the neurosurgical department of the Children's Hospital, back then the most important facility specializing in pediatrics. The public opinion blamed the nursing staff on duty that day, namely nurses and *técnicos* (presumably nursing auxiliaries) for patient neglect. While nurses and midwives refused to tell their names, the questioned auxiliaries were not even interviewed to know their version of the facts.[109]

Finally, the tragic news from the Children's Hospital were some of the few traces to shed light on the professional life of nurses and nursing auxiliaries. One could expect that they blamed the state for the malfunction in the most prestigious sector of the healthcare system. But as seen in other interviews, commentators talked only about technical issues. That would change only in times of economic crises, when it became clear that the new system was not stable enough to fill the gaps the abolition of public social and medical services had left behind.

1.10 Crises: From Economic Pressure to Political Dissatisfaction

External factors helped the resistance movement to ripen. Early in the 1980s, Latin American countries were hit by sharp economic decline.[110] To cover the budget deficit, governments requested loans from abroad. However, by the end of the decade the debt of the subcontinent doubled.[111] State investment remained low, whereas dissatisfaction started to rise.

In Chile, the recovery phase after the economic slump between 1972 and 1977 came to a sudden end. As budget policy depended mainly on export, especially copper, the decline of the sales figures was disastrous.[112] In 1982, Chile's GDP shrank 14.3 percent, while the unemployment rate rose to 23.7 percent.[113] The regime defended cuts in public spending because of the "deep economic crisis."[114] Furthermore, economists who were close to the junta advised for devaluating Chile's currency, nationalizing bank houses, and decentralizing public companies.[115] To pay off the debts abroad, they used tax revenues and then asked for new loans.[116]

The crises affected all kinds of companies. Small entrepreneurs faced existential fear because of the four-year-long shrinking of the purchasing power. All this happened at the moment when (intents of) municipalization had already weakened and fragmented the economic potential of rural and suburban areas.[117] The Minimal Employment Program (*PEM*) for professionals was extended and complemented with a similar program for non-profesional workers, the Occupation Program for Heads of Household (*Programa de Ocupación para Jefes de Hogar*, *POJH*),[118]

The existing deficits in the provision of healthcare either remained acute or worsened because of the crises and the continued intervention on the welfare system. The situation seemed so alarming that, despite the repression, civilians were still willing to take the streets and demonstrate. In fact, the correspondence of the head of the *CNI* (successor organization of the *DINA*) suggests he was not positive about the Ministry of Health's managing of Santiago hospitals, where children suffered unnecessarily.[119]

It became commonplace that people were not willing to accept the dictatorship's plan to solve the crises. Unemployment, or even the fear to become redundant, led to the question of whether Pinochet's refounded state would really be the promised land for Chileans. In the following section, we will discuss the changes nurses faced during reforms and crises, and importantly, how this convoluted environment facilitated the emergence of new resistance movements within nursing and other professions.

2 Nursing the Welfare State

2.1 Poor Payment, Unemployment, and Struggling for Recognition

So far, we have shown the magnitude of changes in political, social, and economic life caused by the state reforms between 1979 and 1982. Some of these realignments did not address precisely academic training in nursing. Nevertheless, changes to auxiliary nursing training fed the reassessment of other health professions. To understand how severe the state interventions were for nursing, it is important to analyze first the number and the distribution of women and men who worked in hospitals and public health by the beginning of the 1980s.

Compared to the 1970s, the administration of the nursing workforce became well documented. This was especially so during the reform process, notably in an early stage, when the NHS became the NSHS. In the winter of 1980, the ministry ran a nationwide data query to assess human resources efficiency of the public system. Payroll and wages were sent to a central registry at the ministry, which helped set the staffing standards of the new NSHS. For the first time, all state-employed nurses, midwives, and social workers alongside physicians, dentists, and biochemists appeared on a single inventory.

Expectedly, most of the registered nurses (about 2500) worked in Santiago, Valparaíso, and Concepción, with a third of them based in the capital.[120] The cities with fewest nurses were in the northern regions; for example, the hospitals and healthcare centers of Tarapacá Region employed as few as 22 professional nurses.[121] But even the centrally located Maule Region, the fourth most populated, had only 174.[122]

Nurses were allotted across seven different grades (12 to 18, from a total of 36) of the Unified Salary Scale. But a striking finding is that 80 percent of them were in the three lowest grades. In checking throughout the first seven years since enforcement, no nurse was sitting at the highest third, as those were ranks reserved for the high bureaucracy, such as regional secretaries, and the beneficiaries of the Law No. 15.076, mostly physicians and dentists.[123] This was a form of embedded institutional discrimination which affected all female professions in the sector, and only one example of the disadvantageous treatment of the female workforce more broadly.[124] As already seen in previous chapters, the asymmetry between high-ranking professions and nurses was mirrored in wage as well as social differences between professional nurses and auxiliary staff. Archives show that a nurse in a hospital in the north of the country earned 11,738.57 *pesos* monthly, while a nursing auxiliary for the same number of weekly hours (probably even more) 6,706.06 *pesos*,[125] while a female hospital clerk earned 8,215.03 *pesos*,[126] all three of them employed at the exact same hospital.

The net salary of the staff within a single salary rank could differ as well. Additional bonuses were granted for specific services or missions, or temporary roles entrusted personally by managers to specific professionals. In 1980, high-profile nurse Peake was contractually registered as an administrative employee, not as a nurse, and earned the handsome amount of 94,000 *pesos*.[127] As she had no offspring and did not work in a rural area, that wage included no extra bonuses. Yet, it was the location of the workplace which provided the most profitable allowances. A physician in Punta Arenas, next to the Strait of Magellan in the far south, earned a base salary of around 47,000 *pesos*. But because of the location allowance, the salary would go up to 87,903.66 *pesos* monthly.[128] And still be below Peake's. Yet Peake was given a special treatment and her privileged contract was not representative of most nurses' material realities.

Another issue was employability. It is unclear how many nurses lost their jobs during the implementation stage of the healthcare reform, whereas nurse-historian R. Núñez, who published a study about nurses' working conditions in the 1970s and 1980s in Chile, reported many voluntary and involuntary dismissals arising from that process.[129] The testimonials she gathered seem to correlate with Salazar and Pinto's conclusion that the reform cost the jobs of some 100,000 healthcare workers from the public system. Even if the numbers may not be backed by primary sources, we can infer that a silent wave of redundancies affected nurses.[130]

However, the increasing number of redundancies was not the only problem nurses faced. In her speeches as the president of the *CECh*, Carmen Oye talked repeatedly about nurses being excluded from the policy-making process, an outcome of additional regulations for other professionals, notably physicians. She also talked about a loss of leading posts in health centers and hospitals and the shrinking political power that resulted from the legal inability of the *CECh* to control the profession.[131] Like other presidents, before and after her, she mentioned an overall shortage of personnel, infrastructure, and supplies in the sector, but she never seemed to attribute all this to the government's policies. As way of an example, in 1982 Oye referred to the negative consequences of municipalization for the working conditions of nurses, though she never formally proposed any alternatives.

Much as problems for the nursing community seemed to grow as the reform went on, the board's politically motivated behavior equated with self-sabotage. Indeed, the employment issue moved down in the list of priorities until the *CECh* board sided with the resistance movement in 1986.[132] Even the closing down of an independent nursing section in the public system, a very threatening outcome, did not even appear once on the agenda.[133] Likewise, such sensitive issue as the closure of nursing schools since 1977 was silenced. But then so was nursing's thinning institutionality.

Behind closed doors, though, things seem to have been talked about more openly. Repeatedly, the *CECh* board kept on complaining about the provisions granted to the physicians. More importantly, between 1979 and 1982 Peake and Oye attempted several times to meet with the highest administrative levels of the Ministry of Health, hoping to prove them wrong in the nursing policy. But every time, *FONASA* rejected their requests.[134]

Winning out in this critical situation, the *CECh* board would boast of success in another conflict. They claimed to have gained nurses' right to apply to some of the highest management ranks. Since 1979, most ward nurses had been under the rule of head physicians creating a technical hierarchy that mirrored a gender hierarchy. For Oye this was a loss of the "rational structure of nursing."[135] In her last speech as president, she informed about various letters she had sent to the Ministry of Health.[136] According to her, their plea was successful. Between 1981 and 1982, health minister Hernán Rivera Calderón agreed to enact a permanent directive (*Directiva Permanente No. 7*), which allowed again the appointment of head nurses in hospitals.[137] Furthermore, Oye encouraged him to appoint nurses in 93 health centers as supervisors of nursing auxiliaries.[138] It is not clear how many physicians respected this directive. In her study, Núñez states that in most cases medical directors neglected appointments for nurses or did not even know about the directive.[139] In the end, Oye's tactic proved highly successful in at least one goal—securing her own job as a head nurse at *Hospital J.J. Aguirre.*

Peake carried on with her work as a health policy lobbyist, and certainly the most influential nurse in public policy more broadly. After the NHS stopped operating, and its nursing section disappeared, she accepted a position in the central bureau of the Ministry of Health. Since 1981, Peake had been overseeing the ministry's efforts to control nosocomial infections. Her lack of expertise in that area—for 30 years, she had worked away from the clinic—suggests that Peake still was a protégée of the government. Büchi and minister Rivera praised her as:

> "skilled, honorable, with excellent interpersonal communication, and of a high professional quality."[140]

Peake still ran the *Enfermería* magazine and by this she controlled the official communication of nurses on the nationwide level. It would seem that she also sought to neutralize any sign of resistance, like the one surrounding the last election. In the course of the 1980s, she, in fact, introduced a content policy so that articles were aligned with the board's political leanings. The number of articles about corporate and social themes shrank, which turned the magazine into a rather technical publication.[141]

The two other nurses working at the former NHS office, Sofía Matus and Lidia Weitzel, were not dismissed either. Matus became the nursing representative in the restructuring commission of the Ministry of Health,[142] while Weitzel was hired in the human resources department[143] and led the Santiago branch of the *CECh*.[144] The career of Oye continued, too. She was still the regional counselor for La Serena and resumed her position at *Hospital J.J. Aguirre* chairing one of the largest nursing departments in the country.

But there was also Pincheira, still active in her 80s, though not in state politics. Her achievements for Latin American nurses in the 1950s and 1960s were not forgotten in Chile, nor in the WHO. Her strong but simple presence, along with her visions for a nationwide nursing policy, created a kind of cult around her person.[145] Assisted by Peake, she maintained the traditional relations with the UN, WHO, ILO, the International Council of Nurses, and the Pan-American Nursing Foundation.[146]

Pinochet's Chile did not hinder cooperation between the *CECh* and international organizations, including matters about labor. That is rather remarkable, because the government did not particularly hide their disdain for worker rights. The International Agreements About the Working Conditions of Nurses, a document published by ILO in 1979, recommended that governments enhanced collaboration with their nurses' organizations,[147] and offered governments a tool to implement the agreements.[148] Pinochet ratified none of them.[149] Given the political oppression, this is no surprise. Also, in 1979, he and his advisors imposed the legal basis to exclude the associations of professionals from political participation.

2.2 From Public to Private

On February 8, 1979, in the high summer, when people usually leave hot Santiago, Pinochet received the boards of the professional associations to discuss his reform plans. Peake was there on behalf of the nurses; one of the few women, perhaps even the only one, in this meeting. But gender was not a topic spoken of openly in those days. The label "professional" was then a neutral term but under male domain. However, most of the attendees felt they were valued as negotiation partners.[150] Peake's and Oye's political statement, documented in *Enfermería*, stands for nurses who also believed that negotiation was still an option. But they misunderstood Pinochet's behavior. In a brief mention soon after the meeting, Oye referred to conservative lawyer Julio Durán in *Enfermería* as follows:

> "There exists a mutual agreement to wake the colegios from their winter sleep, as our friend in combat, Mr. Julio Durán, president of the lawyers, expressed."[151]

Durán was a former presidential candidate (Radical Party, 1964) and president of the lawyers' association, a respected man and tolerated by the junta. Despite his background, it took the *CECh* board quite some time to open up about his speech in front of other fellow nurses. Only in the winter of that year *Enfermería* reported about the futile meeting with Pinochet and their solidarity with Durán. But that came too late. All professional associations had already received the order to be reorganized within 90 days as private associations.[152] Unable to refuse the order, Durán, Peake, and all the others who met with Pinochet, accepted the new terms with bitterness.[153]

Disenchantment was evident in nurses' change of tone. For seven years, the board members had been enthusiastic supporters of the junta and its nationalist discourse, and even accepted unfavorable governmental policy. In exchange, they bargained for better working conditions and more influence in health policy in the late 1970s economic crises. Then, while hitting another economic crisis, even Peake realized that the state reforms would actually terminate their professional autonomy. Disappointed, she wrote:

> "We will no longer be a part of a free guild system as associations often are."[154]

But the association had no choice. To avoid a complete ban, the board accepted all terms. On April 28, 1981, minister of the economy Rolando Ramos Muñoz received the *CECh*'s draft for the new statutes as a private association.[155]

The year 1981 marks really a change in the state administration of professional associations. From one moment to the other, the documentation of the Ministry of Health stopped tracking systematically this aspect of health policy—for nearly a decade the control of the board members had been a task of the ministry of the interior. As the healthcare reform unfolded, the health minister also lost the right to get involved in salary negotiations while overseeing the associations' finances moved to the ministry of economy.

Despite the magnitude of those changes, the Pinochet regime did not set up an entirely new system. It only enacted decrees which complemented the nursing laws from 1952 (NHS) and 1953 (*CECh*). However, the title of "nurse" was no longer required to be an academic degree and somewhat lost its political value.[156] That was probably the reason why Pincheira thought the whole nursing profession was in danger:

> "A new status, gearing towards new legal standards in order to replace law 11.161."[157]

Nevertheless, the associations would not have much else to do. It was the widest delivery of rights in Chilean nursing history, because accepting the legislation meant also accepting all previous measures since 1973.[158]

In March 1981, the new constitution came into force. A half year later, minister Ramos eventually signed off the remaking of the *CECh* as a private law body.[159] And with that, nurses saw the three-decade-long golden age of the associative movement crumble in front of their eyes.

We have seen how academically trained nurses, since the 1970s already in a struggle for survival, had to face more complications for their professional lives. Examples like those of Pincheira, Peake, Oye, or Weitzel have shown that at least the *CECh* board members survived all crises. But their colleagues had problems to stay or to ascend in professional life. More than that, the association of elite nurses, supposed to defend nurses' rights, continued to tolerate the national policies. And that caused political problems.

2.3 *The* CECh *Under Pressure*

Silence. That is what is found when one looks for reactions of nurses toward the changes which occurred between 1979 and 1981. Only the *CECh* board members wrote about their experiences and feelings, but as we have shown, they did so in a very cautious way. Surprisingly quickly, they moved on as if nothing extraordinary had happened.

In April 1982, the general council of the *CECh* held an extraordinary meeting to discuss future policies and elect the first board of the reformed association. Pincheira was 79 years old and Peake 72, and by then they had lived many lifetimes in their outstanding careers. Conversely, those who had recently joined nursing politics or proposed something like a policy for nursing were too young to have witnessed the dictatorship of Ibañez or the revolution in freedom of Frei. They seemed indeed too young to be heard.

But the board had to implement the new regulation. The law required from associations an election involving all members of the national and regional branches, as the new statutes were technically a constitutive act. It became the most extensive poll since the founding of the nurses' association, in 1953.[160] Sonia Garrido Ballerino, already in office between 1971 and 1973, became the first president of the reformed association. Oye went back to the *Hospital J.J. Aguirre*. Peake was no longer the general secretary, but in return, became the first vice secretary (*prosecretaria*).[161]

Everything was settled. But then, an incident boycotted the election. In her last speech as president, Oye said:

> "Despite the reporting done *publically* in the newspapers, trying to convince the public and our associates that the election has been stolen by the electoral commission [...]. [I can assure that] the electoral process has complied with all the required regulations."[162] (emphasis added)

By "reporting done publically in the newspapers" she was referring, reproachingly, to statements made by a group of nurses who were then making their entry into the public sphere as nurse leaders. These were Patricia Talloni, Patricia Grau, Margarita Reusch, and Alfredo Opgaard.

Grau told us in an interview that she learned about the elections from a newspaper and, together with some close friends from work, she decided to run for Santiago's regional council.[163] Talloni, who joined the group after the 1982 elections, explained to us her motivation to get in contact with them:

> "Most of us, nurses, didn't know about the elections from 1982. Later we noticed that as in the years before the regional council of Santiago held meetings regularly with representatives, elected by their peers, from health facilities. And so, we joined those meetings to get information and voice our concerns and problems. The president of this committee was a supporter of the dictatorship [Lidia Weitzel], so she had little or no intention to help us out. Her answer was always 'the law is the law.'"[164]

Grau, Opgaard and Reusch were convinced of the voter fraud. They were told that their list did not have enough votes to make it to the board. Their unrest was evident—Opgaard even spoke of a "non-transparent" and "manipulated" election,[165] terms that back then were uncommon when referring to nurses' business. The group of young nurses consulted *Vicaría de la Solidaridad* to receive legal assistance, where one of its lawyers advised them to make a public statement.

But the complaints of Talloni, Grau, Reusch, and Opgaard had no actual effect. For the election was confirmed and made official. Nevertheless, Oye's own statement suggests that the fraud claim was too serious to be ignored. Additionally, the board members were rather traditional in their doings and thus not used to facing oppositional groups or being challenged. Even less so in public. The worst part for them was that, though being defeated, the forty-years younger nurses stood united in their cause. Without realizing, the 1982 election would represent not only a turning point in the careers of the young activists but also a balance of powers in the history and political culture of nursing in the country.

On closer inspection, that group sought to increase their constituency base and convince others of the fraud claims.[166] They contacted other members of the regional councils, called them by landline phone, wrote them letters, or met them personally. These were lengthy and tiresome tasks in the early 1980s. But that seemed necessary to formalize the opposition front. Talloni explained it as follows:

> "As political parties were persecuted and decimated, and having in mind the number of violations and arbitrary decisions, this required mobilizing large social and political movements."[167]

Firstly, they met in the rooms of *Vicaría*. Later, in 1984, they met in their houses or in the facilities of the medical association and the agriculture engineers' association.

A key way of spreading resistance ideas among nurses and other health professionals was publishing in outlets like *Solidaridad*, *APSI*, *Hoy*, and *Fortín Mapocho*. Grau commented that other actions of resistance, especially those of the Association of Educators (*Asociación Gremial de Educadores de Chile*), inspired them. The group of schoolteachers became in the early 1980s a merger of opposition forces against the boards that were protected or appointed by the Pinochet regime.[168] While fellow campaigners did not mention other sources of inspiration, it was surely an array of ideas and representations about the eventual continuation of a pro-Pinochet board, and the dictatorship itself, which sowed the seed of resistance among other nurses.

The resisting nurses called themselves the Guild Renewal Movement (*Movimiento de Renovación Gremial, MRG*).[169] Their plan was, as they put it, to work for Chilean nurses and do better than the board had done. This aspiration involved further development of nursing and nurses' engagement in politics. *MRG*'s vision went beyond better working conditions. They regarded democracy as the bedrock value of Chilean society and their organization as a flag of resistance against the then decade-long dictatorial rule.[170]

Nevertheless, it was important for Talloni, Grau, Reusch, Opgaard, and their fellow campaigners that their mergers would not establish a parallel organization to the *CECh*. For that, they did not like the schoolteachers' strategy. Opgaard put it this way:

> "We did not want to be like a movement parallel to the association, but rather we were a group of individuals and professionals who wanted to shape the nurses' association differently."[171]

Nurses' *MRG* impacted on other professionals who were unhappy with the happenings in their associations. Similar groups formed across professional associations,[172] but they failed to engage their closest and critical veto players—the student organizations. Many of the leaders of the student movements did not come from medical faculties.[173] For that reason, one might assume that they organized their conferences and demonstrations in other faculties. If this was the case, then Talloni and her colleagues, like the members of the officiating boards, operated in isolation of the student movements.

Until 1986, the *MRG* remained weak, not only because they were "on training" but also because of the political culture in Chile. Whoever held power or sat in a position powerful enough to shape health policy most likely was from the generation of Talloni's parents, or grandparents even. The time was not ripe yet for fundamental changes. Like the civilian-military cooperation, the long-standing *CECh* board was still powerful enough to reject new ideas and to silence new voices. However, for the first time since 1973, the façade had crumbled. Peake needed to prove that everything was still under her control. She had to demonstrate this before the military junta, hoping that Pinochet and his circle would stop reducing nurses' rights. And she had to succeed in the most important conflict for nursing education, the survival of nursing schools in universities.

2.4 Dismantling Academically Trained Nursing

By the beginning of the 1980s, the menu of losses, problems, and conflicts in the nursing profession was manifold, but no other topic was as much discussed among nurses as the university reform and its consequences for nurses. It was demoralizing for nurses that, for the first time since 1953, nursing was no longer a profession of mandatory university-based training. Nurses felt that an academic degree was both a part of the mystique of their profession and an indication of scientific background. But academization was, too, a marker of social standing, which accounted for patterns of collective behavior. Drawing on Ayala's description of Chile's nursing model, we can conceptualize this as a process of "de-academization of nursing." For Pincheira, this was the second wave of de-academization.

During the 1940s, as a PAHO counselor she faced the shutdown of the nursing schools in the Dominican Republic, as decided by Gen. Rafael Trujillo. Like her efforts back then, 1980s Pincheira tried to protect academic training in Chile. In 1981, she proposed an alternative policy branded as a national study plan, alongside a plan for postgraduate degree courses. For her, the only way to impart nursing professionals "their historic and social role" was by doing full academic training.[174] Knowing that Chile's was the heaviest handed of military regimes, Pincheira probably never really thought claims like this would be heard. They were not.

Equally unhelpful were interventions of the *CECh* board members against the university reform. Oye and Peake threatened the government with canceling the celebrations of the International Nurses' Day, in 1981, perhaps aware that this was not going to be taken seriously. As can be expected, Pinochet and the health administrators simply ignored the threat. But celebrations still went ahead, where Oye tried to calm down the other nurses, assuring them that the relevance of academic training would be known and recognized sooner than later. She confidently claimed that the *CECh* board *was* going to persuade the government to change the course of events.

Oye looked for allies in other professional associations. And Peake, in universities. In the annual report for the period April 1980 to April 1981, it reads that the medical faculty of the University of Chile had confirmed it would not close its nursing school. The same guarantee, as they assured, had been given by University of Concepción.[175] Peake promised to make similar alliances with all other universities.[176] For this, she drew on Pincheira's vision. In collaboration with *ACHIEEN*, they proposed a core content program as well as an accreditation project for schools and training programs in nursing. In other words, the *CECh* aimed at having as much control over the profession as they did in the old days, were it not for the new regulation of associations as private entities that made nurses' affiliation optional.

The board failed already in this. A year after Peake announced triumphantly her conquering intervention at the University of Chile, she admitted that making deals with other universities was becoming a never-ending road full of disappointments. What is more, all those actions lacked the necessary legal basis, and so the National Audit Office refused them.[177] Even the University of Chile did not feel bound by their own promises. In fact, two of its three nursing schools were shut, one on the campus in the North and the other in the East of Santiago. Only its medical faculty in the

South of Santiago continued to train nurses.[178] By this, the number of graduates in this institution fell from 724 in 1980 to 448 in 1982.[179] That was the largest fall of nursing students since 1977 (see Chap. 3).

A similar change introduced around that time was the implementation of new curriculums for the remaining nursing schools. A comparison of the courses offered to nurses and midwives revealed one crucial element of state policy, that of aligning academic nursing to vocational training. One step was the suppression of social science classes,[180] which was one of the few subjects which laid a scientific foundation to trigger the development of nursing policies. An analysis of the lesson plan for the nursing students of the University of Chile for the 1980s demonstrates that the already meager contents about nursing history, labor rights, and professional ethics (compared to the midwifery profession) were entirely removed.[181] The same changes were introduced to all other public nursing schools,[182] and certainly to all other female academic professions.

Information is scant about other major universities, such as University of Concepción and the Catholic University in Santiago in this regard.[183] Yet such universities seemed to have less influence on health and nursing politics, studies, and reforms. Neither their medical faculties nor their nursing schools appeared in the archives of the Ministry of Health to the extent the public universities did. Also minor were the reactions about other private academic institutions in the print press and nursing publications.[184]

Shutting nursing schools in universities, despite the commitment of Peake and her colleagues, showed just how easy for the medical faculties was to close them altogether. The loss of the theoretical background was significant, as diminishing the contents weakens a profession technically and also politically. But the most urgent operation was to contact all universities and literally beg their directors and boards not to close their nursing schools. And, as we will explain in the following, this would also imply lobbying with regional authorities not to open further vocational institutes.

2.5 *The Vocational Threat*

PAHO supported governments to recruit more nursing auxiliaries. Nursing was since its inception a diverse field. People from different social backgrounds provided nursing care. Especially in hospitals, they formed nursing crews. Nevertheless, the reform process juxtaposed university-trained nurses to carers of less complex training within a logic of competition for relevance and employment.

In 1978, some 21,000 nursing auxiliaries worked in the public system. As in the previous administrations, top decision-makers did not see them as aids of but as a replacement for the professional workforce. Especially in rural areas policies relied on their work to increase coverage in primary care.[185] Regarding this, a reform authorizing training in private vocational institutes further de-academized the nursing profession in the view of the nurses.

And yet the conditions of training in all vocational institutes improved during the years of the reform. Aspiring nursing auxiliaries then had to complete a two-year study program. That was more than double the time compared to the 1970s, though the emphasis was on practical training just like university-based education. Bedside teaching represented two-thirds of the vocational training,[186] while in universities contents like sociology and ethics remained marginal.[187]

The rise of private institutes encountered strong resistance among professionals. Complaints by laboratory technicians (*tecnólogos medicos*) were accompanied by Peake's awful descriptions of nursing auxiliaries as "inferior competitors" and holders of an "insufficient training at unjustified costs."[188] The animosity was such that in 1979 the *CECh* board sent letters reprimanding the nurse lecturers of the institutes making them aware of their "misconduct."[189]

A movement of professional associations, with Peake probably taking the lead in 1980, intervened in the Ministry of Health and demanded that the government educated society about the differences between institute education and university training. Health undersecretary Cruz agreed to inform citizens through the print media that universities offered a "higher quality" of education,[190] however erroneous that claim was. But training at vocational institutes went on. Even Lidia Weitzel, who had become very influential in the Ministry of Health, could not convince Cruz to intervene in, what she called, the "unrest of the professional associations" about the private institutes. Plans for institutes' statute reform, elaborated together with Peake, were discussed but never implemented.[191] Institute-based training seemed unstoppable as the professionals' protests declined with time.

Once again, we have analyzed the struggle from the point of view of academically trained nurses. Simply the fact that nursing auxiliaries were not often asked their opinion led to an imbalanced argument when making the case of the nursing care needed. This imbalanced assessment anticipates the inequalities embedded in healthcare which become more salient in times of reform.

3 Conclusion

This chapter has shown how nurses reacted to and navigated a wave of different reforms in social policy, including the end of the NHS and the decentralization of the system. More importantly, they faced the enactment of a new political constitution within a national atmosphere of growing dissatisfaction toward Pinochet's dictatorial rule.

When the NHS ceased operating, it looked very different to what it once was, prestigious and powerful. Facing state repression, defenders of the old system like professional associations were ignored. However, this is but one aspect demonstrating that the nurses' association, and professional associations in general, represented only a small social elite. Powerful women at the nurses' board used to control many aspects of their profession and health policy that affected nurses. Furthermore, nursing auxiliaries' expanded training, just when nursing schools in universities closed, shows how social standing intersected with gender in the way nurses as stakeholders were perceived and treated when disagreements with the government rose. In fact, once the replacement of the professional workforce with nursing technicians began, there was no turning back. That was never negotiated or even meant to be negotiated.

Throughout the course of mere three years, from 1979 to 1982, the professional associations lost representation within public law. But they also found themselves in a cultural milieu so different from the one that once applauded their socially oriented ethos. They were now pressured to embrace the principles of an open economy and the work ethics that it carries. The few moments of protest were only an outcry of the professional associations that tended to vanish upon time.

Nevertheless, the reform process was lengthy and uneven, greatly hindered by economic crises from 1982. While politicians were busy deciding on the growing debts and unemployment, nurses as health professionals were the first witnesses of the economic downturn. The effects of the crises did not appear in *Enfermería*, nor in the letters sent by nurses to state authorities. It is probably because of the unabated political control the military junta exerted that we can now only read about vocational institutes and academic career debates, but not about existential crises. Becoming a nurse between 1979 and 1982 also meant to remain silent about structural problems. Or to say it out loud but risk confrontation.

A key premise in critical social science is that where there is power, there is resistance. Particularly, subservient obedience on the part of elite nurses triggered the rise of young nurses' movement within the association. Forty years younger than the board members, they challenged the status quo and wanted to change a culture they considered corrupt and incompatible with their ideal of democracy. On the administrative side, the outcome of their actions was not successful and the nursing association remained under Peake's control. And yet, the seemingly negative outcome of their renovated social movement in the 1982 election did not only test the young nurses' repertoire of action. It also fueled it.

Notes

1. Frei Ruiz-Tagle, Eduardo. Breaking into the Big Leagues: How to Continue the Chilean Miracle, in: *Harvard International Review* 32, No. 3, 2010, p. 12-15.
2. Chile and Brazil (1964–1985) were the only dictatorships in South America which tried to legalize their illegal governments with the implementation of a constitution, in: Agüero, Felipe: Los Civiles (la derecha) en la Repression, in: Represión en la Dictadura: El Papel de los Civiles, in: Nosotros los Chilenos 15, Santiago [LOM] 2005, p. 27.
3. Since 2021, Büchi has been a board member of *Banco de Chile*, one of the country's leading financial institutions, https://portales.bancochile.cl/nuestrobanco/es/gobierno-corporativo/directorio [2022-05-14].
4. Decreto Supremo No. 1.150, 24.10.1980, Texto de la Constitución Política de la República de Chile.

   The drafting of the constitution started already in October 1973, in: Ensalaco, Mark: Chile under Pinochet. Recovering the Truth, Pennsylvania [University of Pennsylvania Press] 2000, p. 133.
5. The plebiscite about the new constitution was sentenced without an electoral register or a ballot secrecy. The former president Jorge Alessandri was one of the authors of the first draft. The final version was elaborated by advisors of Pinochet who belonged to the *gremio* movement (Chaps. 1, 3), in: Bustos, Isidoro: Die Verfassung der Diktatur. Die Entwicklung der Grundrechte in Chile, Berlin [FDCL Verlag] 1987, p.102;

   The so-called Group of the 24, *Grupo de los 24*, addressed proposals and critics to the military junta to generate changes of the new constitution, in: Biblioteca Nacional de Chile: Grupo de Estudios Constitucionales, http://www.memoriachilena.gob.cl/602/w3-article-94389.html [13.05.2022].
6. Sucesos y opiniones, in: *Solidaridad*, No. 126, 15.-31.12.1981, 1981, p. 10-12 [1/4-3/4].
7. Bustos described the dictatorship in the following way: "a provisory government, commanded by the supreme commander of the army who named himself 'President of the Republic,'" in: Bustos (1987), p. 102.

8. Decreto Ley No. 2.448, 09.02.1979, Modifica regímenes de pensiones que indica;

   Decreto Ley No. 3.500, 13.11.1980, Establece nuevo sistema de pensiones.
9. Witte, Lothar: Die Entwicklung eines Modells: 20 Jahre Rentenreform in Chile, in: Chile Heute (2004), p. 417-432, 419.
10. ¿Quién gana y quién pierde? El Nuevo sistema de pensiones, in: *Solidaridad*, No. 108, 01-1981, p. 17 [1/3].
11. Biblioteca Nacional de Chile: Mujeres de Elite y Caridad, http://www.memoriachilena.gob.cl/602/w3-article-100704.html [22.05.2022].
12. The following decree laws were decisive for the implementation the new labor law:

    1. Decreto Ley No. 2.756, 03.07.1979, Establece normas sobre organización sindical;

    2. Decreto Ley No. 2.757, 04.07.1979, Establece normas sobre asociaciones gremiales;

    3. Decreto Ley No. 2.758, 06.07.1979, Establece normas sobre negociación colectiva.
13. Pérez Ahumada, Pablo: Why is it so Difficult to Reform Collective Labour Law? Associational Power and Policy Continuity in Chile in Comparative Perspective, in: *Journal of Latin American Studies*, Vol 53, No. 1, 2021, p. 81-105.
14. Quote: "personas naturales, jurídicas, o ambas, con el objeto de promover la racionalización, desarrollo y protección de las actividades que les son comunes, en razón de su profesión, oficio o rama de la producción o de los servicios, y de las conexas a dichas actividades comunes," in: Decreto Ley No. 2757, 04.07.1979, Establece normas sobre asociaciones gremiales.
15. Only one public criticism from the professional associations could be found. It was signed by the Confederation of Professional Associations, in: *El Mercurio*, 11.02.-17.02.1979, 11.02.1979, p. 7.
16. Quote: "los profesionales a quienes afecten tales normas pueden pactar libremente honorarios superiores o inferiores a los máximos o mínimos fijados en los aranceles que rijan la actividad de su profesión," in: Decreto Ley No. 2.516, 30.01.1979, Dispone normas sobre aplicación de los aranceles de honorarios de profesionales y exigencia de títulos para el desempeño de determinados cargos.
17. Five professions had predominantly female members. The government and the media referred to them only in marginal notes. For the leaders of the professions dominated by men, they served as an argument for their claims to speak for all professions. For example, in: S.E. designó comisión: Reestudiarán decreto de aránceles profesionales, in: *El Mercurio*, 04.02-10.02.1979, 08.02.1979, p. 1.

18. Quickly after the announcement, a commentator described the decree law as a "blitzkrieg" against the professionals, in: Por donde pecas pagas, in: Análisis, No. 32, 03-1981, p. 9-12 [1/5-5/5].
19. Decreto Ley No. 3.621, 07.02.1981, Fija normas sobre colegios profesionales;

    The basis for the abolition of the obligatory membership was Article 19 of the new constitution, which enshrined a general interdiction for every kind of obligatory membership, in: *Revista Chilena de Derecho*, Vol. 21, No. 1, 1994, p. 83-132, 84.
20. Member surveys undertaken in the associations of the physicians, social workers, civil engineers, dentists, lawyers, and technical engineers showed that a majority (88 to 95 percent) refused to change their statutes, in: Sucesos y opiniones, in: *Solidaridad*, No. 126, 15.-31.12.1981, 1981, p. 12 [4/4].
21. Asociaciones: unidad gremial a prueba, in: *Solidaridad*, No. 39, 01-1981, p. 5.
22. Gobierno: "Una realidad que no se va transar", in: El Mercurio, *El Mercurio*, 05.02.-11.02.1981, p. 6.
23. Colegios profesionales: unidad gremial a prueba, in: *Solidaridad*, No. 39-1981, 01-1981.
24. Navarro, Arturo: La rebellion de los Profesionales, in: APSI, No. 95, 24.03.-06.04.1981, p. 2-3 [3/6-4/6].
25. It would appear that *FENATS* became less important in the struggles about labor law. For the years 1979 to 1982, we only found only one mention in the documentation of the Ministry of Health. It was a criticism against the unsuccessful adaption of NHS employment contracts to the NSHS, in: Ministerio de Salud, Asesoría Jurídica: Min. Salud (O) No. 59, Mat. Descuentos en las remuneraciones del personal de los Servicios de Salud, 59-2423-1982, 07.01.1982, p. 1-2 [20-21/30];

    It appears that only the Confederation of Professional Associations was still a legitimate partner in negotiations with the Ministry of Health. See, for example, in: *El Mercurio*, 11.02.-17.02.1979, 11.02.1979, p. 7.
26. *El Mercurio*, 19.03.-25.03.1981, p. 6;

    Until 1986, the leadership of the teachers' association was in the hands of teachers who were loyal to the military junta. The first criticism against the government made by teachers in the media appeared in 1981 and did not represent the opinion of the board members, in: Navarro (1981), p. 2-3.

    The teachers who joined the resistance movement called themselves Command for Democratization (*Comando por la Democratización*), in: Guzmán (2012), p. 40.
27. It came to a dispute with the government about the validity of the members' votes, in: Sí, al Colegio, in: *Solidaridad*, No. 111, 15.-31.03.1981, p. 7 [2/2];

At first, Pinochet refused to talk with the professional associations. He entrusted the Minister of Justice, Mónica Madariaga (mandate: 1977-1983), his cousin, to deal with this task, in: *El Mercurio*, 29.03.1981, 26.03.-01.04.1981, p. 4.

28. S.E. recibió a presidentes de colegios, in: *El Mercurio*, 16.04.1981, 16.04.-22.04.1981, p. 4.
29. Ibid., p. 4.
30. Asociaciones: Colegios ratifican posiciones, in: *El Mercurio*, 09.05.1981, p. 6.
31. According to the consulted archives, it would seem that none of the professional associations were sentenced by the military junta. Therefore, we can say that all professional associations accepted the new terms.
32. Examples for criticism of professional associations not against the military junta but against their politics related to professionals:
    1. Detención de Luis Navarro, Triunfo de la Solidaridad, in: *Solidaridad*, No. 111, 15.-31.03.1981, S. 7 [2/2];
    2. Editorial. Transmisión e indiferencia, in: *APSI*, No. 95, 24.03.-06.04.1981;
    3. Navarro (1981), p. 2-3.
33. Arturo Navarro stated that the Chilean society ignored the struggle, in: Navarro (1981), p. 2-3.
34. Decreto con Fuerza de Ley No. 1-3063, 13.06.1980, Reglamenta aplicación iniciso segundo del artículo 38 del Decreto Ley No. 3.063 de 1979;

    The decree was described, in: *El Mercurio*, 13.06.1980, 12.06.-18.06.1980, p. 1.
35. Ibid, p. 1.
36. Licitación de los mercados, in: *Fortín Mapocho*, 07-1981.
37. Decreto Ley No. 3.477, 02.09.1980, Establece normas de carácter presupuestario, de administración financiera y de personal.
38. Miranda states that mayors were not elected but instated by the central government, in: Miranda R., Ernesto: Descentralización y Privatización del Sistema de Salud Chileno, in: La Salud en Chile [Ed. Miranda, Ernesto], Santiago 1994, p. 5-66, 49-50.
39. ¿Municipalizar o privatizar?, in: *Solidaridad*, No. 129, 1982, p. 11 [1/1].
40. Ibid., p. 64.
41. Ministerio de Salud, Oficina Minsal-BID: M.S. Ord No. 1609, Mat. Comunica adjudicación Licitación No. 4C-1/80, 1609-2244-1981, 18.02.1981, p. 1-6 [11-16/20];

    Responding to petitions of the mayors, the Ministry of Health justified the delay in the implementation process as a necessary break to analyze the impact of the measures in the previous months, in: Ministerio de Salud, Depto. de Planificación: Ord No. 3B/3991, Mat. Solicitud de traspaso de establecimientos, 3991-2448-1982, 20.07.1982, p. 1-1 [1/24].

42. Ministerio de Salud, Subsecretaría: Min. Salud, Ord. No. 2405, Mat. Convenio Fondo Nacional de Salud-Municipalidades para venta de órdenes de atención, 2405-2252-1981, 10.03.1981, p. 1-22 [8-29/29].
43. Quote: "La autonomía y la libertad académica no autoriza a las universidades para amparar ni fomentar acciones o conductas incompatibles con el orden jurídico, ni para permitir actividades orientadas a propagar, directa o indirectamente, tendencia político partidista alguna," in: Decreto con fuerza de Ley No. 1, 03.01.1981, Fija normas sobre Universidades.
44. Ley de Universidades. El saber entra al mercado, in: *Solidaridad*, No. 108, 01-1981, p. [3/3];

    Since 1983, a treasurer and a vice-rector formed with the director a new executive committee for the University of Chile. They were advised by a team of nine counselors, the so-called Board of Directors (*Junta Directiva*), appointed by the director since 1983. Each one of the ten faculties sent a representative, in: Autoridades superiores de la Universidad de Chile, in: Anales de la Universidad de Chile, No. 4, 03-1984, p. 9-15;

    As in the case of the University of Chile, the biggest and most important technical college in Santiago was reduced to its faculties in the capital and was named University of Santiago (*Universidad de Santiago*), in: Decreto con Fuerza de Ley No. 23, 15.04.1981, Sustituye denominación de la Universidad Técnica del Estado;

    In 1981, the *Solidaridad* quoted a study from the oppositional think tank *FLACSO*. Their authors criticized that, different to the guaranteed freedom of education, state surveillance continued. Since 1973, the delegated directors only reported to the Pinochet regime. Furthermore, *FLACSO* suspected a continuous wave of redundancies because of the new legislation, in: *Solidaridad*, No. 108, 01-1981, Ley de Universidades. El saber entra al mercado, p. [3/3];

    The dismissal of teaching staff because of political engagement, common practice since September 1973, became legal. Even the governments beyond dictatorship would have to deal with the decision to dismiss an employee in case of "engagement as a political activist" (participación como activista político), like in this case from the Education Ministry, in: Ministerio de Educación, Universidad de Chile: Oficio No. 2516, Materia. Informa Situación Funcionaria de Eduardo Núñez Madrid, 2516-48284-1980, 08.08.1980, p. 1-1 [1/18].
45. Pinedo Castro, Francisco Javier: El Nacimiento de una Universidad en el Valle Central y la Amputación de las Sedes Regionales de la Universidad de Chile: El Caso de la Universidad de Talca, in: *Revista Anales*, Vol. 7, No. 4, 2012, p. 57-79, 72.

46. The liberalization of the finance policy began in 1981. One year before, the project was presented in a solemn ceremony, also attended by the vice president of the finance department of Harvard University and the US-American ambassador, in: Financiamiento Universitario: El Sector Privado debe participar, in: *Revista de la Universidad de Chile*, No. 167, 21.08.1980, p. 1 [1/2-2/2];

    In a parallel process, all employees had to adapt their employment relationship to the new legislation, including a recalculation of every salary according to the Unified Salary Scale of the state or to a private employer, in: *El Mercurio*, 23.01.1980, p. 4;

    In case of the most important institution in charge of training health professionals (Chap. 3), the medical faculty of the University of Chile in North Santiago, those agreements could be traced for the first time in 1981, which means right after the implementation of the reform. The agreements set the regulations about how many students, university professors, professionals, and auxiliary workers of the university–owned Hospital J.J. Aguirre could practice dental treatment, vaccination, and the care of pregnant women and newborn children. They also defined the invoicing procedure for those treatments, in: Ministerio de Salud, Asesoría Jurídica: Ord No. 743, Mat. Convenio de atención de beneficarios del Servicio de Salud Metropolitano Norte con la Universidad de Chile, 743-2236-1981, 26.01.1981, p. 1-13 [18-30/39].
47. Obreque, Williams; Andrés, Guido: Régimen Jurídico de las Universidades Privadas de Chile, Santiago [Biblioteca del Congreso Nacional de Chile] 2014, p. 4-7.
48. Only three of the new private universities were accredited by the government, in: Zurita P., Matías; Brzovic Y., Daniel: Un paso al frente. Una historia del Frente Patriótico Manuel Rodríguez (FPMR), Santiago [Universidad de Chile] 2010, p. 133.
49. In 1980, for the first time, a health minister reported a job shortage in the public healthcare system: Ministerio de Salud: Min. Salud, No. 0134, Campo acupacional de los profesionales de salud, 2091-0134, 22.01.1980.

    For example, the number of job offers in the public health system for midwives shrank in 1979, in: Ministerio de Salud: M.S. Ord No. 1337, Mat. Presentación de 4 de junio de 1979, Matronas egresadas, 1337-2028-1979, 20.07.1979, p. 1- 9 [74-82/108].
50. The number of registered students fell from 20,669 to 17,405 between 1980 and 1982. This decrease of 16 percent was imposed on almost every faculty of the University of Chile. Exceptions were the numbers of students in mathematics, chemistry, physics, and pharmacy and a even more drastic reduction of the architecture students (1563 to 773) in the same time span, in: Actas de la Junta Directiva de la Universidad de Chile, 1982, 1-17.

An article that appeared in the university's bulletin explained that the cuts in state funding affected the enrolment numbers. The universities had to decide by themselves the number of professionals they wanted to employ. Same for the number of students, in: Velasco Rayo, Carmen: Formación de Recursos Humanos en el Area de la Salud y Educación continuada, in: *Revista de la Universidad de Chile*, No. 152, 15.03.1979, p. [1/8-4/8].

51. The following professions continued to have only an academic curriculum:
    a) Biochemist (Licenciado en Bioquímica)
    b) Dental surgeon (Licenciado en Odontología)
    c) Physician (Licenciado en Medicina)
    d) Veterinarian (Licenciado en Medicina Veterinaria).
    e) Psychologist (Licenciado en Psicología)
    f) Pharmacist (Licenciado en Farmacia), in: Decreto con Fuerza de Ley, No. 03.01.1981, Fija normas sobre Universidades.
52. Called as such because they were meant to "professionalize" manual workers and de facto technicians as the country industrialized. Secondary schools offering different paths of technical training arose from the same process.
53. *Solidaridad* did not mention the job shortage. Only *Hoy* published precise criticisms, in: El "no" de las bases, in: *Hoy*, No. 111, 05.-11.09.1979, p. 22 [2/2].
54. As per some accounts, the first vocational institute began to operate back in 1906, in: Rivera, Anny: Educación técnico-profesional privada: Atajo dudoso pero honorable, in: *APSI*, No. 96, 07.04.-04.1981, p. 2-4 [1/4-4/4];

    Documents found in the archive of the Ministry of Health suggest that the catholic church trained healthcare auxiliaries already before the reform took place. The first accreditation of training by one of its institutes we could find dates back to 1981, in: Ministerio de Salud: M.S. Ord No. 335, Mat. Formación de Auxiliares de Enfermería, 335-2232-1981, 15.01.1981, p. 1-1 [7/9].
55. Las transformaciones educacionales bajo el régimen militar, in: Programa interdisciplinario de investigación en educación, Vol. 1, Santiago [PIIE] 1984, p. 205.
56. Ministerio de Salud: M.S. Ord. No. 1086, Control de instituciones capacitadoras de personal paramédico, 1932-1086, 04.05.1976.
57. In 1977, *PROPAM* offered training for some 400 students in three cities (Santiago, Viña del Mar, and Antofagasta), mostly in agriculture. For Rocha, this was only the beginning. In an interview published by *Hoy*, he talked about his plans to create a university and even open a hospital in partnership with the health and education ministries, in: Cursos. El examen de los institutos, in: *Hoy*, Año 1, No. 2, 08.-14.06.1977, p. [7/7];

Rocha claimed that he already received permit notice from somewhere in Ohio (US) and from the Federal Republic of Germany. We found no evidence for this statement (2022).

58. Example for an attempt of Gerardo Rocha to receive a state recognition for his training programs for nursing auxiliaries, in: Ministerio de Salud, Depto. Recursos Humanos: M.S. Ord No. 1904, No autoriza lo solicitado por *PROPAM* de acuerdo a Circular No. 118/78, 1904-1997-1978, p. 1-1 [39-81].
59. Cursos. El examen de los institutos, in: *Hoy*, No. 2, 08.-14.06.1977.
60. Quote: [...] "este Ministerio estima no procedente la autorización de estas personas, cuyas carreras pseudo médicas sólo tienden a producir confusiones con las carreras existentes y problemas con los colegios profesionales," in: Ministerio de Salud Pública, Secretaría Ejecutiva Comisión Mixta: M.S. Ord No. 2091, Mat. Programas de Formación de Personal del Área de Salud, 2091-1998- 1978, 28.11.1978, p. 1-3 [55/57-57].
61. Cruz Mena, health undersecretary, approved at least for one institute a training program for nursing auxilairies, in: Ministerio de Salud, Depto. Recursos Humanos: M.S. Ord No. 509, Mat. Autorizaciónpara curso de Auxiliares que se efectúa en el Instituto Zipter, 509-2024-1979, 22.03.1979, p. 1-2 [11/12-33];

    In 1977, he decided not to ban them, despite "operation anomalies," because of "hundreds of thousands in the need of training in order to improve their own living," in: Cursos. El examen de los institutos, in: *Hoy*, Año 1, No. 2, 08.-14.06.1977, p. [5/7].
62. After the rejection of his training offers, Rocha founded a new kind of holding, probably to valorize his concepts and methods. He called the company the Rocha Corporation for Development and Culture (*Corporación Rocha para el Desarrollo de la Educación y la Cultura, CREDUC*). It included *PROPAM*, the Chiropody Institute Gastonia College (*Instituto de Podología Gastonia College, CIDEC*), the Institute of the Worker *(Instituto del Trabajador*), and the *Fundación Opus Vitae*, obviously all directed by himself, in: Educación técnico-profesional privada: Atajo dudoso pero honorable, in: *APSI*, No. 96, 04-1981, p. 3 [3/4];

    To initiate his training programs Rocha applied for a accreditation from the education minitsry, in: Ministerio de Educación: Anexo No. 1, Coloca organización y medios Fundación Opus Vitae a disposición Ministro de Educación, 1-48284-1980, 17.06.1980, p. 1-5 [2-6/18];
63. Especially the launch of new healthcare centers in rural areas was planned with auxiliary nurses in the first place, in: Ministerio de Salud, Oficina de Asuntos Internacionales, Dr. Juricic T., Jefe Oficina Asuntos Internacionales: No. 1950, Mat. Se solicita la asesoría técnica de dos enfermeras, 1950-1997-1978, 08.11.1978, 1-1 [25-81].

64. Even the nurses could not deny that they needed auxiliary nurses in order to meet the requirements in the services they offered, in: Ravera P., Enfermera, Div. Ciencias Médicas Occidente, U. de Chile, Servicio de Cirurgía, Hospital San Juan de Dios et al.: Factores de Variación en Ausentismo de Personal, in: Enfermería, Nos. 84-85, 04-09-1985, p. 53–60, 53.
65. One of the results of the nursing topics discussed in the PAHO conference of 1982 was the recognition that the expansion of nursing services was only possible by expanding nursing auxiliaries' availability and increasing their education level, in: La Enfermería en América Latina, in: *Enfermería*, No. 76, 04-05-06-1983, p. 6.
66. Decreto con Fuerza de Ley No. 5, 16.02.1981, Fija Normas sobre Institutos profesionales;

    A precise description of the procedure: Estado tendrá institutos profesionales, in: *El Mercurio*, 14.02.1981, p. 8.
67. In 1981, *APSI* magazine reports about the opening of 30 new vocational institutes only in the metropolitan area of Santiago "within the last years." The state administration would approve once they fulfilled three conditions: registration process due to the internal revenue system, provision of an adequate infrastructure, and fulfillment of the sanitary standards, in: Rivera (1981), p. 2-4.
68. The education and Ministry of Health supervised training programs in podiatry, laboratory assistance, cosmetics, and optics only for the final examen, not during the training phase, in: Ministerio de Salud, Depto. Recursos Humanos: Min. Salud (O) No. 631, Mat. Informe de Salud sobre carreras solicitadas por Institutos Formadores, 631-2426-1982, 28.01.1982, p. 1-3 [15-17/17].
69. Ministerio de Salud: M.S. Ord No. 1937, Egresados en el año 1980 de cursos de formación y nivelación de auxiliares paramédicos, 1937-2248-1981, 26.02.1981, p. 1-2 [1-2/2].
70. Interviews with Teresa Aburto (medical-laboratory auxiliary) and Ivette Cap de Ville (nursing auxiliary), Santiago, March 2016.
71. In 1978, the Ministry of Health set up a commission formed by members of the medical association and employees of the University of Chile, which was meant to determine an extension of the work profile of nursing auxiliaries, in: Ministerio de Salud, Jefe de Gabinete: Ord No. 1868, Mat. Preparación Programa Ministerial 1978, Sector Salud, 1868-1963-1977, 13.10.1977, p. 1-22 [39/60-92].
72. Ministerio de Salud, Asesoría Jurídica: Ord No. 0352, Mat. Contratación como Médicos de Auxiliares Técnicos, 0352-1989-1978, 05.03.1978, p. 1-2 [5/6-26].

73. Ministerio de Salud, Depto. Apoyo a los Programas Química y Farmacia: M.S. Ord No. 0333 Mat. Descripción funciones de Auxiliares de Farmacia, 0333-1989-1978, 13.03.1978, p. 1-5 [9/13-26].
74. Ministerio de Salud: M.S. Ord No. 1937 Egresados en el año 1980 de cursos de formación y nivelación de auxiliares paramédicos, 1937-2248-1981, 26.02.1981, p. 1-2 [1-2/2].
75. This statement was also formulated by Bustamante et al. They found evidence for similar healthcare reforms in Colombia and Mexico, in: Bustamante, Arturo Vargas; Méndez, Claudio A.: Healthcare privatization in Latin America: Comparing Divergent Privatization Approaches in Chile, Colombia, and Mexico, in: *Journal of Health Politics, Policy and Law*, Vol. 39, No. 4, 2014, p. 841-886, 851;

    Labra and Marchiori Buss (1995) accused "radicalism" of the cuts on public healthcare compared to similar policies in Spain, Argentina, Brazil, US, Mexico, and the Canadian province of Quebec, in: Labra, María Eliana; Marchiori Buss, Paulo: Introdução, in: Sistemas de Saúde: continuidades e mudanças [Ed. Labra, María Eliana & Marchiori Buss, Paulo], São Paulo-Rio de Janeiro [Hucitec] 1995, p. 9-28, 25.
76. Miranda (1994), p. 5-66, 34.
77. Chanfreau (1979), p. 94.
78. Traslado se hará en dos etapas – Hospital San Borja al Paula Jaraquemada, in: *El Mercurio*, 25.11.1976, p. 5.
79. Ministerio de Salud: Ord No. 397, Mat. Solicita proposición que indica, 397-2233-1981, 16.01.1981, p. 1-1 [1/10].
80. Decreto Ley No. 2.763, 03.08.1979, Reorganiza el Ministerio de Salud y crea los Servicios de Salud, el Fondo Nacional de Salud, el Instituto de Salud Pública de Chile y la Central de Abastecimiento del Sistema Nacional de Servicios de Salud.
81. Furthermore, two other institutes were founded, the National Institute of Public Health (*Instituto Nacional de Salud Pública*), a health department to control sanitary standards, occupational safety, and so on, and *CENABAST*, a logistic center to provide construction and equipment in: Ministerio de Salud: Decreto No. 296, Aprueba el Reglamento Del Ministerio de Salud, 296-2011-1979, 10.09.1979, p. 1-15 [1/15-34].
82. Labra, Maria Eliana: La reinvención neoliberal de la inequidad en Chile: el caso de la salud, in: *Cad. Saúde Pública*, Vol. 18, No. 4, 2002, p. 1041-1052, 1046.
83. Miranda (1994), p. 37;

    In 1978, the Ministry of Health confirmed that the upcoming reform was inspired by the System of Free Election, in: Ministerio de Salud, Jefe de Gabinete: Ord No. 1868, Mat. Preparación Programa Ministerial 1978 - Sector Salud, 1868-1963-1977, 13.10.1977, p. 1-22 [39/60-92];

Those who had a certain income received a *Medicina Curativa* pass (*Carnet de Medicina Curativa*), in: Ministerio de Salud, Subsecretaría: Min.Salud (O) No. 2405, Mat. Convenio Fondo Nacional de Salud-Municipalidades para venta de órdenes de atención, 2405-2252-1981, 10.03.1981, p. 1-22 [8-29/29].

84. The major difference was that the salaries were no longer managed by the centralized NHS, but, for example in the case of the Hospital J.J. Aguirre, by the University of Chile, according to its contract with the NSHS of North Santiago, in: Actas de la Junta Directiva, Sesiones 61-75, 1984, Sesión 65a, Exposición del Director del Hospital José Joaquín Aguirre, p. 2-47, 11.
85. Example of the privatization of a public health facility in central Santiago, in: Ministerio de Salud, Asesoria Jurídica: M.S. Ord No. 1395, Mat. Autorización de conenio con la Corporación Privada de Desarollo Social con el Servicio de Salud Metropolitano Central, 1395-2242-1981, 10.02.1981, p. 1-3 [5-7/7];

    Example of the transmission of healthcare to a church-owned institution: The contract of the *Fundación Hospital Parroquial De San Bernardo* with the NSHS in the South of Santiago, in: Ministerio de Salud, Secretaría Ministerial Regional, Asesoría Jurídica: Ord. No. 90, Mat. Convenio entre Fundación Hospital Parroquial de San Bernardo y Servicio Salud Sur, 90-2238-1981, 14.01.1981, p. 1-8 [2-9/9].
86. Ministerio de Salud, Subsecretaría: Min.Salud (O) No. 2405, Mat. Convenio Fondo Nacional de Salud-Municipalidades para venta de órdenes de atención, 2405-2252-1981, 10.03.1981, p. 1-22 [8-29/29].
87. The public pharmacies of the urban sector of Maipú, in: Aumentan las enfermedades infecto-contagiosas, in: *APSI*, No. 95, 24.03.-06.04.1981, p. 8-9 [5/6-6/6].
88. In March 1981, Büchi informed the director of *FONASA* about the corporations agreed between private companies and the NSHS pinnacles since November 11, 1980—eight new contracts had been signed. One of the new partners was the German sect Colonia Dignidad in the region of Maule. It was the only one of the eight organizations ran predominantly by foreigners. Twenty-three already existing contracts (*convenios*) were prolonged. Three of them had no private origin. They pertained to the Chilean Army and Carabineros, the Red Cross, and the Catholic University in Santiago. The conventions mainly defined the status of hospitals and healthcare centers in Santiago, but also in the regions of Maule and Valdivia, as well as in some areas in the North and South (i.e., La Serena, Araucanía and Puerto Montt). Generally, the state was represented by an authority of one of the 27 NSHS. Only in one of the eight cases a hospital, the Psychiatric Hospital of Santiago, autonomously signed a contract with a private company, in:

Ministerio de Salud: Min. Salud (O) No. 2356, F.M.S. Mat. Convenios, 2356-2252-1981, 09.03.1981, p. 1-6 [2-6/29].

89. The statements of several mayors, stored in the archive of the Ministry of Health during the 1980s, proved that only some urban areas executed the new rules before 1987. Even the basic program for the NSHS, which included the consultation of a physician or his visit in case of inability to leave home, involving the staff of public health centers, could not be provided in the poor sectors of the country. Another important component of a medical treatment, the second opinion of a physician in case of a difficult diagnosis, existed mostly just on paper. Office hours in ophthalmology and psychiatry were only accessible in urban areas and sometimes only in private clinics, in: Ministerio de Salud, Subsecretaría: Min.Salud (O) No. 2405, Mat. Convenio Fondo Nacional de Salud Municipalidades para venta de órdenes de atención, 2405-2252-1981, 10.03.1981, p. 1-22 [8-29/29].
90. Ministerio de Salud: Min.Salud (O) No. 2357, Mat. Convenio Colonia Dignidad, 2357-2252-1981, 09.03.1981, p. 1-1 [6/29];

    The subsidy was reduced to 8.4 million *Pesos* in January 1982, in: Ministerio de Salud, Asesoría Juridíca: M.S. Ord No. 145, Mat. Comunica aprobación de convenio que indica, para regir en 1982, 145-2423-1982, 12.01.1982, p. 1-1 [30/30].

    Decreto Ley No. 2.763, 03.08.1979, Reorganiza el Ministerio de Salud y crea los Servicios de Salud, el Fondo Nacional de Salud, el Instituto de Salud Pública de Chile y la Central de Abastecimiento del Sistema Nacional de Servicios de Salud.
91. Decreto con Fuerza de Ley No. 3, 19.05.1981, Fija normas para el otorgamiento de prestaciones y beneficios de salud, por instituciones de Salud previsional.
92. The state contribution to public health budget had declined from 50 percent in 1980 to 40 percent in 1990, while the beneficiaries' share had increased from 36 percent to 47 percent, in: Manuel, Annik: The Chilean health system: 20 years of reforms, in: Salud Pública Mex, Vol. 44, No. 1, 2002, p. 60-68, p. 65.
93. González Toro, Nicolás; Infante Barros, Antonio: Programas de Alimentación Complementaria del Sector Salud en Chile, in: *Boletín de la Oficina Sanitaria Panamericana*, Vol. 89, No. 6, 1980, p. 565;

    In addition to that, there were about 20,000 nursing auxiliaries and other auxiliary workers. Furthermore, there was the non-medical staff like drivers, housekeepers, security guards, and so on.
94. Ministerio de Salud, Depto. de Planificación: M.S. Ord No. 498, Mat. Evaluación AREAS/UOS, 498-2024-1979, 20.03.1979, p. 1-3 [16/18-33].

95. Ministerio de Salud, Comisión Central de Reestructuración: Ord No. 2008, Mat. Encasillamiento, 2008-2031-1979, 15.10.1979, p. 1-4 [42-45/64].
96. It is probably because of the job shortage that the Ministry of Health allowed the NSHS of Talca to re-employ dismissed healthcare professionals, in: Ministerio de Salud, Depto. Recursos Humanos: M.S. Ord No. 2679, Mat. Responde consultas formuladas por el Consejo Técnico de la Región del Maule, 2679-2255-1981, 17.03.1981, p. 1-1 [6/8].
97. Labra (2002), p. 1045.
98. Greve (2001), p. 69.
99. Salazar, Gabriel; Pinto, Julio: Historia Contemporánea De Chile IV. Hombría y Feminidad - Gabriel Salazar y Julio Pinto, Santiago [LOM] 2002, p. 195.
100. Ministerio de Salud, Asesoría Jurídica: Circular No. 3, Instrucciones relativas a indemnización especial establecida por la letra E) del artículo 29 del Decreto Ley No. 2879, de 17 de octubre de 1979, 3-2081-1980, 11.01.1980, p. 1–3.
101. Only for the already mentioned private healthcare provider Paula Jaraquemada a job shortage was found in the department of internal medicine, in: Ministerio de Salud, Servicio Salud Central: Ord No. 629, Mat. Becados en Medicina Interna 1981, Hospital Paula Jaraquemada, 629-2236-1981, 04.12.1980, p. 1-1 [1/39].
102. For example, complaints about the health reform, written by a delegation of the nursing staff of the *Hospital Clínico Regional de* Concepción, in: Ministerio de Salud, Asesoría Jurídica: M.S Ord No. 0146, Mat. Situación de las Sras. Hilda Vera Placencia y Helia Arriagada, funcionarias del Hospital "Dr. Guillermo Grant Benavente," de Concepción, 0146-2249-1981, 20.02.1981, p. 1-5 [1-5/8].
103. Ministerio de Salud, Asesoría Jurídica: Decreto No. 30, Modifica Decreto Supremo No. 110 de 1963, Reglamento de la Ley 15.076, 30-2339-1982, 23.02.1982, p. 1-8 [1-8].
104. Only *Solidaridad* reported that during the first six months 15,000 schoolteachers and an unidentified number of employees of the public system of Santiago (referred to as "numerous") had been dismissed, in: Sucesos y Opiniones, in: *Solidaridad*, No. 126, 15.-31.12.1981, 1981, p. 10 [1/4].
105. Report of the *Solidaridad*: The companies received the legal means to end employment contract because of "necessities of the company." This was not applicable for the employment contracts concluded before the publication of decree law No. 2.200 (Chap. 3), in: Nuevas Normas laborales. El contrato de Trabajo, in: *Solidaridad*, No. 118, 15.-31.08.1981, p. 8 [1/2].

106. The names of some peaceful opposition groups can be found in: Corporación de Estudios Nacionales, Grupo de los 24, Los 8, Nueva Democracia, in: *El Mercurio*, 22.03.1981, 19.03.-25.03.1981, p. 4;

   Also at the beginning of the 1980s, violent resistance became a serious problem for the government: Between 1977 and 1981, the number of terrorist attacks against state institutions and transportation facilities increased from 15 to 212 per year, in: Ensalaco (2000), p. 147.
107. Monreal was also a member of the Health Circle of the Academy of Christian Humanism. That was another think tank of the Catholic Church. However, the most important one during the 1980s was *Vicaría de la Solidaridad*.
108. In 1980, social workers were mentioned for the first time in *Solidaridad*, but not representing any kind of labor organization, in: Mujeres: conquistar la dignidad, in: *Solidaridad*, No. 105-1980, 15.-31.11.1980, p. [1/2].
109. According to the interview partners of *Hoy*, the neurosurgical department of the Children's Hospital was in the early 1970s one of the ten best in the world. At the end of the decade, it has disappeared from all rankings. The authors of *Hoy* also used this dramatic incident to criticize the deficient equipment of the neurosurgical department. Examples were the lack of a computer tomograph or the shortage of sheets for the beds, in: Salud. Los muertos en Neurocirurgía, in: *Hoy*, No. 115, 03.-09.10.1979, p. 18 [2/6].
110. Bustamante, Arturo Vargas; Méndez, Claudio A.: Healthcare Privatization in Latin America: Comparing Divergent Privatization Approaches in Chile, Colombia, and Mexico, *Journal of Health Politics Policy and Law*, Vol. 39, No. 4, p. 841-884, 843;

   Nohlen and Thibaut compared the economic crises of 1982–1986 with the Great Depression of 1929–1933 in North America and Europe, in: Nohlen, Dieter; Thibaut, Bernhard: Trotz alledem: Demokratie – Zur politischen Entwicklung Lateinamerikas in den neunziger Jahren, in: Lateinamerika am Ende des 20. Jahrhunderts [Ed. Junker, Detlef, Nohlen, Dieter, Sangmeister, Hartmut], München [Beck] 1994, p. 235-261, 248;
111. Sangmeister, Hartmut: Verschuldung und soziale Schuld, in: Chile heute, München [Vervuert] 1994, p. 104-123, 105.
112. The Economy is bad, but 1982 was worse, in: New York Times, 20.01.2009.
113. Thibaut, Bernhard: Soziale Entwicklung und Demokratie in Lateinamerika zu Beginn der neunziger Jahre, in: Lateinamerika am Ende des 20. Jahrhunderts, 1994, p. 124-148, 131.

114. Presidente Pinochet anunció: Disminuición del gasto público para enfrentar la recesión, in: *El Mercurio*, 11.03.-17.03.1982, p. 8.
115. Biblioteca Nacional de Chile: Crisis económica 1982, http://www.memoriachilena.gob.cl/602/w3-article-98012.html [2022-05-13].
116. Sangmeister (1994), p. 110-111.
117. *Fortín Mapocho*, No. 76, 02-1982.
118. The Program of Minimal Employment existed since 1974 (Chap. 3) and the Program for the Head of the Household until 1982.
119. Labra (2002), p. 1045.
120. For example West and North Santiago, places of some of the largest hospitals in the country:

 1. West-Santiago: Ministerio de Salud: Decreto No. 325, Encasilla a Funcionarios del Servicio de Salud de Metropolitano - Occidente, 325-2055-1980, 31.07.1980, S. 1–26.;

 2. North Santiago: Ministerio de Salud: Decreto No. 0320, Encasilla a Funcionarios del Servicio de Salud de Metropolitano - Norte, 0320-2056-1980, 31.07.1980, p. 1–35.
121. This information results from two documents:

 1. Ministerio de Salud: Decreto No. 0332, Contrata a Funcionarios del Servicio de Salud de Iquique, 0332-2057-1980, 31.07.1980, p. 1–13;

 2. Ministerio de Salud: Decreto No. 0305, Encasilla a Funcionarios del Servicio de Salud de Iquique, 0305-2052-1980, 31.07.1980, p. 1–3.
122. This information results from two documents:

 1. Ministerio de Salud: Decreto No. 340, Contrata a Funcionarios del Servicio de Salud de Maule, 340-2058-1980, 340-2058-1980, p. 1–7;

 2. Ministerio de Salud: Decreto No. 313, Encasilla a Funcionarios del Servicio de Salud de Maule, 313-2053-1980, 31.07.1980, p. 1–14.
123. The Unified Salary Scale is valid until today (May 25, 2022).
124. Further information about the unequal treatment of women in employment, in: Zárate (2013), p. 145.
125. An example of a salary of a nurse (Sara Hammad Torres), in: Ministerio de Salud, Servicio de Salud Coquimbo, IV Región: Ord. No. 411, Mat. Informa Solicitud de Desahuicio de D. Sara Hammad Torres, 411-2249-1981, 27.01.1981, 1-1 [8/8];

 An example of the salary of nursing auxiliaries. In this special case for the Region of Coquimbo, in: Ministerio de Salud, Servicio de Salud Coquimbo, IV Región: Ord No. 371, 371-2246-1981, 23.01.1981, p. 1-1 [5/5].
126. Ministerio de Salud, Servicio de Salud Coquimbo, IV Región: Ord No. 366, Mat. Informa solicitud de desahúcio de D. María Pilar Vega Mallea, 366-2247-1981, 23.01.1981, p. 1-1 [1/20].

127. Ministerio de Salud: Decreto No. 599, Contrata Sobre la Base de Honorarios, Suma alzada, A.D. Gladys Peake Guevara, 599-2068-1980, 31.12.1980, p. 1-5 [1-5].
128. As Punta Arenas is in one of the most distant areas of the country, as seen from Santiago, health professionals working there received the highest salaries. For the physicians it meant a 60 percent extra payment due to the incentive allocation *(asignación estímulo)* and another 35 percent due to the incentive professional allocation (*asignación estímulo funcionario*). One example is the contract of the physician Eric Román: Ministerio de Salud: Resolución No. 048 Contrato para D. Eric Román Carasco [working title], 048-2071-1980, 29.10.1980, p. 1–2.
129. Núñez (2012), p. 19.
130. Especially in the southern provinces there was a shortage of nurses. For example, the few health professionals in the area of Llanquihue (1982) could not assure the healthcare coverage for all inhabitants, in: Ministerio de Salud, Depto. Salud Rural: Ord No. 3J/4128, Mat. Indica medidas a tomar en el desarollo Plan Específico Salud Rural, Provincia de Llanquihue, 4128-2448-1982, 26.07.1982, p. 1-2 [23-24/24];

    Grau, Talloni and Reusch in an interview with *Análisis* (1988) confirmed the job reduction in the nursing sector, in: Colegio de Enfermeras: Defender la Salud, Defender la Profesión, in: *Análisis*, 22.-28.02.1988, S. 29 [Fondo Patricia Talloni, Museo de le Memoria, Santiago 00003-03];

    All midwives employed after 1982 received only jobs in the *PEM* program, in: Interview with Anita Román Morra, Santiago, January 2020.

    The Enfermería confirmed "some" cases, in: Carmen Oye González en la sesión solemne del "Día Mundial de la Enfermería" 12 de Mayo de 1982, in: *Enfermería*, No. 73, 07-08-09-1982, p. 3–4, 3.
131. Quote: "El traspaso de Consultorios Periféricos de los Servicios de Salud a las Municipalidades [...] significa cambiar de previsión y perder derechos y beneficios adquiridos [...]. Al comenzar de nuevo como empleado particular se pierden los beneficios inherentes a la calidad de empleado público, ya que se incorporan a un nuevo sistema," in: Memoria Anual del Colegio de Enfermeras, in: *Enfermería*, No. 72, 04-05-06-1982, p. 35–46, 40;

    Carmen Oye González en la sesión solemne del "Día Mundial de la Enfermería" 12 de Mayo de 1982, in: *Enfermería*, No. 73, 07-08-09-1982, p. 3–4, 4.
132. The employment issue became a side note in the annual reports, for example, in: Memoria Anual del Colegio de Enfermeras, in: *Enfermería*, No. 72, 04-05-06-1982, p. 35–46, 40.

133. Until 1979, nine nurses had worked in the management level of the NHS. By this, they had also been in charge of the departments of human resources, program development, and professional development. It seems that each one of the nine nurses continued to work in the management level of the new NSHS system. For example, Sofia Matus Lagos, in: Matus Lagos, Enfermera Asesora, Depto. Apoyo a los Programas, Ministerio de Salud: Análisis y Proyecciones de Investigación en Enfermería, Ministerio de Salud, in: *Enfermería*, No. 61, 07-08-09-1979, 27-31.
134. Memoria Anual del Colegio de Enfermeras, in: *Enfermería*, No. 72, 04-05-06-1982, p. 35–46, 35, 41.
135. Carmen Oye González, en la sesión solemne del Día Mundial de la Enfermera, in: *Enfermería*, No. 68, 04-05-06-1981, p. 26–28, 28.
136. Carmen Oye González en la sesión solemne del "Día Mundial de la Enfermería" 12 de Mayo de 1982, in: *Enfermería*, No. 73, 07-08-09-1982, p. 3–4, 4.
137. Carmen Oye González, en la sesión solemne del Día Mundial de la Enfermera, in: *Enfermería*, No. 68, 04-05-06-1981, p. 26–28, 29;

    Pincheira mentioned the directiva permanente No. 7 in her editorial, in: Pincheira: Editorial, in: *Enfermería*, Nos. 81-82, 07-12-1984, p. 2.
138. Carmen Oye González en la sesión solemne del "Día Mundial de la Enfermería" 12 de Mayo de 1982, in: *Enfermería*, No. 73, 07-08-09-1982, p. 3–4, 3.
139. Núñez (2012), p. 21.
140. Quote: "una persona idónea, honorable, con excelentes relaciones humanas y gran calidad profesional," in: Ministerio de Salud: Decreto No. 599, Contrata Sobre la Base de Honorarios, Suma alzada, A.D. Gladys Peake Guevara, 599-2068-1980, 31.12.1980, p. 1-5 [1-5].
141. Peake reduced the already low number of articles about the interaction between the nursing organization and Chilean society from 34 percent in the 1970s to 21 percent in the 1980s (editorials and the internal announcements were not included in this analysis). Since then, information about nursing policies only appeared almost exclusively in the annual reports.
142. It was a commission to decide about the approval of scholarships for health professionals, in: Ministerio de Salud: Decreto Exento No. 014, Crea Comisión Redactora Reglamento de Concursos DFL. 338/60, 014-2069-1980, 13.06.1980, p. 1 [9/16].
143. Ministerio de Salud: Decreto No. 18 Contrato a honorarios de D. Lidia Weitzel Trincado, 18-2125-1981, 06.01.1981, 1-2 [3-4/17]
144. Interview with P. Talloni, Santiago, January 2020.

145. An example of the cult around Sofía Pincheira: Since 1984, the general council met in the *Centro de Conferencias Sofía Pincheira*, in: Garrido Ballerino, Presidente CECh: Discurso de la Presidenta del Colegio de Enfermeras de Chile A.G. en la Ceremonia Solemne con que se Conmemoró "El Día Mundial de la Enfermera," Mayo 1984, in: *Enfermería*, Nos. 81-82, 07-12-1984, p. 36–38, 38.
146. For example in 1981, the participation of *CECh* members in the 17th Congress of the ICN in Los Angeles, USA, in: Pincheira: Editorial, in: *Enfermería*, No. 69, 07-08-09-1981, p. 3;

    Pincheira mentioned mostly the cooperation with *FEPPEN*. In 1982, she started to revise their ethical guidelines, in: Memoria Anual del Colegio de Enfermeras, in: *Enfermería*, No. 72, 04-05-06-1982, p. 35–46.

    An example of the constant information about ICN activities, in: Noticias del Consejo Internacional de Enfermeras, in: *Enfermería*, No. 71, 01-02-03-1982, p. 41–45, 44.
147. ILO: Nursing Personnel Convention No. 149, 1977.
148. ILO: Nursing Personnel Recommendation No. 157, 1977.
149. Memoria Anual del Colegio de Enfermeras, in: *Enfermería*, No. 72, 04-05-06-1982, p. 35–46, 35.
150. That is the impression given by the anouncments of the professional associations' delegates, in: *El Mercurio*, 04.02-10.02.1979, 08.02.1979, p. 1.
151. Quote: "ya que existe el compromiso de sacar a los colegios de su 'hibernación,' como lo denominó nuestro amigo de lucha don Julio Durán, presidente de los abogados," in: Carmen Oye González, en las sesión solemne del Día Mundial de la Enfermera, in: *Enfermería*, No. 68, 04-05-06-1981, p. 26–28, 28.
152. Nueva ley redifine papel de los colegios profesionales, in: *El Mercurio*, 05.02.-11.02.1981, p. 6.
153. Besides all discussions, the members of the professional associations confirmed explicitly their loyalty to the military junta, in: Ibid., p. 6.
154. Quote: "No pasaremos a un sistema libre y gremialista como parecen ser las asociaciones sino más bien a una regulación estatal," in: Memoria Anual Del Consejo general Del Colegio de Enfermeras de Chile Correspondiente al Periodo 1980-1981, in: *Enfermería*, No. 68, 04-05-06-1981, p. 29–38, 29.
155. Colegio de Enfermeras de Chile (A.G.) Informa, in: *Enfermería*, No. 68, 04-05-06-1981, p. 18–19, 18.
156. Article No. 4, Quote: "In order to allow membership, it is necessary to have the title of a professional nurse issued by a university or a vocational institute." (*Para ser asociada del Colegio será necesario poseer el título profesional de enfermera otorgado por una Universidad o Instittuto Profesional*);

Other central points were:

1. Article 8 confirmed the major influence of the Santiago branch (4 of 17 members in the consejo general)

2. Article 9 obliged the national board to exercise a partial election of their members every two years; in: Acta Constitutiva Colegio de Enfermeras de Chile A.G. (Asociación Gremial), in: *Enfermería*, No. 68, 04-05-06-1981, p. 20–25.

157. Pincheira, Sofía: Editorial, in: *Enfermería*, No. 72, 04-05-06-1982, p. 3.
158. Decreto con Fuerza de Ley No. 630, quoted in: Colegio de Enfermeras de Chile (A.G.) Informa, in: *Enfermería*, No. 68, 04-05-06-1981, p. 18–19.
159. Memoria Anual del Colegio de Enfermeras, in: *Enfermería*, No. 72, 04-05-06-1982, p. 35–46, 41.
160. Ibid., p. 35.
161. Primer Congreso Nacional de Enfermería Pediátrica, in: *Enfermería*, No. 78, 10-11-12-1983, p. 3–7, 6.
162. Quote: "A pesar de la pública acusación apareció en la Prensa, para hacer creer al público y a las Colegiadas que el Acto Eleccionario estaba viciado a Comisión Calificadora de Elecciones [...] el acto eleccionario estaba ajustado a la Reglamentación vigente [...] que las tareas a cumplir en una entidad como la nuestra exigen dirigentes y colaboradores de la mayor honestidad, idoneidad y dedicación," in: Carmen Oye González en la sesión solemne del "Día Mundial de la Enfermería" 12 de Mayo de 1982, in: *Enfermería*, No. 73, 07-08-09-1982, p. 3–4, 4.
163. Interview with Patricia Grau, Santiago, March 2017.
164. Quote: "La mayoría de las enfermeras, no supimos de las elecciones del 82, pero luego sí se puso atención a que el consejo de Santiago, (como antes siempre había sido), estaba haciendo reuniones periódicas con Delegadas de establecimientos de salud (representantes de las enfermeras elegidas por sus pares). Así empezamos a llegar a esta instancia, para informarnos, plantear las inquietudes y problemas de sus respectivos servicios. La presidente de este Consejo era adepta a la dictadura, por lo que la acogida a los problemas era mínima (La respuesta histórica fue: ¡La Ley es la Ley!)," in: Email from Patricia Talloni to Markus Thulin, 17.03.2017.
165. In 2012, Guzmán Riquelme interviewed Talloni, Grau, Reusch, and Opgaard for a study about the opposition work of the professional associations in the 1980s, in: Guzmán (2012), p. 89.
166. The new board of the *CECh* was put together by people to whom Oye considered of a "high degree of honesty, ability and dedication";

     Quote: "A pesar de la pública acusación apareció en la Prensa, para hacer creer al público y a las Colegiadas que el Acto Eleccionario estaba viciado a Comisión Calificadora de Elecciones [...] el acto eleccionario estaba ajustado a la Reglamentación vigente [...] que las tareas a cumplir en una entidad como la nuestra exigen dirigentes y colaboradores de la mayor honestidad, idoneidad y dedicación," in: Carmen Oye González en la sesión solemne del "Día Mundial de la Enfermería" 12 de Mayo de 1982, in: *Enfermería*, No. 73, 07-08-09-1982, p. 3–4, 4;

For Talloni, Grau, Opgaard, and Reusch, the members of the national board had been "mere officers of the government's policy," in: Interview with Patricia Grau, 15.03.2017.

167. Quote: "Con los partidos políticos perseguidos y diezmados, la organización de la resistencia ante el cúmulo de violaciones y arbitrariedades demanda el surgimiento de nuevos colectivos político-sociales amplios," in: Guzmán (2012), p. 92.
168. Ibid, p. 95.
169. Colegio Médico: investigan 4 casos de médicos torturados, in: *Fortín Mapocho*, No. 299, 02.08.1984, p. 5.
170. Ibid.
171. Quote. "Ahora, nunca nosotros nos planteamos como movimiento paralelo al colegio, sino un grupo de personas o profesionales que queríamos un colegio distinto," Ibid., p. 93.
172. Interview with Anita Román Morra, Santiago, January 2020.
173. Actas de la Junta Directiva: Sesiones 61-75, 1984, Sesión 65a, Síntesis sobre actual situación estudiantil universitaria, p. 27-31, 27;

     The documentation of the *Junta Directiva* did not mention to which faculty the protesting students belonged. It seems that most of them studied medicine, in: Actas de la Junta directiva: UCH 06-02, Sesiones 1-17, 1982, p. [2-5/5].
174. Pincheira: Editorial, in: *Enfermería*, No. 68, 04-05-06-1981, p. 3.
175. Carmen Oye González, en la sesión solemne del Día Mundial de la Enfermera, in *Enfermería*, No. 68, 04-05-06-1981, p. 26–28, 26-27.
176. Memoria Anual del Consejo general del Colegio de Enfermeras de Chile Correspondiente Al Periodo 1980-1981, in: *Enfermería*, No. 68, 04-05-06-1981, p. 29–38, 29, 33, 35.
177. Memoria Anual del Colegio de Enfermeras, in: *Enfermería*, No. 72, 04-05-06-1982, p. 35–46.
178. Peake was not precise about the date of the closure. It could also have happened in 1983, in: Resumen de la Memoria Anual del Consejo general del Colegio de Enfermeras de Chile A.G. 1983-1984, in: *Enfermería*, Nos. 81-82, 07-12-1984, p. 42–47, 42.
179. Universidad de Chile : Actas de la Junta Directiva: Uch 06, 1982.
180. In 1972, the curriculum of the nursing school of the University of Chile in North Santiago included such subjects as the social sciences Nos. 1, 2, and 3 (Ciencias Sociales I, II, III) in the first three semesters, in: Resoluciones del Rector Delegado, Primera Parte, Oct. 73 – Ene. 74, p. [1-6/6].

181. Midwives but not nurses dropped the following courses: Social-Cultural Anthropology (*Antropología Social Cultural*) and Development in Contemporary Society (*Desarollo de la Sociedad Contemporánea*), in: *Revista de la Universidad de Chile*, No. 57, 05-1977, p. [1-4/7].
182. For example the nursing school in Talca. In 1975, the curriculum included the subjects "Philosophy of Humanity," "Social Development," "Philosophy of Sciences," "Latin American Culture", "Dynamic Structure, Chilean social structure," and "Sociocultural Anthropology" (*Filosofía del Hombre, Desarollo Social Contempráneo, Filosofía de las Ciencias, Cultura Latino Americana and Estructura Dinámica, Estructura Social Chilena, Antropología Socio Cultural*), in: Asesoría Técnica de la Prorrectoría, Universidad de Talca: Decreto No. 1044, Aprueba plan de estudios transitorio, Carrera de enfermería, Sede Talca, Santiago, 22.05.1975, p. 1-2;

    In 1986, the curriculum of the nursing school in Talca experienced fundamental changes. Except for the subject Foundations of Nursing (*Fundamentos de Enfermería*), only technical subjects were taught, in: Robertson Herrera, Juan: Promulga Acuerdo No. 102 tomado en la Sesión No. 28, de fecha 27 de enero de 1986 de la Junta Directiva que aprueba el Plan de Estudios de la Carrera de Enfermería y Obstetricia, Talca, 30.01.1986, p. 1-6.
183. Compared to the public system, much fewer nurses were trained in the private system (70 against 30 per cent). Behn et al. stated for the time span 1978 to 1982, "progress in the professionalization"; hence they did not give details. They celebrated the first master's program in nursing studies, offered in 1980 by the University of Concepción, in: Behn et al. (2009), p. 76.
184. With one exception: Until 1986, the teachers of the nursing school in Concepción authored most of the articles published in *Enfermería*. Until closure, the northern branch of the University of Chile ranked second;

    Peake's preference for authors of the University of Concepción can also result from personal connections, as she was the first director of the nursing school between 1948 and 1952 (Chap. 1).
185. Ministerio de Salud, Asesoría Jurídica: Ord. No. 2C/3931, Mat. Informa sobre presentación de D. Luis Alberto Quezada Leiva, 3931-2447-1982, 15.07.1982, p. 1-4 [13-16/22].
186. Ministerio de Salud, Asesoría Jurídica: Ord No. 2.C/3952, Mat. Ejercicio de Acupuntura. Normas de autorización de profesiones auxiliares paramédicas, 16.07.1982, p. 1-2 [17-18/22].

187. Nursing students had only a five-hour seminar about the development of the nursing profession, in: Ministerio de Salud: Ord No. 547, Mat. Aumenta fondos Programa de Expansión de Recursos Humanos 1986, para incorporar empleos que indica, 547-3101-1986, 23.01.1986, p. 1-15 [17-31/38].
188. Quote : "because of the titles they give, the deficient preparation and the high costs of these institutes" (por el tipo de títulos que entregan, la deficiente preparación y los elevados precios de estos institutos), in: Ibid, p. 35-36.
189. Quote: "They are not supposed to work with such organizations [...] a fraud against people interested in a short training instead of university studies." (en sentido de que no deben colaborar con esa organización [...] engaño de las personas que se interesen por seguir carreras cortas al margen de la Universidad), in: Memoria Anual del H. Consejo General del Colegio de Enfermeras correspondiente al periodo 31 de mayo de 1978 al 1 junio 1979, in: *Enfermería*, No. 61, 07-08-09-1979, p. 36–44, 41.
190. Ministerio de Salud, Depto. Recursos Humanos: M.S. Ord No. 496, Mat. Personería Jurídica, 496-2024-1979, 20.03.1979, p. 1-2 [19/20-33].
191. Memoria Anual del Consejo general del Colegio de Enfermeras de Chile Periodo Mayo 1976 y Abril 1977, in: *Enfermería*, No. 55, 01-02-03-1978, p. 33–44, 35-36.

CHAPTER 5

Nursing in Times of Transition and Distinction (1982–1990)

1 Introduction

Social policy during the military regime progressively replaced the notion of rights for that of "help for self-help." Healthcare was possibly the area that gained more notoriety during this shift in approach, with "self-care" as a commonplace term that spread easily among users and professionals alike. And yet, not everything was a total rupture with the past. The timespan from 1982 to 1990 witnessed further continuities in Chilean healthcare and revealed the impact of the state reform initiated at the beginning of the decade. Even though the number of people with public health insurance did not shrink, the private sector was rapidly expanding. The government still dominated the system's framework. Yet, by the end of the decade it became clear that there would be no returning to the society and politics of the early 1970s. The ministries, supervised by the Armed Forces on one hand, and civilian collaborators on the other, still gave the most important impetus to healthcare. The professional associations were losing ever more power and struck back by forming broader movements and alliances. Actors with new ideas and commitments, especially in political terms, demanded co-determination.

For women, who were heavily represented in healthcare by nurses, midwives, social workers, and auxiliary staff, the institution of patriarchy still limited self-organization and autonomy. Yet now that a number of

© The Author(s), under exclusive license to Springer Nature Switzerland AG 2023

M. Thulin, R. A. Ayala, *Nursing, Policy and Politics in Twentieth-century Chile*,
https://doi.org/10.1007/978-3-030-90835-5_5

biographies of these female actors have reached a wider audience, they have demonstrated that women in such fields not only had political opinions but that these opinions were politically varied and even clashing. In saying that although women still worked mostly in public health areas, it is clear that for the first time, national examinations, rankings, and international foundations amplified the perception of the trained female professions as technically necessary and as players in society. Due to this pivotal role, female staff, especially auxiliary workers, were a very important pillar of healthcare policies.

If social policy has always been linked to the shaping of the nation, during the 1980s health policies moved toward an intricate state ideology, that is, civilian-military cooperation, *gremialismo*, and private entrepreneurship. Especially the municipalization process, but also job creation schemes like the *PEM* and new private healthcare providers, changed working conditions and payment schemes for nurses, which became evident in both the cities and the country. Until 1984, only those who served in state politics had a voice. This eventually changed, however, when, in 1986, the board of the nurses' association shifted leftward. For the first time since its foundation in 1953, the *CECh* developed a different voice and a different policy toward state authority.

As a way of securing proper staffing of a growing health system, training for nurses in privately owned institutions expanded. As the entrepreneurial mentality and terminology infiltrated nurses' day-to-day life, nursing policy accentuated existing differences in a society that grew obsessed with social class.

2 Crises, Political Conflicts, and Transition

2.1 *The Rise of a New Female Resistance Movement*

By the beginning of 1982, economic recession had hit Chile with its full strength.[1] The declining number of available jobs affected mostly low-income groups like auxiliary workers and female professionals more generally. As a result of family commitments, women were more inclined than men to work part-time and undertake less stable, more temporary employment. For women, who represented the majority of state employees in healthcare, it was only a matter of time before this reality would manifest. In the years before, right-wing and conservative female leaders had failed to challenge the civilian-military cooperation, but the time was now ripe for a new female oppositional movement.

In 1984, social worker María Luz Ibarra declared in *Solidaridad* magazine that 70 percent of her colleagues were working without contracts.[2] Figures in relation to this are difficult to find,[3] but what is clear is that the number of staff with stable working conditions in public healthcare had declined rapidly since 1982.[4] In some cases, especially in the cities, unemployed nurses, midwives, and social workers found jobs in religious and other charity organizations, most prominently in the facilities of *Vicaría de la Solidaridad*. But these could accommodate only a small number of applicants. As in the 1970s, hundreds of thousands of individuals relied on precarious governmental employment schemes, most importantly *PEM* and *POJH*.[5] By contrast, a job in the NSHS was still prestigious and offered generally decent working conditions and wages. Even bearing this in mind, the economic downturn reduced the net income of employees. In 1986, *Solidaridad* magazine quoted a member of the medical association who calculated that the purchasing power had fallen by 50 percent during the previous ten years.[6]

Although the economic downturn ended in 1986, forty percent of the workforce remained in precarious employment, most notably in manual labor.[7] The experiences they lived in the 1980s, between financial security and existential fear, marked them for the rest of their lives and triggered a reaction similar to the one seen in 1972 and 1973—losing faith in both the government and its policies. As a result, the opposition gained protagonism and was at the center of social life.[8] Over the course of the 1980s, more and more people gradually regained the courage to gather and reenter the public sphere. Much as it first represented a strong minority, one of the most outstanding examples was the resistance movement of nurses.

In the early 1980s, progressive activists like the nurses of the Guild Renewal Movement (*Movimiento de Renovación Gremial, MRG*) did not get support from the other health professionals. This, however, was not uncommon and a similar lack of support was experienced by other left-wing women in social work and midwifery. The resistance movement was fragmented and operated mostly through isolated groups, except in some specific instances, like physicians' Assembly of the Civility (*Asamblea de la Civilidad*). Sources about the activities of women in the resistance are rare, which would lead us to conclude that their interaction with political actors on national and international levels remained rudimentary.

It was from the middle of the decade that protests developed into strikes and strikes into widespread movements. They culminated in the foundation of the Joint Action of Political Parties for "No" Vote

(*Concertación de Partidos por el No*) in 1988. The Christian Democrats were key instigators in this, growing stronger and more effective as a party than they were back in the early 1970s. The various political movements, parties, unions, and associations all had specific ideas on the principles of democracy, hence the reason why numerous different opinions spread in society. These can be viewed in catholic-influenced publications like *Solidaridad* where opinions were more virulent, while in left-wing papers like *Fortín Mapocho* they remained of a more secular persuasion.[9] Only their peaceful approach to negotiation and their intent to put an end to the dictatorship united them within *Concertación*.

It is also true, however, that other groups were more prepared to respond to the political repression in a more abrasive fashion. These came to the surface in 1983 with the "National Days of Protest" (*Jornadas Nacionales de Protesta*).[10] During those days there arose an aggressive face of opposition from initially peaceful marches. Nurses had a disastrous and challenging work experience when violence broke through.[11] The first peak of the violent confrontations was reached in August of that same year. Several people died and the spiral of violence, mostly covert since 1974, became visible again.

With the ultimate aim of overthrowing Pinochet by force, some of the protesters underwent an even more severe radicalization and organized terror cells, like the Manuel Rodríguez Patriotic Front (*Frente Patriótico Manuel Rodríguez, FPMR*).[12] Their targets being mostly state institutions and officials.[13]

Leftist ideas like those of the *FPMR* were common in the environment of female health professionals. But there were also nurses and social workers who had strong ties to the Christian Democratic Party, as we have seen in the example of Irene Frei Montalva. Resulting from this clash of ideas, nursing became once again highly politicized.

At first glance, national policy on female health professions did not encounter violent resistance. This first impression is, to a large extent, true, as the majority of nurses simply followed Pinochet's leadership until the mid-1980s, though whether that be by conviction or fear is more difficult to determine. The fact that they did not provoke violent confrontations does not, however, mean that nurses were not affected by the climate of hate and destruction that surrounded them. Violence was part of Chile's landscape in the 1980s, as Pinochet's secret police, *CNI*, or the secret service of *Carabineros* could not force an end to the troubles.[14] The attempts to end the dictatorship went on, despite the constant fear that violence could break out even through the most minor advancements in negotiation with the military junta. Professional women, however, opted for a more peaceful approach.

Unlike in the protests against the Popular Unity, in these events women were not loudly showcased in the print media. Christian Democrat and Socialist women met in low-profile venues, as a way of non-confrontational demonstration of the female presence in politics and society. The number of women was impressive considering the absence of overt female movements for over a decade. A striking example was a gathering of 10,000 females on December 23, 1983, for a conference in Santiago's *Teatro Cauplicán.* [15] From then on, female healthcare professionals would be either shunned or talked against in the pro-government media every now and then, but never depicted as a threat to the political order.

When analyzing the development of a female resistance movement in times of dictatorship, it would appear that this began in the healthcare professions. Even though women also worked as schoolteachers, accountants, and clerks, only when referred to as nurses, midwives, or social workers were females mentioned as leading the movements, which gives a hint of nurses' involvement in mass movements. Such spectacular events as the 1983 gathering did not reoccur until 1986, and in the timespan in between the press communicated rather sporadic expressions of overt female power.

As the referendum approached, many nurses took sides in the upcoming conflict as if mirroring a schism in broader society loaded by words like ideology, justice, and democracy. Further nursing planning, and even new divisions like the NSHS and *FONASA*, developed in a climate where decisions once again became highly political, with the state under pressure both nationally and internationally.

2.2 *Universities and the Development of Political Diversity*

During the twentieth century, the University of Chile, the Welfare Board, and the Catholic University in Santiago had a near monopoly on training for female healthcare professionals. Even though the 1980s witnessed the growth of semi-private and private universities, healthcare policy was still under the strong influence of those who had become lecturers during an era of a strong anti-Communist approach propagated by the US. The question was whether traditional institutions were able to keep their monopoly in shaping political opinion despite the private property mentality gaining ground.

Since the 1940s, conservative ideas dominated the policies of the elite female health professionals. However, that started to change during the 1980s crises as left-wing ideas spread and resistance groups emerged. For many health professionals, their training in university had been the cultural background of their political opinions, especially when the climate of political confrontation reached the schools of midwifery, social work, and nursing.

Throughout the 1980s, the University of Chile remained one of the hubs where intellectuals and students contested Pinochet's regime. Other academic centers followed its example. Much to the dismay of the university directorate, even the Catholic University, which had been considered the primary think tank of *gremialismo* since the early 1970s, hosted oppositional student movements.[16] This was a development the military junta could not leave unsolved.

Medical students were expelled over the course of the protests in universities, traces of which can be found in the University of Chile's directorate's reports about medical care being provided in rural areas by physicians who had not yet graduated. Members of the directorate, who were designated by the military, feared the development of a parallel healthcare system run by oppositional students and professionals.[17] But it was not only students who were suspected of carrying out oppositional activities. This is illustrated by the fact that in 1983, Gen. Roberto Soto Mackenney, appointed provost of the university (1983–1987), prohibited university staff from any kind of participation in oppositional movements.[18]

Female healthcare students (i.e., nursing, midwifery, and social work) did not appear in the reports about the strikes and demonstrations. Even if we assume that most of these students did not actually support Army officers on the campus, they were well aware of military intervention in the university board. What is more, at least in the first two years of their degree program, nursing and midwifery students not only attended the same faculty as oppositional medical students, but they also shared the same seminar rooms, listened to the same teachers, and ate in the same canteens; they lived in a common milieu where cross-pollination of ideas took place.

This means that during the 1980s, multiple generations of nurses, midwives, social workers, and others who worked in traditionally female professions were socialized in this climate of protest, even those who had not experienced September '73. Between the ages of 18 and 25, arguably some of the most decisive years of one's professional and private life, students and young professionals experienced a brutal regime while simultaneously entering into contact with leftist literature and gaining exposure to different ideas. For certain, many female healthcare professionals and workers refused to be turned from conservative opinions, but even still the foundations for political diversity had been laid.

2.3 *State Problems and Private Solution*

The rise of the resistance among female health professionals, academic staff, and students was unmissable for the military. The only sustainable method to stop those movements from spreading was to resolve the understaffing issues in the healthcare sector. But the gap was so large that engagement with the private sector seemed vital to bridge it.

In January 1983, health minister Hernán Rivera Calderón (1980–1983) wrote a report about the healthcare sector for the minister of finance. He described the insufficient medical care for the population and demanded more funding be allocated to healthcare, finishing his urgent request with the following summary:

"The situation has come to a critical point, which could undermine the political goals of His Excellency, the President."[19]

The most alarming emergency calls Calderón received came from the hospitals in the East and Southeast of the capital.[20] During the 1980s, the director of the southeastern district (*Servicio de Salud Metropolitano Sur Oriente*) wrote various letters to the health ministry asking for a budget increase because of a general shortage of staff and material.[21] The director of the NSHS in the East of the town became more precise when he reported that the hospital *Del Salvador* was short of approximately 100 beds due to "bad physical conditions" caused by the earthquake of 1985.[22]

Healthcare underwent two significant changes during the 1980s. The first concerned its geographic reach. From the beginning of the modern public system in the 1920s, healthcare policies had only focused on urban projects. But then, decrees, moratoriums, reports, bulletins, and correspondence also addressed the situation of healthcare centers in rural areas. Medical treatment and care outside of the urban settings, which was still disadvantaged compared to the urban hospitals, came more to the fore.

The second change was a nursing issue and effectively the only specific measure taken by the dictatorship about nursing. It consolidated a reality which had shaped the healthcare system since its foundation: nursing auxiliaries, undervalued and ignored, yet working nationwide, became the most important partner outside of the urban hospitals. An exemplary case of such focus on auxiliary work was a 1978 contract with the Inter-American Development Bank, one of the most prestigious international projects of the new NSHS.[23] By contrast, as we will show in the following section, it had been decided that the profession of the academically trained nurse was to disappear in the future design of the healthcare system. This meant that they were meant to lose their place in public health, the most salient project involving nursing, midwifery, and social work since the 1920s.

For all previous governments the expansion of public health, which in the 1980s mostly meant rural health, was one of their main policy focal points, a point that Pinochet never questioned. The difference, however, was that his government provided very little investment for the sector when compared to the financial resources it had at its disposal. In January 1983, an interdisciplinary commission of inquiry initiated by nurses, nutritionists, and midwives (described as a "multiprofessional team") presented the results of a three-day study carried out in 1982 that examined medical care in Chile's Region of Biobio, where Concepción is located. The team had visited the cities of Arauco, Talcahuano, and the Ñuble Province. The evaluation of treatments at NSHS facilities was mainly positive and highlighted the decrease in infant mortality. However, Concepción's NSHS director lamented in an interview that health education still remained rudimentary and that an unknown number of villages were yet to be integrated into the public healthcare system. In addition to this, the provision of medical treatment was not centrally organized as supplies were scarce, an issue that burdened the entire public system.[24]

The commission's report only became specific concerning problems when it illustrated the situation in the *Hospital de Cañete* (133 km South of Concepción). There, no physician was available during night shifts, hygiene standards were insufficient, and the vaccination program had been discontinued due to a lack of supplies.[25] Two other studies we found underline this observation,[26] which led us to the view that the deficiencies in healthcare services were more widespread than the NSHS recognized.

That moment, private medicine seemed to be the solution to every system failure.

Information about private hospitals and healthcare centers is rather scant. In 1981, the private sector counted only 3855 beds compared to the 33,692 in public healthcare facilities. By 1992, this number had risen to 10,600 beds compared to 32,279.[27] Starting in the mid-1980s, the health ministry signed between 18 and 20 contracts annually authorizing private enterprises to take over public hospitals or to open new private clinics and healthcare centers.[28]

Private initiatives had settled in some healthcare areas. In 1985, physician López stated that private facilities did not suffer from supply or staff shortages.[29] This was confirmed in a similar observation by the directorate of the University of Chile regarding the private *Clínica Las Condes* (founded in 1982) and the health centers ran by *Banmédica S.A.* (founded in 1983). Deans realized that those new private entities had "better economic horizons" than the public facilities.[30] The previously quoted article in *Hoy* about the deaths in Santiago's Children's Hospital in 1979 (Chap. 3) confirmed this assessment; authors stated that the lack of technical equipment, such as computed tomography, which was a piece of "standard equipment" in private clinics, only affected people insured through *FONASA*.[31] Unsurprisingly, healthcare staff did not always aim to work in public health and *poblaciones*.

The case of the *J.J. Aguirre* hospital illustrates that most of the physicians would leave the NSHS facilities by 2 o'clock in the afternoon to go and treat patients in private clinics. Then, some nurses and midwives, but most importantly auxiliary workers, covered patients' care in the wards. It is therefore not surprising that Ricardo Vacarezza, one of the leaders of the medical association's opposition movement, criticized the loss of the solidarity principle in 1985, however stating in the same *Solidaridad* article that he was not totally against private medicine.[32]

All in all, the private sector was still too incipient to cover the major gaps that existed. And there was another problem – when Vacarezza mentioned the word "solidarity" he probably did not mean to collaborate with other professional groups to find a solution for problems like understaffing. He quite possibly viewed his own association as having climbed to the political height that was required to counter the will of the military junta in any negotiation.

2.4 *Physicians' Fight, Female Health Professionals' Inspiration*

The pay gap is probably the most prominent sign of inequality in a healthcare system. For Chile the discussion about the right to cash in hand for medical services was the initial point of a much bigger and more permanent conflict between the physicians and the military junta, with 1986 being its most strained period. This fight paved the way for other resistance movements, but also showed that even the powerful medical association relied on the help of the female professions.

Besides a general shortage of supplies and staff, the biggest problem for the healthcare system was the deficit in secondary and tertiary medicine. Only professionals were able to treat complex clinical matters and chronic diseases, but most of them did not work in rural areas or even in the periphery of the cities. If patients were lucky and found a hospital or a healthcare center with nurses, physicians, or midwives, many times they had to make an additional payment (Chaps. 2–4). Although we found no statistical survey of this illegal practice, it certainly seems to have been more of a rule than an exception. Finally, in November 1985, the Pinochet government reacted. It implemented a law including a "regulation to enforce the right to protect health" with the promising clearance contained therein:

> "The facilities of the NSHS are not allowed to reject people nor request additional payments for a treatment."[33]

But statements like this were not meant to abolish additional payments, but rather to direct fresh money into the state treasury: the second part of the law introduced a sliding scale staggered system, the so-called Regime of Health Benefits (*régimen de prestaciones de salud*): all of the insured by *FONASA* were ranked according to four different categories (A through D) based on their monthly income.[34] After the free choice of the physician, the government also adopted the flat fee system (*cheque bono*) from *Medicina Curativa* for *FONASA*.[35] Llambias-Wolff (2013) described it as a "new co-payment."[36] Juan Luis González Reyes, who was president of the medical association in 1986, used more drastic words in an interview published in *Solidaridad*. He considered the law to be the beginning of "economic liberalism" in health care and absolutely contrary to the idea of public healthcare coverage.[37] In 1990, the *CIEPLAN* author Pilar Vergara voiced the same opinion, stating that she considered the year 1986 to be the culmination of privatization and mercantilism in healthcare.[38]

On the other hand, *Coordinadora de Salud*, or Health Coordinator, which was a conglomerate of professional associations from Santiago, was founded. The actions of its leader, Ricardo Vacarezza, attracted so much attention that even the international press, most prominently the *New York Times*, reported on the story.[39]

In 1983, the regional council of journalists in Santiago moved to the oppositional side.[40] The regime responded to the leftward move with intimidating measures,[41] but those measures failed to have the same impact as they had had in the 1970s. In fact, they even helped to confirm and promote critical opinions. In 1984, the adversaries of the dictatorship also gained the majority on the national board.[42] As with the lawyers, the new political reorientation did not go undisputed,[43] but it served as an example for the democratic movement in other associations. Indeed, as early as 1985, the opposition won the majority in the general councils of five other associations; in healthcare these were the associations of midwives and of social workers.[44]

However, the opposition movements in other associations are not as well documented as the cases of journalists, lawyers, and physicians.[45] Political science student Gabriel Guzmán Riquelme provided a broad picture of all movements in 2012 based on the archives of the Memory and Human Rights Museum. His analysis supports the reporting by *Solidaridad* about the events in the teachers' association.

At the time, the *Association of School Teachers* was by far the largest organization of professionals, with some 80,000 members.[46] The first free elections since its foundation in 1975 took place only in October of 1985. The pro-government board had successfully postponed elections until then. The Command for the Re-democratization of the Association (*Comando por la Redemocratización del Colegio*)[47] was founded in 1984 and successfully gained the majority in the general council.[48] However, a group of disappointed teachers (mostly adherent to left-wing parties and movements) had already left the association in 1984 and founded their own association. For the first time, members of a private association decided to go separate ways. The Guild Association of Educators of Chile (*Asociación Gremial de Educadores de Chile, AGECH*) was then being watched by the Pinochet regime, just like the journalists' general council.[49]

On March 20, 1985, three bodies were found beheaded on a street near Santiago. The remains belonged to men associated with the *AGECH*.[50] This assassination was generally referred to as the Case of the Decapitated (*caso degollados*) and would become one of the biggest political scandals of the Pinochet regime during the 1980s. The generals first disseminated misinformation to protect the murderers, but investigations uncovered the involvement of the secret service of *Carabineros*.[51]

The assassination took place during a state of siege. However, the pressure from civilians on the streets and the reporting on the part of the oppositional press forced the regime to start a trial. On August 2, 1985, the investigation led to the resignation of Gen. Mendoza, director of *Carabineros* and member of the military junta since 1973.[52] But despite that the accused police were dismissed, the unrest about the assassination did not wane. The disturbing Case of the Decapitated became a turning point across the entire opposition. In the case of the associations, it enabled them to delegitimize the regime with respect to its credibility in serving justice.

Upon learning about such shocking events, several unions and associations implemented human rights departments to protect their members and clients and, in case of healthcare, their patients. Exactly one year after the Case of the Decapitated, the most powerful umbrella association of professionals, the Federation of Professional Associations (*Federación de Colegios Profesionales*) headed by González, founded a Human Rights Department.[53] From that moment on, *Solidaridad* documented each step González took; their interest was likely due to this push to elevate the fight for human rights as well as González's affinity to the Christian Democracy (he was former CD president and Frei's family doctor).[54]

The government would not listen to them, González initiated three strikes between January and March 1986. Their impact was minimal because nurses, midwives, social workers, and other female professionals could not identify with the goals advanced by the physicians and continued to work. To meet this challenge González had to amplify and diversify the movement. For this, he added claims of female professionals to his agenda and adopted the strategy of civil disobedience.[55] Finally, he invited everyone who wanted to bring an end to the dictatorship to join his protest movement.

González' Assembly of Civility (*Asamblea de la Civilidad*), founded on April 26, 1986, united a vast range of healthcare professionals and other peaceful oppositional groups.[56] He became its first president.[57] This time, the impact on national politics, at least from González' perspective, was far-reaching. Thus, González felt confident enough to demand a return to democracy.[58] The government continued not to respond, and so he called for a general strike on July 2nd and 3rd of 1986.[59]

A week after, a unit of *Carabineros* arrested 14 members of the assembly, including González.[60] Once again, the regime tried to revive the dictatorial might of the 1970s. From our research it seems impossible locating detailed sources with information on how the assembly then continued to work. It is clear, however, that González must have been well suited to play the role of a martyr and that Pinochet had to backpedal. On August 13th, he dismissed health minister Winston Chinchón (1983–1986) and replaced him with Juan Giaconi Gandolfo, who became the first civilian to head the health ministry since 1973.[61] González was eventually released on bail. Three weeks later, the *FPMR* attacked Pinochet's motorcade in an assassination attempt.

The regime then imposed the state of siege for the second time since passing the new constitution. Yet this could not stop the loss of its authority. Shortly after the repeal of censorship, information about a group of physicians and nurses who had treated injured members of the *FPMR* after the September attack reached the press.[62] Their destiny did not become as publicized as the Case of the Decapitated, but the imprisonment of *CECh* members, to be analyzed below, was of particular importance for nurses. It was a milestone on nurses' way to the front line in the fight against the dictatorship.

Pinochet could not weaken the opposition, but it paralyzed its manifestation in the Assembly of Civility: although González's movement resumed its activities in 1987, it would never again reach the impact it had the previous year.[63] The same happened to the movement within the associations.[64] Over the next two years, it mostly merged into the *NO* campaign.

Another reason for the inactivity of the Assembly of Civility in 1987 must have been the crises which shook the medical association that same year. The members of Santiago's regional council could not agree on a new strategy after the end of the state of siege.[65] This situation affected the regional council with the largest number of members in particular. Vacarezza had already achieved his reinstatement as the director of the *Hospital Del Salvador* on October 16, 1986.[66] This success, however, did not solidify his position within the association. In 1988, the council was still unable to agree on a new board.[67] Athough González remained in office, national and international news outlets took less and less notice of him.[68]

The temporary weakness of the medical association was the moment in which a group of female healthcare workers, namely from the *CECh*, started to operate. After the election of a new general council in 1986, the nurses crossed the red line set by the military. Physicians never stopped demonstrating,[69] but in the year before the plebiscite, their leaders lost their exclusive representative status.[70] Although the new board of the *CECh* adopted a number of doctors' demands, such as the claim for better healthcare coverage, they also raised new issues. In a way, physicians' movements set the tone for the resistance of female health professionals.

Like most associations, during the 1980s female movements seemed less powerful than in the early 1970s. However, by 1986, the physicians had noticed that they would be unable to overthrow Pinochet without them. González needed the women to lead the Assembly of Civility to success. This was the moment when the new movement of left-wing nurses appeared on the political stage. This development was not unproblematic, because many elite professionals remained loyal to the Pinochet regime. Their left-wing nurses did not agree with the physicians about all aspects of health policy, but most important was the common goal to end the dictatorship. As a result, female and male professionals started to cooperate, inspiring each other, while at the same time also learning to differentiate their professions and their self-conceptions.

Before leaving the general view and move on to nursing politics, we point out some of the events that we consider to be important for the development of healthcare in the last ten years of the twentieth century, the years in which democracy in Chile was restored.

2.5 Team Players Still Missing: Healthcare in the 1990s

The constant economic growth favored in the 1990s the stabilization of the political system and the state funding for healthcare. Political oppression ended, so conflicts between government and professionals returned to public life. This very quickly opened old wounds, most importantly when it came to the negotiation of salaries. The medical association reinvigorated, but made the same mistakes as in the 1970s and 1980s. Its board failed to engage the opinion of other healthcare professions.

The *NO* had won in the 1988 plebiscite, with 54.71 percent of the population voting against Pinochet's rule to expire.[71] The victory strengthened the union of moderate conservatives, Catholics, liberals, left-wing factionists, and some of their peaceful splinter groups.[72] Pinochet accepted the outcome and left the government, but not the headquarters of the Armed Forces.[73]

What followed was the first of five coalition governments of the Joint Action of Parties for Democracy (*Concertación de Partidos por la Democracia*) coming to power on March 11, 1990. Those who had hoped for deep structural changes were quickly disappointed. For although the Armed Forces, still under the supreme command of Pinochet,[74] handed the government over but did not release the state.

Despite the backwardness in politics, during the 1990s, Chile became the economic role model for Latin America. For conservatives, this was clearly a sign of democratic success. If we observe only the macro-economic growth, which had already started in 1986, it was indeed an impressive outcome. Due to the combination of increased exports, increased state investments, and low inflation, the government coalitions were able to present a balanced state budget.[75] For many Chileans and Latin Americans, the Pinochet regime had bequeathed a successful economic model. However, this was a one-sided interpretation.

Although the poverty rate decreased between 1987 and 1998 from 45.1 to 21.7 percent,[76] 3.61 million Chileans still lived below the poverty line.[77] Most of the new jobs created since 1990 existed only in temporary employment and the low-wage sector. Precarious working conditions and payment did not improve and the real wages for most of the population remained low.[78]

In the healthcare sector, the *Concertación* governments inherited various abuses from the dictatorship: the reduction of state investments, the inefficient administration, and the deficient distribution of state funding, as seen in the region of *Concepción* and the *Hospital J.J. Aguirre*, which had institutionalized health inequalities. As opposed to their counterparts in prosperous communities, various NSHS facilities that provided healthcare in poor neighborhoods had to pay their staff lower wages and ran the services with insufficient or outdated equipment. This situation affected female employees[79] and patients in rural areas and in *poblaciones* in particular.[80]

President Aylwin (1990–1994) decided not to attempt to implement fundamental healthcare reform.[81] Instead he aimed to bring in changes to enhance the regulatory role of the state[82] and improved funding for the NSHS. Furthermore, just as under the dictatorship, their major concern was the provision of primary care,[83] which would be expanded to nearly 80 percent of the population by the end of the century.[84]

Although post-dictatorship governments increased public spending on healthcare during the 1990s, they could not improve the quality of the healthcare being provided.[85] This was due to the numerous structural problems described above and also in part to developments within the medical association.

In one of his first measures upon coming into office, Jorge Jiménez de la Jara, the first health minister of *Concertación* (1990–1992), tried to solve what he considered to be one of the most urgent problems: care in emergency rooms. His methods, though, were contested by the medical association leading to the first conflict between the state and the medical profession of the democratic era.[86] At the height of the confrontation, in October 1992, Jiménez resigned from office.[87] By 2014, ten other ministers had already followed him out of office, making it the highest turnover at the head of a ministry.[88]

As the most powerful leader of the physicians and president of the medical association since 1993, Vacarezza vowed he would act strictly within the sphere of civil society.[89]

Surprisingly, an overarching merger of all healthcare workers and professionals did not seem to have occurred with the restoration of democracy. The most important strikes of the medical association in 1992, 1993, and 1999[90] took place without the participation of female health professionals and workers. Fragmentation at the level of representation started again to characterize lobbying work of professional and auxiliary groups. This suggests that only the threat of a common enemy could trigger collaboration to such a significant extent.

3 Nursing Becomes Political

3.1 *The Distinction Continues: Professionals and Auxiliaries*

Just as the physicians struggled to bring the health professionals together, nurses also failed to become spokespersons for all caregivers. They were far too busy dealing with all the damage to their university programs to focus on strenuous team building work. And this is why the following analysis of working conditions, training, and lobby work is divided once again into a section about professionals and a section about auxiliaries. It is only with regard to issues such as gender policy and political resistance that common points will come to light.

During the 1980s, nursing was mainly taught in civil universities under military supervision. In 1983, the nursing school of the University of Chile defined the following characteristics for the profession:

> "Teaching nursing means educating a health professional with scientific and humanistic knowledge. It entitles the graduate to apply their nursing skills to treat healthy and sick individuals at every stage of life, aiming for the greater goal of the health of the country."[91]

The method most commonly resorted to accomplish this goal since the 1920s was the public health concept, with the health unit of *Quinta Normal* (Chap. 1) as a paramount example. Nurses, social workers, midwives, and nursing auxiliaries cared for women and infants, taught disease prevention, cooperated with physicians, and, most importantly, joined forces to assure health status improvement.

However, as the preceding chapters have shown, this was the reality of only a few. In many communities, buses and bicycles continued to be the only means of transportation for an ill person to reach a health facility, however underequipped.[92] The case of the *Hospital J.J. Aguirre* has demonstrated that even in the most prestigious facilities of the state-funded system the staff and supply shortages were part of the daily routine. Two midwives who had worked in NSHS healthcare centers in the *poblaciones* of Santiago recount that even in the late 1980s the infrastructure for women in labor and child delivery was poor.[93]

But in 1986, the labor legislation passed in 1978 (Chap. 3) was applied to nurses: that year, Rodríguez Palacios, Büchi's successor as undersecretary of health, instructed that nurses were hired under the terms of Law No. 2.200,[94] which meant longer working hours, less pay, and limited labor rights compared to the existing contracts in the public system. Similar treatment of nursing auxiliaries was not documented, but it can be assumed that these conditions and circumstances also applied to their profession.[95]

According to Figueroa, in healthcare there was a staff shortage of nearly 50 percent in Santiago. And although there is no precise data, it can be assumed that this also affected other areas, especially in the countryside. In 1983, only 36 percent of all employed nurses worked outside of urban settings.[96] One impact of the second wave of closures of nursing schools (Chap. 4) was that the number of annual graduates went down from 610 (1982) to 310 (1990); this was especially obvious in the case of the University of Chile where two-thirds of nursing schools had closed by the end of the 1970s.[97] Two research papers, from 1982 (Concepción)[98] and 1985 (Santiago),[99] were evidence of the consequences of labor shortages in professional and auxiliary nursing.

Although the *CECh* repeatedly demanded these policies be changed,[100] in studies with wording as drastic as the one found in the documentation of the Ministry of Health its board avoided relating the nursing crises with the social grievances.[101] Considering the fact that its authors never even used the word "*población*,"[102] the whitewashing also continued during times of social upheaval like the National Days of Protest. If chief editor Peake allowed articles to be published about the experience of her colleagues in rural areas, like Chaitén (1.250 km south of Santiago) in 1975[103] or Casablanca (close to Viña del Mar) in 1980,[104] only some details were criticized while health coverage went unquestioned.[105]

It was only in 1987, with Peake out of the editorial board, that this undertone changed. The first indication of this was an article by four nurses addressing nursing shortages in the Araucanía Region (600 km south of Santiago). The analysis was a project of the *CECh* regional council in Temuco (*Consejo Regional de Temuco*), making it the first to be independently published without the supervision of a university or a nursing school. In comparison to previous years, the nurses who did the investigation took on a more objective position. This is indicated by the information they provided about the ethnic characteristics of the people living in this region, the misconduct of the local authorities, and the working conditions of the nursing auxiliaries.[106]

Like in previous decades, supervising nursing auxiliaries was an important part of nurses' professional identity. But health ministry documentation shows that the lack of nurses in rural healthcare centers had led to an autonomously operated, albeit underpaid and exploited, nursing system run by auxiliaries.[107]

It is clear that if nurses and nursing auxiliaries worked together, they seldom formed a team, as the examples of Ivette Cap de Ville (Chap. 1) and other records illustrate. It can thus be determined that the wish for better communication with the nursing auxiliaries and their inclusion in the healthcare team, as a group of healthcare professionals demanded in 1986,[108] was more likely an exception.

Distinction had also increased during the time of the civilian-military cooperation, which depended on the nursing auxiliaries to achieve improvements in rural areas. Noticeably, it was only with international aid, like the Inter-American Development Bank, that Chile was able to build a comprehensive network of healthcare centers throughout entire regions, which health professional healthcare workers visited only sporadically to check and keep some form of control.

The era of rapid expansion of vocational institutes, between 1982 and 1986, reflects a period of auxiliaries' relative autonomy. Plus, the demand for nursing auxiliaries was too high for it to be satisfied with trained workers, which is why it was not hard for self-taught auxiliaries to find jobs. This came along with a number of vocational institutes which had no legal permission to operate,[109] fueling nurses' argument about low standards in the education of nursing auxiliaries, and reinforcing their own image in the public eye as professionally-trained women.

The gender distribution within the workforce of nursing auxiliaries remains unclear. As nursing was seen as a job ascribed to women, it is more likely that most of them were in fact women who had to manage a much more demanding work schedule than other healthcare professionals.[110]

The examples of Chaitén and Casablanca show there were only two shifts, one starting at 8 a.m. and one starting at 8 p.m; there was no allotted vacation time. In areas that were difficult to reach, nursing auxiliaries lived in the communities, perhaps even together with some of patients and their relatives. They had to provide what we would categorize today as a type of on-call service. Nursing auxiliaries did not have access to seminars, workshops, or other types of further education, and did not have what one would refer to as a professional career.[111]

In retrospect, one might anticipate a strong spirit of resistance towards oppression, especially in the mid-1980s, when strike movements in healthcare exploded. While it is not completely clear whether nursing auxiliaries joined the oppositional movements—these were dominated by professionals after all—their participation had been important in the seizure of power of the national strikes in 1970, 1972, and 1973. It is unlikely that nursing auxiliaries refused to join the opposition if they worked in hospitals, not because all of them necessarily agreed with the demands that led to the protests, but in order to avoid confrontation with their direct supervisors, the nurses or other health professionals. If there was a spirit of resistance, it was more subtle than overt and did not come to the surface.

As we have suggested, there has been no one time when modern nursing has looked like a unified professional model. It has rather been like a mosaic of different carers and training paths arising out of different eras, policies and reforming ambitions. The fierce criticism of the vocational institutes on the part of nurses has had clear consequences as nursing auxiliaries have continued working for low wages and having limited access to the privileges of the university-trained branch, such as funds for specialization or the right to self-determination. Chile has never had a school of paramedic science, for instance, and as a result the training relies on, and is controled by, nurses. As professional nurses embrace new responsibilities, especially in management, a great workload keeps being transferred to auxiliaries, and so industrial action sometimes goes through some negotiations with nurses as their superiors. In their process of differentiation, technical as well as social, university-trained nurses and nursing auxiliaries have interfered in each other's plans, with the latter group being subservient to the former, a process that itensified as vocational training expanded in the early 1980s. Hence the political tension between these two groups, which surfaces episodically and is explained by its historical construction throughout the century.

3.2 The Left-Wing Nurses: On the Fast Lane From Victory to Imprisonment (1984–1986)

Besides criticism and adverse publicity in 1982, the distribution of power in the *CECh* board remained steadfast. Only a small circle around Peake decided on nursing policy, which means that they mostly executed the government's guidelines. All this changed in 1984 when the Guild Renewal Movement gained its first victory and entered direct confrontation with the military junta. By the end of the year, it was clear that nursing policy and politics could no longer use a one-sided approach.

In 1984, the *CECh* had 3000 members, 48 percent of whom worked in Santiago.[112] Like in other associations the general council passed no decision without the agreement of Santiago fellows. Since the foundation of the *CECh* in 1953, nurses based in Santiago had been either the innovators or the supporters of the national board's politics. But as in the case of the physicians, the controversy surrounding their attitude toward the dictatorship changed the distribution of power within the nursing association.

1984 was also the year when the members of the 12 *CECh* councils were asked to return to the ballot box. The written sources, however, paint an unbalanced picture of this event considering that an announcement for the elections only appeared in *El Mercurio*,[113] and the results only in *Fortín Mapocho* – ignoring results outside Santiago. However, it marked one of the most memorable turning points in the history of nursing in Chile. The author of the article in *Fortín Mapocho* must have known this because he chose the headline "Opposition wins the majority in the regional council: Triumph of the nurses." Patricia Talloni, Patricia Grau, Alfredo Opgaard, and the new president of the regional council, Margarita Reusch of the Guild Renewal Movement, had climbed the most important rung on her way to the top of the nursing association.[114] Considering the oppositional goal of the new board, it was only a matter of time before the conflict with the Pinochet regime would escalate.

On March 18, 1986, *El Mercurio* reported that the military prosecutor in Santiago had ordered the immediate imprisonment of nurses Gladys Corral and Margarita Reusch.[115]

The grounds for the arrest of Corral and Reusch were an open letter they had published in their council's bulletin. It was addressed to the chief investigator of the case of the decapitated teachers and criticized the acquittal of the accused *Carabineros*.[116]

The imprisonment was either a warning shot fired by Pinochet or that his government had simply not anticipated the strong media response: after only one day in prison, Corral and Reusch were released on a 20,000 pesos bail, which was double the average monthly salary for a nurse at the time.[117] But the government did not drop the charges, and the members of Santiago's regional council addressed the *CECh*'s national board. The acting president Elizabeth Gudelhoefer[118] and Peake had kept out of this affair thus far, but now they had to either show their support or officially cut ties with their colleagues. According to *El Mercurio*, on March 22, Gudelhoefer and other high ranking *CECh* members intervened and met with then health minister Chinchón. The article in *El Mercurio* revealed the dilemma they had taken themselves into:

> "[*CECh* members] assured the fundamental intention of their organization was only dealing with professional, gremial and scientific tasks. [...] They expressed their concern about the accused leaders [of Santiago's council]. They had addressed unjustified accusations against *Carabineros*."[119]

Even though Peake and Gudelhoefer disagreed with Santiago's board members, the *CECh* hired a lawyer to help them. In order to avoid appearing complicit, they published another statement regarding this event two days later in which the directory once again emphasized its pro-government position:

> "The general council of the Chilean Association of Nurses emphasizes its firm gremial position in order to supervise the ethical and professional practices of its members, as well as improve these practices. The council therefore distances itself from any kind of political activity."[120]

In the same article, the *CECh* board stated that their engagement with the authorities had caused the pending charges against Corral and Reusch to be dropped.[121] *Solidaridad* authors gave another explanation. They quoted González, president of the medical association, who awarded those achievements to the human rights department of the Federation of Professional Associations and the support of all its members.[122]

At first glance, 1984 was not going to be a year of political diversity within the *CECh*. The military junta had successfully demonstrated its power, and the national nursing policy was still under the control of the conservative nurses. Nevertheless, the election in Santiago's council and Peake's (undesired) commitment for Corral and Reusch caused ruptures in the foundations of the long-standing conservative model for Chilean nursing. It would be up to Santiago's new elected board to prove that they could effectively lead the organization and gain the sympathies of fellow nurses in other regions.

3.3 A New Spirit Under Old Circumstances (1986–1990)

Five months after Reusch and Corral were imprisoned, in September 1986, *CECh* members once again were called to cast their ballots. This time, the opposition won the majority in almost all local councils and in the general council as well.[123] Only the members in Rancagua (85 km south of Chile) voted for the acting board.

Peake and Gudelhoefer had published an announcement of the election in *El Mercurio*. They presented themselves as a movement named "Nurses for the Profession," or "List No. 1." They claimed that the principles they presented were "strictly professional," with "no ideological influence," and that they only "focused on service-related objectives." The three most important goals they wanted to reach were the exclusivity of academic training, better working conditions, and higher salaries.[124]

The goals of the opposition, on the other hand, went unchanged, but they made their demands part of a political vision. In October 1986, Talloni, sitting as the president of the *CECh*, summarized the goals as follows:

> "[Our goal is] the defense of the university and the threatened professions. Each organization follows its own guidelines but without losing track of a common strategy. [The approach] has to be coordinated, firm and uninterrupted, and be realized within a specific time frame. [...] The fight for healthcare and education means helping the re-establishment of democracy in Chile."[125]

With Pinochet still in power, the installation of the new board had a twofold significance: for the second time since 1972/1973, the *CECh* entered into a political conflict with the goal of overthrowing a government. And for the first time since its foundation, the association moved toward the left of the political spectrum.

The new directory consisted mostly of former Santiago board members. Talloni became the president, Opgaard the vice president, Grau the general secretary, and Elba Contreras the treasurer.[126] Reusch was confirmed as the president of Santiago's regional council. But List No. 1 had also obtained some votes and its members took on positions in the general council, too. Peake sat as the representative for Santiago, and with that she became the direct contact person for Reusch,[127] although bearing little influence.

Contrary to the former *CECh* boards, Talloni and her board tried to stave off decline by distancing itself from the dictatorship. With the tailwind of international ratification, they started preparing for confronting the health ministry. In order to extend its sphere of influence, the new board tried to find a common denominator with other associations by organizing a meeting of all healthcare professionals.[128] In doing so, the *CECh* used the connections they had already established with Vaccarezza's Health Coordinator as well as with González's Federation of Professional Associations.

On October 2, 1987, some 1500 professionals met at Teatro Cariola in Santiago. It was not recorded which groups participated or what subjects they discussed. However, the outcome was another gain in prestige for the

CECh as Talloni became vice president of the Federation of Professional Associations. The first march organized by the *CECh* took place on October 22, which was followed by a 24-hour strike two days later.[129]

The impact of the two actions was strong enough to force the health ministry to enter into dialogue. Once again, however, it did not lead to an agreement.[130] As a direct consequence, the *CECh* organized a new one-day strike on December 15th. Talloni and the board demanded the end of the second wave of municipalization (since 1986) as well as the release of the incarcerated physicians and nurses who had supported the *FPMR*.

The nurses did not seem to have achieved the goal of mobilizing all professional associations. Various photos of the protests archived at *Fortín Mapocho* suggest that only other nurses followed the call. The attempt to reactivate *FENATS* is even more difficult to portray.[131] National and international newspapers did not add the nurses' demands to their agenda, which may indicate the absence of physicians. It was the reaction of the Pinochet government which attracted the attention of a broader audience.

On November 28, 1987, Talloni received an anonymous telephone call with a death threat.[132] She therefore contacted the *Vicaría,* where lawyers advised her not to leave her house,[133] but as the telephone calls continued Talloni was put under police surveillance for 15 days.[134]

The situation eventually calmed down, but worsened again in February 1988, when other *CECh* members were also affected by similar anonymous calls. Talloni therefore organized a press conference of the Federation of Professional Associations chaired by González in Santiago. Physicians and nurses found themselves working together again, years after collaborating for legal protection for Reusch and Corral in March 1986.[135] On February 13th, *Fortín Mapocho* and *El Mercurio* published parts of Talloni's speech in the press conference:

> "We received several anonymous calls with death threats against members of the *CECh.* They also threatened to destroy the association. [...] In recent times we have also seen unidentified individuals loitering around the headquarters in a provocative and conspicuous manner."[136]

El Mercurio reported that machine gunfire could be heard in the background of the anonymous callers.[137] Those threats did not fail to work.

The author of *El Mercurio* noted that Talloni and other members of the *CECh* board appeared visibly affected at the press conference.[138]

The *CECh* hired lawyer Julio Barría.[139] He was able to get Talloni and two of her colleagues under police surveillance through the Appeal Court for a thirty-day period. During that same timespan, *Carabineros* secured the *CECh* headquarters on Miraflores street with periodic patrols.[140] The threats ceased at once, but the callers were never identified.

The threat against the *CECh* board caused a media response. It attracted the attention of the public, but nurses from other regions did not react publically in this and other events. One of the male nurses from Talca interviewed for this research, Luis Campos, stated that in 1988 he still had not noticed any changes in *CECh*'s policies. He presented himself as one of the leaders of Talca's regional council and reported about demonstrations and strikes against the dictatorship, but underlined the disconnection of his office from the national board in Santiago.[141] Two nurses who had worked in Iquique confirmed his resentment toward the national headquarters.[142] They told us that they felt removed from the actions of the national board and felt left alone with their own problems.

Those critical voices were not isolated cases. The loss of members continued even though the new board vehemently tried to stop it.[143] Therefore, the board's renewed victory in the elections for the general council in 1988 was only a partial success.[144] The press did not comment on the election, which was likely because the presidency did not change. Furthermore, all of the events taking place around this period stood in the shadows of the imminent plebiscite,[145] for which the *CECh* took the side of the *NO* campaign. Talloni remembered:

> "We went out onto the streets for the plebiscite, for life and the health system. For us, everything was interrelated. We were part of a bigger ensemble, part of a collectivity."[146]

In 1988 and 1989, the *CECh* benefited from the increasing international interest in the Chilean system transformation. For the first time, PAHO supported profession-specific campaigns, like *CECh's* fighting the closing of nursing schools in university.[147] Thanks to the financial support of a Spanish partner organization, Talloni was able to participate in the ICN conferences in New Zealand, Panama, Mexico, Spain, and Ecuador, in 1988 and 1989.[148]

In addition, the *CECh* intensified their cooperation with other international organizations. In May and June of 1988, a Canadian group of labor organizations and NGO members visited the *CECh* headquarters in Santiago. Nurses from France, Canada, South Africa, Argentina, Peru, Venezuela, Denmark, Panama, Switzerland, and Sweden wanted to learn about the situation in Chile.[149] Even the cooperation with *FEPPEN*, which had ceased in 1986, was re-established.[150] However, only a few cases of such cooperation led to personal contacts, as seen in the case of ICN and OXFAM.[151]

The interest of the international actors also increased due to the virulent discussion about protecting human rights. Eric Stover's research on the participation of healthcare professionals in the torture of dissidents motivated authors elsewhere to write international reports, even if these did not raise discussion within the *CECh*. Although nurses had pledged their commitment to protecting human rights in 1986 (Santiago's regional board) and 1987 (national board),[152] corresponding statements only referred to cases in which nurses had become victims.[153] This marked nurses' narrative as victims under the dictatorship. It fit the image of the defeated in the fight for an academic career and for the position of head nurse.

Until she became sick and died in 1987, Oye was the head nurse at the University Hospital *J.J. Aguirre*.[154] Although it was the healthcare facility with the largest number of professional nurses in the country,[155] this high position in the hierarchy was not exemplary for other NSHS hospitals and healthcare centers. The Permanent Directive No. 7, negotiated during Oye's presidency (Chap. 4),[156] was implemented in only 13.5 percent (1985) of the public health facilities.[157] This situation was comparable to that in the private sector.[158]

During all those years of fundamental changes in policies and self-determination, the prioritization of the work fields remained constant. Universities, vocational institutes, the *CECh*, and the health ministry dedicated most of their staff and supplies to *materno-infantil*. It is not clear how deep the impact of the corresponding expert association, the Chilean Society of Paediatric Nursing, was. The same problem arises when assessing the three specialist nursing associations (surgery, intensive care, and infectiology) founded during the 1980s.[159] It is likely that the participation was low, however.

A more urgent matter concerned the place of nursing in universities and the *CECh* policy regarding the vocational institutes. The Peake administrations had not developed adequate strategies, although the number of private institutes had steadily been growing since the early 1980s. Talloni was very critical about this development.[160] She responded to the opening of the training centers in articles she wrote for several regional and national journals.[161] On September 14, 1987, she organized a press conference during a visit to Talca, which, according to sources, up until then was nurses' only event of this kind in the history of the *CECh* to take place outside the capital. Talloni argued for a common strategy across all associations in the health sector to address the vocational institutes issue. She also threatened the nurses working for these institutes with exclusion from the *CECh*. Above all, she criticized *PROPAM*. The company had recently opened another vocational institute in Talca.[162] However, Talloni could not stop the wave of creating new institutes between 1986 and 1987.[163]

The new vocational institute in Talca continued to operate, whereas the nursing school at the University of Talca closed in 1989.[164] This shows that the voices of the nurses could not outweigh state policies or stop the private initiatives. Also nursing students did not become very active in relation to this in their movement.[165] However, the biggest problem was a lack of cooperation with other health professionals. As seen in the case of the medical association, collaborative work was essential, especially during the dictatorship. Talloni's engagement in the Federation of Professional Associations and the support of González when she was threatened with death were steps in this direction. However, it would seem that the leaders of professionals'organizations feared to dilute their goals, or even their identities, when they engaged too much with each other.

3.4 Nursing After Dictatorship: Transition and Distinction

In the early 1950s and 1970s, nurses had chosen a political camp to strengthen their voice in healthcare and nursing policy. While the outcome had been clearly promising in 1952, but disastrous in 1973, the redemocratization of the nation between 1988 and 1998 had its ups and downs. The greatest challenge was to keep nursing training in academia and find a way to collaborate with the growing number of nursing auxiliaries.

In 1993, health minister Jorge Jiménez de la Jara stated that Chile needed 1300 more professional nurses. Eight years later, there were 18 nursing schools that belonged to a university, more than ever before.[166]

However, the number of nurses had not increased significantly (3500 in 1990 and 4000 in 2000).[167]

The change that Talloni and the rest of the board had hoped for would not happen until the 2010s, when the number of nurses rose from 4177 (2007) to 7428 (2015).[168] Between 2007 and 2014, the number of nursing students grew from 1233 to 3875. The same holds true for workplace policy, part of a general increase in the enrollment numbers for the 12 healthcare professions.[169]

In 1992, the first government of *Concertación* met another demand of the *CECh* and prolonged the nursing studies from four to five years.[170] At the same time, the differentiation of the qualification programs increased at an unprecedented rate. While in the year 2000 the 18 existing nursing schools offered 18 different degree programs in nursing, the 38 schools in 2010 offered 110.[171] Master studies and BA theses became an inherent part of academic nursing.[172] The next important step occurred in 1997, when the national standards for nursing studies were adopted meeting modern technical and educational standards.[173]

The issue of the increasing enrollment numbers, the longer period of study, and the adoption of higher technical standards was the question of how comparability could be guaranteed. As a consequence of the 1979/1980 university reform, since the late 1980s Chile had seen an enormous number of new universities being launched; there were, however, no standardized assessment measures to regulate them.

Between 1979 and 1982 the nursing programs in private universities focused on technical aspects, therefore neglecting what they regarded as inherent in nursing and university education: namely the forming of critical thinking and being an active citizen.[174] But it is highly questionable that such a sharp separation of profiles was new. Even in times of the welfare state, the geographic and financial gaps in society were reflected in the nursing schools. For example, over the course of the entire twentieth century, the renowned and cosmopolitan University of Chile differed from any kind of religious or secular private institutes.

One of the most important topics discussed in Chile's nursing policies during the first two decades of the twenty-first century was the development of a standardized national nursing examination. *ACHIEEN*, the most active player in this regard, had started lobbying for this around 1980 and continued to do so also in newly founded democracy. The medical association took on the lead once again by implementing a centralized nursing test during the first administration of Michelle Bachelet, in

2009.[175] At the time, the University of Chile was still the most important player in academia; that same year it introduced the *ACHIEEN* guidelines for its national nursing examination (*Examen Nacional de Enfermería, ENENF*), which led to a certificate the students received.

However, no successor governments of the dictatorship with its *gremialismo* philosophy tried to limit the freedoms of educational institutions by forcing all universities to adopt this exam. Therefore, in 2011 only 17.2 percent of all nursing schools were accredited according to *ACHIEEN* guidelines. Three of the 18 universities that had become accredited were the Catholic University in Santiago, the University of Santiago, and the University of Concepción.[176] These three universities, together with the University of Chile, still trained the majority of the country's nursing professionals.[177] But quantity was no longer synonymous with quality.

Despite the enormous differences in quality, the revitalization of the notion of a career in nursing after the dictatorship is a story of success. At the beginning of the twenty-first century, nursing was one of the most popular degree programs, with some 40,000 students (8.1 percent of all people who studied in university in Chile).[178] However, this development did not increase nurses' lobbying in national politics. The most important reason was probably the fragmentation of employee representation between 1973 and 1990.

In contemporary narratives, the dictatorship overshadows all aspects of Chilean society and politics. One important example is the self-organization of the nurses. The *CECh* no longer represents all nurses, nor does any one organization. More than 30 years after the transition of the state from civilian-military cooperation to democracy, the fragmentation of the professional associations advanced rapidly. Many federations, associations, and umbrella organizations appeared. This development weakened the nursing association further. Therefore, the confrontation with other professional associations is not always led by the *CECh,* but by new organizations like the National Federation of Associations of Nurses, which is a labor union of university-trained nurses working in public hospitals.[179]

Another legacy from the dictatorship is the fight for the reintroduction of management positions for nurses in hospitals and healthcare centers. At the time of writing, nurses are still waiting for a landmark decision by the Ministry of Health to re-establish the former authority of head nurses.[180] The liberalization and deregulation of the sector under the Pinochet regime make it difficult to assure comparable nursing standards both nationally and internationally.

But there are also continuities that were not at all affected by the deep political changes. The role of the nursing auxiliaries was not—and still is not—on any policy agenda, with respect to either ideological discussions or health reforms and political crises. In 1994, some 26,972 nursing auxiliaries worked for the NSHS.[181] The quality of their work primarily depends on their equitable integration into healthcare teams.

Furthermore, in 1994, the title used for the nursing auxiliaries was finally changed to paramedical technician (*técnico paramédico*). The length of their training program was increased to 1800 hours[182] and then again to 2500 hours (2.5 years) in 1994 and 2017, respectively.[183] Even their standing improved during the 1990s,[184] although recognizing the importance of their work is not common in the professional class.[185]

In 1997, after a new nursing law was passed, the health ministry expanded the field of paramedical technicians' application by introducing the training program called Higher Education Nursing Technician (*Técnico de Nivel Superior en Enfermería, TENS*).[186] The differentiation became necessary because of the growing mechanization of healthcare professions. Thereby, individuals who were trained in vocational institutes are still relevant to the system and, important for this book's argument, including their representatives in policy-making could greatly contribute to the democratic process and quality of care.

During the 1990s, many nursing auxiliaries transferred to the expanding private sector. But outside the public system, with its tradition of workers' unions, their representation appeared to be weaker.[187] Their work within healthcare teams, however, remains disproportionately important, considering that in 2016 some 104,621 *TENS* and 42,698 paramedical technicians were registered, compared to 44,473 university-trained nurses.[188]

Despite the expansion of the infrastructure and the further development of medical care (in both supplies and methods), the provision of healthcare remained the biggest challenge for the decision-makers after 1990. Nurses, paramedical technicians, and *TENS* are the only group of healthcare personnel who work in every town in the country. Therefore, for an important portion of the population access to care largely relies on them. University-trained nurses run preventive care; on top of this however they also informally diagnose and treat, but despite this reality they still get paid less than physicians, dentists, biochemists, and pharmacists, all of whom are the only beneficiaries of Law No. 15.076.[189]

Despite their growing number, the urgent lack of nurses[190,191,192] is another worrisome effect of the staffing policy of the twentieth century, its lowest point having been reached during the dictatorship. Although professional nursing has been re-established in the healthcare system, the danger of a new nursing crisis has yet to be averted. The most important issue might be not only lacking funds for opening up nursing jobs but also improving the attractiveness of the profession as a way of persuading candidates and keeping them interested in this field.[193]

Protecting academic training in nursing in 1990 was a last-minute resort. From the very beginning, the new democratic government made it clear that it wanted to guarantee healthcare staffing for both professionals and technicians. The distinction between professionals and auxiliaries remained a segregating perspective to describe caregivers in that country. As the new millennium approached, patients learned to distinguish them and in the process were given a picture of nursing divided into two distinct social classes. "Distinction" can be a good word to describe interactions within a nursing workforce made up of professionals and "workers." Collaboration thus remained more of a view on how future versions of Chile's nursing would look like.

4 Conclusion

As the troublesome decade of the 1980s closed, the nursing profession had undergone radical transformation. In a mere 60 years of formal existence, nurses had witnessed the rise of scientific medicine, embedded the shift from monastic apprenticeship to university education, consolidated its institutionalization within the state bureaucracy, opened up to foreign ideas, and navigated the radically shifting winds in national politics. Probably unaware of its long-term effect, they never really turned away from policy-making, especially in healthcare and higher education.

Indeed, few nurses in the 1990s would realize the political importance of their involvement in social policy: for themselves, for nurses reading in the twenty-first century, and for women's integration in society more broadly. That lack of a political consciousness in nursing worsened in the decades to follow owing to an educational blackout in history and social science alongside a self-imposed silence on national politics. Policies united nurses, but politics divided them. Silence helped to bring stability for a while.

This chapter, however, has highlighted continuity amidst change. Throughout that long-standing transformative process that shaped the nursing profession, nurses learned to develop networks with other women, participated in broader political movements, moved along high-profile politicians, drafted policy papers, bargained with contending groups, and monopolized a title and training.

Unused to a private-property approach, an entire nation learned the hard way that state protection was a thing of the past. The 1980s language had invented a new social currency and in the public imagination healthcare no longer equated to a right.

Despite some *loci* of resistance, nurses were not immune to such change. Training as well as employment expanded in the private sector. Even nursing activities were monetized. Equally, the new normal was to pay for a university education and healthcare, as democratic politicians owned businesses in both areas and at the same time ran the country. One might thus wonder how nursing made sense in the broader socio-economic order. Nurses seemed useful in pro-growth policies, as history had shown that nursing was central to a healthy workforce. And so the industry-like production of staff grew unregulated, one nurse at a time. And with that, even the most selfless of professions became infused with the ideas of capitalist welfare.

Notes

1. Within one year, the (registered) unemployment rate rose from 11 percent to 20 percent. In Santiago, still by far the largest city (3.98 million inhabitants), the number of job seekers doubled between 1979 (167.000) and 1983 (342.000), in: Banco Central de Chile: Indicadores Económicos y Sociales de Chile 1960-2000, Santiago 2001, p. 523, 576, https://www.bcentral.cl/documents/33528/133439/bcch_archivo_098139_es.pdf/9c630e90-825a-0e4a-1508-d215cd808413?t=1573279634953 [20.05.2022].
2. "Profesionales jóvenes. Profesional para qué..." in: *Solidaridad*, No. 180, 30.06.-13.07.1984, p. 16-17; The professional association of the social workers refused to be treated like that. It is not clear how far they went with the petition they sent to the health ministry, in: Ministerio de Salud, Depto. Recursos Humanos: Ord Nr. 7821, Mat. Información sobre profesionales que trabajan en el Sector Salud, 7821-3041-1985, 23.12.1985, 1-2 [1-2/12].

3. Manzano Chávez documented a wave of redundancies in all sectors of the public system but gave only numbers for the Santiago metropolitan area, in: Manzano Chávez, Liliana: Estratos y clases sociales en Chile, in: *Revista de Sociología*, Vol. 20, No. 0716-632x, 2006, p. 97-130, 112.
4. In the health ministry archives only dismissals of professionals are recorded. Dismissals of auxiliaries were perhaps not considered important enough to remember. For 1983, more dismissals under the label "early retirement" were found. A special law passed in the same year was frequently applied, in: Ministerio de Salud, Depto. Recursos Humanos: Ord Nr. 3E/6147, Mat. Sobre proposiciones fundadas de contratación de personal jubilado en el sector y nominación de funcionarios afectos a las causales del Art. 236 letra f) del DFL 338/60, 6147-3041-1985, 04.10.1985, 1-3 [3-5/12].
5. Graham, Carol L.: Safety Nets, Politics, and the Poor: Transitions to Market Economies, Washington D.C. [The Brookings Institution Press] 1994, p. 34.
6. "Médicos. No hay Salud," in: *Solidaridad*, No. 230, 29.08.-17.09.1986, p. 2.
7. Thibaut, Bernhard: Soziale Entwicklung und Demokratie in Lateinamerika zu Beginn der neunziger Jahre, in: Lateinamerika am Ende des 20. Jahrhunderts [Ed. Junker, Detlef; Nohlen, Dieter; Sangmeister, Hartmut], München [Beck] 1994, p. 124-148, 129; A study from 1986 demonstrates that in four regions during the second half of the 1980s the wage gap increased, in: Contreras, Dante: Pobreza y Desigualdad en Chile: 1987-1992, in: *Estudios Públicos*, No. 64, 2016, p. 57-94, 92, https://www.cepchile.cl/cep/site/artic/20160303/asocfile/20160303184217/rev64_contreras.pdf [20.05.2022].
8. Huneeus, Carlos: La democracia semisoberana: Chile después de Pinochet, Santiago [Taurus] 2014, p. 67.
9. *El Mercurio* and *La Tercera*, also reported about the opposition movement, Ibid., p. 73.
10. Masivas protestas. Panfletos del período de la dictadura militar (1973–1988), in: Biblioteca Nacional de Chile, http://www.memoriachilena.gob.cl/602/w3-article-96595.html [20.05.2022].
11. In mid-1983, the government concentrated the largest military contingent in Santiago since the coup d'état, in: Ensalaco (2000), p. 136.
12. Zurita (2010), p. 122.
13. Figueroa Clark, Victor: The Forgotten History of the Chilean Transition: Armed Resistance Against Pinochet and US Policy towards Chile in the 1980s, in: *Journal of Latin American Studies*, Vol. 47, Cambridge [Cambridge University Press] 2015, p. 491-520, 508.

14. Ensalaco (2000), p. 146.
15. Biblioteca Nacional Digtal de Chile: Colectividades, http://www.memoriachilena.gob.cl/602/w3-printer-92915.html [17.05.2022]. [31] Ensalaco describes "search and destroy operations" executed by the CNI, in: Ensalaco (2000), p. 146.
16. Villagrán (2005) states that the political repression was less severe at the *Universidad Católica* of Santiago, in: Villagrán, Fernando: Cuando el verdugo vistió de paisano, in: Represión en dictadura: el papel de los civiles [Ed. Délano, Manuel; Vera, Richard; Aguilera, Silvia], Nosotros los Chilenos 15, Santiago [LOM Ediciones] 2005, p. 4-25, 16-18.
17. The *Junta Directiva* reported about the existence of illegal practicing physicians. The *Junta* gave no numbers but considered it as a threat to the profession, in: Actas de la Junta Directiva, Sesiones 61-75, 1984, Sesión 71a, Sumario a un alumno de la Facultad de Medicina, p. 2-16, 11.
18. For example, the dean of the Faculty of Arts was dismissed in 1983. Gen. Roberto Soto Mackenney (1983–1987) described his politics as "vindictive" and "against the university" (*antiuniversitaria*), in: Actas de la Junta Directiva, Sesiones 18-35, 1983, Sesión 26a, Sesión Especial Privada de la Junta Directiva de la Universidad de Chile, 11.04.1983, p. [6/27]; The members of the *Junta Directiva* had heard about the participation of academic staff in the protests but could not verify this, in: Síntesis sobre la actual situación estudiantil universitaria, in: Actas de la Junta Directiva, UCH 06-04, Sesiones 61-75, 1984, Sesión 65a, p. 27-31, 31; In 1984, the impact of an oppositional movement was impossible to ignore. *Solidaridad* reported about an *Asociación de Académicos de la Universidad de Chile*, founded to face the forthcoming wave of redundancies, in: *Solidaridad*, No. 171, 01-1984, Académicos. En la defensa de la "U," p. 19; In 1985, an unknwon number of students elected a new dean for the Faculty of Physics and Mathematics without the permission of the university's directorate. The *Junta Directiva* did not accept their election, in: Actas de la Junta Directiva, Sesiones 76-87, 1985, Sesión 85a, Ultimos acontecimientos en la Facultad de Ciencias Físicas y Matemáticas, p. 9-10, 9; In 1985 there were protests in the Faculty of Education, probably also with the participation of teachers, in: Actas de la Junta Directiva, Sesiones 76-87, 1985, Sesión 85a, Entevista del señor Rector con su Excelencia el Presidente de la República, p. 10-11, 10.
19. Quote: "la situación supera un nivel crítico tal que hace peligrar los objetivos políticos establecidos por su Excelencia el Presidente de la República." It was not the first time he gave it such an embellished look. This suggests the expression that "His Excellence," using his words, had rejected previous similar proposals "emphatically," Quote: "los objetivos

del Sector [...] nuestros planteamientos que su Excelencia ha sido enfático en rechazar," in: Ministerio de Salud, Subsecretaría: Ord Nr. 2A/12, Mat. Situación Presupuestaria del Sector Salud, 12-2556-1983, 03.01.1983, 1-3 [6-8/37].

20. This does not mean that the state of healthcare in the West of Santiago was better: In December 1986, the health director of this area reported to the ministry that the state funding for medical treatments was "absolutely insufficient," in: Ministerio de Salud, Servicio de Salud Occidente: Res. Nr. 773, Mat. Informa Situación Financiera del Subtítulo 24, 773-3097-1986, 18.12.1985, 1-2 [6-7/32].
21. Ministerio de Salud, Servicio de Salud Metropolitano Sur Oriente: Reservado Nr. 276, Mat. Programa Financiero 1986, 276-3098-1986, 10.01.1986, 1-1 [4/75].
22. Ministerio de Salud, Servicio de Salud Metropolitano Oriente: Ord Nr. 091285, Mat. Presupuesto Colocación de Embarazadas de Alto Riesgo, 091285-3096-1986, 06.12.1985, 1-2 [1-2/25].
23. Ministerio de Salud, Depto. de Planificación, Jiménez Vargas, Coronel de Aviación (A), Ministro de Salud: M.S. Ord Nr. 1884, Mat. Preparación Programas Ministeriales 1979. Respuesta a cuestionario, 1884-1997-1978, 05.11.1978, 1-31 [40/70-81]; Inter-American Development Bank, in: *El Mercurio*, 01.-07.10.1978, p. 8.
24. Ministerio de Salud, Depto. Programa de las Personas: Ord Nr. 3F/58, Mat. Informe de visita de supervisión a VIII Región, 58-2556-1983, 05.01.1983, 1-11 [11-21/37].
25. Ministerio de Salud, Depto. Programa de las Personas: Ord Nr. 3F/58, Mat. Informe de visita de supervisión a VIII Región, 58-2556-1983, 05.01.1983, 1-11 [11-21/37].
26. Second study, released in 1982, in: Specific Plan for Rural Health Care (*Plan Específico de Salud Rural)* for the province of Llanquihue, in: Ministerio de Salud, Depto. Salud Rural: Ord Nr. 3J/4128, Mat. Indica medidas a tomar en el desarollo Plan Específico Salud Rural, Provincia de Llanquihue, 4128-2448-1982, 26.07.1982, 1-2 [23-24/24]. Third study, in: Ministerio de Salud, Depto. de Programación: Ord Nr. 3F/7896, Mat. Indica se efctúe asesoría y supervisión a establecimientos traspasados a la Municiplalidad, 7896-3042-1985, 27.12.1985, 1-3 [8-10/19].
27. Hernández, Teresa; Weintraub, Marcela: Enfermeras universitarias en hospitales públicos y clínicas privadas: percepción de su situación laboral, in: Reforma Sectorial y Mercado de Trabajo. El caso de las enfermeras en Santiago de Chile [Hrs. Weintraub, Marcela; Hernández, Teresa; Flores, Verónica], Serie políticas sociales, No. 31, Naciones Unidas, Comisión Económica para América Latina y el Caribe, Santiago de Chile 1999, p. 9-46. 10.

28. República de Chile, Junta de Gobierno, Secretaría: Acta No. 11/85, 28.05.1985.
29. La Salud. Diagnóstico reservado, in: *Solidaridad*, No. 213, 16.-30.11.1985, p. 12-14, 12.
30. Actas de la Junta Directiva, Sesiones 36-48, 1983, Sesión 39a, Análisis de Proyecto de fundación "Hospital Clínico de la *Universidad de Chile*," p. 2-27, 13.
31. Salud. Los muertos en Neurocirurgía, in: Hoy, No. 115, 03.-09.10.1979, p. 18 [2/6].
32. La Salud. Diagnóstico reservado, in: *Solidaridad*, No. 213, 16.-30.11.1985, p. 12-14, 14; One year later, criticism against *ISAPREs* appeared in the same magazine, in: Ley de Salud. En este mundo, todo se paga, in: *Solidaridad*, No. 217, 31.01.-27.02.1986, p. 4-5, 4. In 1990, Francisco Quesney Langlois, who had been the undersecretary of the health ministry in 1979, then working for *Banmédica S.A.*, labeled the privatization process as a positive outcome. He referred to a 1988 survey conducted with people who were insured by *ISAPREs*. Only 85,000 out of 1.5 million people surveyed complained about the healthcare quality. Langlois acknowledged systemic problems in the public sector, but for him they had nothing to do with the private entities which "fairly operated within the legal framework." But Quesney also admitted that most of the *ISAPREs* users had higher wages than those the *FONASA* assured, in: Quesney L., Francisco: Algunas ideas en torno al sistema *ISAPRES*, in: Estudios Públicos, No. 38, Santiago 1990, p. 193-216, 212.
33. Article No. 2, Quote: "Los establecimientos asistenciales del Sistema Nacional de Servicios de Salud no podrán negar atención a quienes la requieran, ni condicionarla al pago previo de las tarifas, o aranceles fijados a este efecto, sin perjuicio de lo prescrito en los artículos 16 y 28," in: Ley Nr. 18.469, 23.11.1985, Regula el ejercicio del derecho constitucional a la protección de la salud y crea un régimen de Prestaciones de Salud.
34. The employees of the NSHS were exempted from paying additional fees, except in case of dental treatment, in: Ministerio de Salud, Asesoría Jurídica: Ord Nr. 2C/406, Mat. Informa sobre Ley Nr. 18.469, 406-3099-1986, 20.01.1986, 1-3 [14-16].
35. The deductible was 25 percent for the assured of the groups A, B, and C. For the group D, the maximum was 50 percent, in: Article No. 25, in: Ley No. 18.469, 23.11.1985, Regula el ejercicio del derecho constitucional a la protección de la salud y crea un régimen de Prestaciones de Salud.
36. Llambias Wolff, Jaime: The Rise and the Fall of Welfare Health Legislation in 20th Century Chile: A Case Study in Political Economy of Law, York (Canada) 2013, p. 180; Annick Manuel saw it as a completion of the 1979/1980 healthcare reform, in: Annick, Manuel: The Chilean Health System: 20 Years of Reforms, in: *Salud Pública*, No. 44, 2002, p. 60-68, 65.

37. Ley de Salud. En este mundo, todo se paga, in: *Solidaridad*, No. 217, 31.01.-27.02.1986, p. 4-5, 4.
38. Vergara criticized in a CIEPLAN study that municipalization caused several problems. Many did not know about the categories of the additional payments and forced the patients' families to make a pro forma additional charge. Vergara described them as "irregularities and insufficiencies." She stated that such payments restricted access to check-ups, in: Vergara, Pilar: La política social y los programas hacia la extrema pobreza del gobierno militar chileno, in: Papers 35, Santiago [CIEPLAN] 1990, p. 27-60, 46.
39. Dorman, Ariel: The Challenge in Chile, in; New York Times, 29.06.1986. Vacarezza's leadership and the activity of the health coordinator are only documented for the year 1986. For example, in the newsletter from January 1986 Vacarezza accused additional payments for *FONASA* patients, in: Coordinadora de Salud: A los trabajadores de salud, Santiago 1986 [Museo de la Memoria, Módulo B8 Estante 14 Caja 4, Fondo Patricia Grau]; The health coordinator started operating in 1984, in: Boletín Coordinador de Salud. Año 1, N°2. 25.05.1984 [Museo de la Memoria, Módulo B8 Estante 14, Caja 4, Fondo Patricia Grau].
40. Guzmán (2012), p. 31.
41. In February 1984, the offices of the regional council were searched. The report does not provide information as to whether it was a secret service or *Carabineros*, in: Colegio de Periodistas. Allanamiento sin precedentes, in: *Solidaridad*, No. 195, 16.02.-01.03.1985, p. 2.
42. Guzmán (2012), p. 31.
43. Ibid., p. 32.
44. Associaciones privadas eligen Directivas, in: *Solidaridad*, No. 201, 18.-31.05.1985, p. 17; Information about the elections in the councils of psychologists, midwives, and social workers, in: Psicólogos, matronas y asistentes sociales, in: *Fortín Mapocho*, 07.06.1984, 291, p. 9.
45. These were between 25 and 30 different private associations.
46. Guzmán (2012), p. 78; Accounts vary and report up to 100,000 teachers, in: "Colegio de Profesores. En busca del tiempo perdido," in: *Solidaridad*, No. 215, 15.-27.12.1985, p. 17; According to the website of the teachers' association, there were 76.551 members in 1977, in: Colegio de Profesores de Chile. Historia, in: https://www.colegiodeprofesores.cl/historia/ [21.05.2022].
47. Quote: "Comando por la democratización del Colegio," in: Colegio de Profesores. En busca del tiempo perdido, in: *Solidaridad*, No. 215, 15.-27.12.1985, p. 17.
48. On March 3, 1986, the new board was elected, in: *Colegio de Profesores de Chile*. Historia, https://www.colegiodeprofesores.cl/historia/ [21.05.2022];

49. In March 1984, the rooms of the national board of the association were searched by *Carabineros*, in: Ensalaco (2000), p. 141.
50. Al concluir asamblea plenaria: Obispos llaman a la reconciliación y a la paz entre los chilenos, in: *Fortín Mapocho*, 20.06.1985, p. 5.
51. The intelligence service of the Carabineros (*Dirección de Comunicaciones de Carabineros*).
52. Only in 1991, one year after the end of dictatorship, legal proceedings started, in: Lúnecke (2000), p. 114; Six effectives of *Carabineros* were sentenced to prison in 1993, in: The Whole World was watching: The 1988 Plebiscite. The Observer Group of the Latin American Studies Association, in: The Chile Reader, 2014. p. 512-519, 514.
53. Asociaciones privadas crearon Departamento de Derechos Humanos, in: *Fortín Mapocho*, 24.03.1986, p. 11.
54. Délano, Manuel: Juan Luis González, in: El País, 12.07.1986.
55. Women's organizations were represented, in: Valdés E., Teresa: Las mujeres y la dictadura militar, Santiago [FLACSO] 1987, p. 37; The blueprint for González's strategy of civil disobedience was the movement against dictators Jean-Claude Duvalier in Haiti and Ferdinand Marcos in the Philippines, in: Bastías Saavedra, Manuel: Sociedad civil en dictadura: relaciones transnacionales, organizaciones y socialización política en Chile (1973-1993), Santiago [Universidad Alberto Hurtado] 2013, p. 242.
56. Ibid., p. 189.
57. Ibid., p. 56-57.
58. Quote: "satisfecho y orgulloso por el éxito de la huelga general y el refuerzo que ello significa para la lucha pacífica y la desobediencia civil por el retorno a la democracia," in: El País, 12.07.1986.
59. Ibid.
60. Stover, Eric: The open secret. Torture and the medical profession in Chile, Washington (American Association for the Advancement of Science) 1987, p. 57.
61. Winston Chinchón possibly resigned to the health ministry following pressure from the medical association.
62. The clinic operated in Las Condes district. The following nurses worked there: Patricia Herreros, Elba Salinas, and Gina Cerda Yeomans, in: Palomera Valenzuela, Adriana; Rosas Aravena, Pedro: Presencia e impacto de las mujeres en la lucha armada contra la dictadura en la prensa oficialista. La Tercera 1978–1989, in: *Cuardernos de Historia*, Nr. 48, S. 89-125, Santiago [Universidad de Chile, Departamento de Ciencia Históricas] 2018, p. 115; The *Fortín Mapocho* reported about the destiny of the nurses: Largo y dramático relato hizo *enfermera* al juez – En tres horas revivió su drama, in: Fortin Mapucho, June 6, 1987 [Museo de la Memoria, Fondo 00000617, Talloni Valdés Patricia].

63. In an interview with the newspaper *El Mostrador*, Patricio Basso, vice president of the *Federación de Asociaciones de Académicos* from 1986 to 1987, named two reasons for shrinking activity of the *Asamblea de la Civilidad* – the imprisonment of its leaders and the missing solidarity within the movement, in: Dimter, Hugo: José Luis Federici, la primera gran derrota del régimen, in: *El Mostrador*, 28.08.2017.
64. Only *El País* documented the imprisonment of the nurses after the exposure of the secret clinic in Las Condes, in: Délano, Manuel: Huelga de hambre de los presos acusados del atentado contra Pinochet, in: *El País*, 18.03.1987.
65. Guzmán (2012), p. 60.
66. Cuatro meses de estado de sitio. Los hechos consumandos, in: *Fortín Mapocho*, No. 379, 12.01.1987, p. 12-13, 13.
67. Médicos a la deriva, in: *Fortín Mapocho*, No. 816, 18.06.1988, p. 7.
68. Since 1987 González appeared only a few more times in the national press, for example in the case of the imprisoned nurses Reusch and Corral.
69. Archivo Fortín Mapocho: Paro de Médicos becarios en el Hospital J.J. Aguirre, https://www.archivofortinmapocho.cl/imagenes/paro-de-medicos-becarios-en-el-hospital-j-j-aguirre-2/ [22.05.2022].
70. Boletín Informativo, Colegio de Enfermeras, No. 1, 1987, p. 12 [Museo de la Memoria, Fondo 00000617, Talloni Valdés Patricia].
71. Supported by the international partners, in: The Whole World was Watching: The 1988 Plebiscite, in: The Chile Reader, 2014, p. 512.
72. Some continued on the way of violence, in: Krumwiede (2004), p. 264.
73. Ensalaco (2000), p. 179.
74. Nohlen et al. (1994), p. 243.
75. Ibid., p. 243.
76. Banco Central de Chile: Indicadores Económicos y Sociales de Chile 1960-2000: Encuesta de Caracterización Socioeconómica Nacional, Santiago 2006, p. 968.
77. The definition of "poor" varies. For example, the *Banco Central* distinguishes between "poor" (*pobre*) and "indigent" (*indigente*). In 1998, some 820,021 people fell into the second category, in: Ibid., p. 968.
78. Bastías (2013), p. 301.
79. Rotarou, Elena S.; Sakellariou, Dikaios: Neoliberal reforms in health systems and the construction of long-lasting inequalities in healthcare: A case study from Chile, in: *Health Policy*, No. 121, 2017, p. 495-503, 499.
80. Castiglioni, Rossana: The politics of social policy change in Chile and Uruguay: retrenchment versus maintenance, 1973-1998, Abingdon-on-Thames [Routledge] 2005, p. 2.

81. Bossert, Thomas J.; Villalobos Dintrans, Pablo: Health Reform in the Midst of a Social and Political Crisis in Chile, 2019-2020, in: *Health Systems & Reform*, Vol. 6, No. 1, p. 1-10, 1.
82. Llambias-Wolff (2013), p. 252.
83. Jeong, Hanbeom: Political Dynamic and the Welfare State in Chile under Economic Globalization, in: Chile under Economic Globalization, in: *The Korean Journal of International Studies*, Vol. 11, No. 1, p. 201-234, 220.
84. Domínguez-Cancino, Karen A; Palmieri, Patrick A.; Martinez-Gutierrez, Maria Soledad: National Health Policy Reform for Primary Care in Chile: A Qualitative Analysis of the Health Program Documents, in: *Journal of Primary Care & Community Health*, Vol. 11, 2020, p. 1-11, 2.
85. Annick (2002), p. 66.
86. Strikes took place in Santiago, notably in the *Hospital J.J. Aguirre*. The medical association gave unacceptable work conditions as the reason for the work stoppage, in: Aprobada Ley de Servicios de Urgencia, in: *Colegio Médico de Chile*: Boletín Mesa Directiva Nacional, No. 1, Santiago 1993, p. 6.
87. Carta de Jorge Jiménez de la Jara dirigida al S.E. Presidente Patricio Aylwin, 29.10.1992, in: Archivos Históricos, *Universidad Alberto Hurtado*, https://archivospublicos.uahurtado.cl/index.php/carta-de-jorge-jimenez-de-la-jara-dirigida-s-e-presidente-patricio-aylwin [22.05.2022].
88. "El complejo Ministerio de Salud: 11 personas a cargo desde 1990," in: 24 horas, 31.12.2014, https://www.24horas.cl/nacional/el-complejo-ministerio-de-salud-11-personas-a-cargo-desde-1990-1543629 [22.05.2022].
89. "Un Proyecto de Salud para Chile," in: *Colegio Médico* de Chile: Boletín Mesa Directiva Nacional, No. 1, Santiago 1993, p. 1-3.
90. Description of the strikes, in: Azolas A., Patricio: 70 años con la salud del país, in: *Vida Médica*, 04.12.2018;
91. Quote: "La carrera de Enfermería prepara a un profesional universitario, con conocimientos científicos y humanísticos, que lo capacitan para proporcionar atención de Enfermería al individuo sano o enfermo en cualquier etapa de su vida, o a la familia y comunidad, de acuerdo con las necesidades de salud del país," in: Facultad de Medicina, Descripción de carreras y programas académicos. Descripción de Carreras. Enfermería, in *Anales de la Universidad de Chile*, No. 3, 11-1983, Serie 5, p. 236.
92. A nurse commented in 1977 that home visits helped to attain positive outcomes of the therapy, but because of invalid address or relocation these activities often required a great deal of time, in: Atención Esforzada de Médicos Urbanos, in: *El Mercurio*, 14.11.1977, p. 6.

93. Interview with the midwives Ernestina Valdebenito and María Inés Zavala, Santiago, February 2017.
94. Ministerio de Salud: Ord Nr. 515, Mat. Empleos Médicos Programa de Expansión afectos al DL 2.200, de 1978, 515-3100-1986, 22.01.1986, 1-23 [14-35/87].
95. Various municipalities could not afford hiring professionals and so they used mostly staff to be paid in the lowest groups of the Salary Scale, in: Flores et al. (1999), p. 64.
96. Figueroa, María: Rol de la Enfermería Profesional, Concepción [Universidad de Concepción] 1991, p. 8 [Museo de la Memoria, Fondo Patricia Grau, 1-10/81].
97. Primer Congreso Nacional de Enfermería Pediátrica, in: *Enfermería*, No. 78, 10-11-12-1983, p. 3–7, 6; No precise numbers found. Garrido counted in 1984 about 800 nurses working in hospitals but gave no numbers for the rural areas, in: Garrido Ballerino, Presidente CECh: Discurso de la Presidenta del Colegio de Enfermeras de Chile A.G. en la ceremonia solemne con que se conmemoró "El Día Mundial de la Enfermera," Mayo 1984, in: *Enfermería*, No. 81-82, 07-12-1984, p. 36–38, 36-37.
98. Ibid., p. 9.
99. Ministerio de Salud, Depto. Programa de las Personas: Ord Nr. 3F/58, Mat. Informe de visita de supervisión a VIII Región, 58-2556-1983, 05.01.1983, 1-11 [11-21/37].
100. The *CECh* constantly complained about unemployment and difficult work conditions, but compared themselves to the medical association in a very cautious way. One example, in: Resumen de la Memoria Anual del Consejo General del Colegio de Enfermeras de Chile A.G. 1983-1984, in: *Enfermería*, Nos. 81-82, 07-12-1984, p. 42–47.
101. For example, in *Enfermería*, in: Schálchli V.: Recursos de Enfermeras del Servicio Nacional de Salud – Diciembre – 1973, in: *Enfermería*, No. 40, 04-05-06-1974, p. 36–47.
102. Like in *El Mercurio*, until 1987 *Enfermería* editors did not use the term "*población*." The only article which reports about the work done by nurses in "peripheral health centers" (*consultorios periféricos*) refers only to technical aspects and avoids a critical view of the system, in: Salomon, Enfermera Docente, Departamento de Salúd Pública y Medicina Social, Facultad de Medicina, U. de Chile Santiago Norte et al.: Condiciones de Eficiencia de los Servicios de Enfermería en Consultorios Periféricos S.N.S. de la Región Metropolitana, Santiago 1977, in: *Enfermería*, No. 52, 04-05-06-1977, p. 5–12.
103. For 4500 people in the zone of Chaitén, a fishing and farming village, there were one hospital and three health centers. One physician, one midwife, and three nursing auxiliaries but no nurse were employed. The hos-

pital did not have a kitchen; a woman from the neighborhood was in charge of cooking the meals for the patients. Nursing auxiliaries were self-taught, and there was an overall shortage of supplies, in: Acevedo, Enfermera docente, Depto. de Enfermería, Sede Norte, U. de Chile et al.: Enfermera en un programa de salud rural, in: *Enfermería*, Nos 43-44, 01-06-1975.

104. Reyes A., Enfermera Atención Rural, Servicio de Salud, Viña del Mar and Herrera L., *Enfermero* Atención Rural, Servicio Salud, Valparaíso, San Antonio: Experiencias en la implantación de las normas técnicas para el programa de postas de Salud en Casablanca—V Región, in: *Enfermería*, No. 66, 10-11-12-1980, p. 52–58.
105. Two studies from 1984 described the work of nurses in rural areas with a focus on pediatrics: 1. Anabalón, Enfermera de Salud Pública del Hospital de Lautaro, Temuco, IX Región de la Araucanía: Participación de Enfermería en Atención Primaria y Secundaria de Salud del niño con Síndrome Diarreico a niveles ambulatorio, rural y urbano e intrahospitalario, in: *Enfermería*, No. 79, 01-02-03-1984, p. 2–9; 2. Atención primaria y secundaria ideal que debería recibir al niño con Síndrome Diarreico dentro del Sistema de Salud existente en Chile, vía posta rural, Consultorios Urbano de Salud, Hospital Comunidad, in: *Enfermería*, No. 79, 01-02-03-1984, p. 22–27.
106. In 1986, the Araucanía Region had 720,964 inhabitants. Some 224 nurses worked there in the public sector and 20 in the private sector. No information about nursing auxiliaries was found, in: Gallegos Morales, Miembro Depto. de Ejercicio Profesional y Gremial del Consejo Regional Temuco, IX Región et al.: Práctica del Ejercicio Profesional en la IX Región de la Araucanía, in: *Enfermería*, Nos. 90-91, 06-12-1987, p. 29–33.
107. Figueroa (1991), p. 8.
108. The already described case of a commission which had visited the Viña del Mar Region in 1986, in: *Enfermería*, No. 66, 10-11-12-1980, p. 52–58.
109. Not all of them operated legally. In 1986, health minister Chinchón briefed his colleagues in the ministries of finance and labor about several of those new institutes diffusing "propaganda" which would "confuse" those who wanted to undertake training as nursing auxiliaries. Several programs and courses did not seek state approval. The graduates could not easily find a job or accepted informal employments. Chinchón asked the two other ministries to run an information campaign about this problem in the schools, in: Ministerio de Salud, Depto. Recursos Humanos: Ord Nr. 3E/56, Mat. Sobre instituciones que imparten cursos de Auxiliares Paramédicos sin la autorización correspondiente, 56-3096-1986, January 6, 1986, 1-4 [19-22/25].

110. In only one article found in *Enfermería* auxiliaries were referred as women, in: Ravera P., Enfermera, Div. Ciencias Médicas Occidente, U. de Chile, Servicio de Cirurgía, Hospital San Juan de Dios et al.: Factores de Variación en Ausentismo de Personal, in: *Enfermería*, Nos. 84-85, 04-09-1985, p. 53–60, 53.
111. We found only one seminar for nursing auxiliaries, which was about care for alcoholic patients, in: Ministerio de Salud, Depto. Programación: Ord. Nr. 3F/7767, Mat. Prórroga plazo de aplicación al programa de Educación a Distancia para Auxiliares de Postas, 7767-3040-1985, 19.12.1985, 1-2 [4-5/16].
112. Elecciones en Colegio de Enfermeras, in: *El Mercurio*, 24.07.1984, p. 4.
113. *El Mercurio* announced the elections in Santiago, Iquique, Antofagasta, La Serena, Valparaíso, Rancagua, Talca, Concepción, Temuco, Valdivia, Puerto Montt, and Punta Arenas but did not publish the outcome, in: Elecciones en Colegio de Enfermeras, in: *El Mercurio*, 24.07.1984, p. 4.
114. Oposición gana mayoría en el Consejo Regional: Triunfo de enfermeras, in: *Fortín Mapocho*, No. 299, 02.08.1984, p. 5.
115. Encargaron reos a dirigentes de las enfermeras, in: *El Mercurio*, 18.03.1986, p. 2.
116. The accusation against the police was signed by Reusch and the president of the psychologists' association, in: Latorre Gaete, Patricia, Directora del Colegio de Sicólogos; Reusch, Margarita, Secretaria Consejo Regional Santiago: [Letter to] Juan Luis González [Mueso de Memoria, Fondo 00000617, Talloni Valdés Patricia].
117. Fallo de Corte Marcial: Concedida libertad a dos dirigentes de enfermeras, in: *El Mercurio*, 19.03.1986, p. 6.
118. Memoria Anual del Consejo General del Colegio de Enfermeras de Chile A.G. Periodo Junio 1984 a Junio 1985, in: Enfermería, No. 86, 10-11-12-1985, p. 37.
119. Quote: "a quienes expresaron que las asociadas de la Orden tienen como fundamental objetivo dedicarse a asuntos estrictamente profesionales, gremiales y científicos. Deploraron las actividades que significaron trastornos en los establecimientos asistenciales, porque ellos van en perjuicio de los enfermos. También manifestaron su preocupación por las dirigentes procesadas por presuntas injurias a *Carabineros*," in: Ante Fiscal Militar: Apelaron por las Enfermeras Procesadas, in: El Mercurio, 22.03.1986, p. 7.
120. Quote: "El Consejo general del Colegio de *Enfermeras* A.G. reiteró su irrestricta posición gremial, orientada a velar por el desempeño ético-profesional de los colegiados y su permanente perfeccionamiento y, por lo tanto, su posición al margen de cualquier acontecimiento relacionado con política contingente," in: Enfermeras fijan posición gremial, in: *El Mercurio*, 24.03.1986, p. 3.

121. Ibid, p. 3.
122. Profesionales y derechos humanos. Hacia un trabajo concertado, in: *Solidaridad*, No. 220, 28.03.-17.04.1986, p. 2.
123. Announcement of the elections for the board of the Santiago regional office, in: Revista del Consejo Regional Santiago, No. 8, 08-09-1986, p. [3/6]; Elections of the other boards, in: Colegio de enfermeras: Defender la salud. Defender la profesión, in: *Análisis*, 22.-28.02.1988 [Museo de la Memoria, Fondo 00003, Talloni Valdés Patricia].
124. Quote: "estrictamente profesionales, sin postulados ideológicos y únicamente con objetivos de servicio," in: Elecciones en el Colegio de Enfermeras, in: *El Mercurio*, 07.08.1986, p. 4.
125. Quote: "Defender la Universidad y las profesiones amenazadas, cada organización con su propia modalidad, estilo y acciones, pero sin perder de vista los objetivos principales, es la tarea de hoy que deberá comprometer el esfuerzo de todos y (de) cada uno, en forma coordinada, decidida, sin desmayos y por el tiempo que sea necesario,[…] porque luchar por la salud y la educación es ayudar a conquistar la democracia en Chile," in: Discurso de la Presidente Nacional del Colegio de *Enfermeras*, Sra. Patricia Talloni Valdés, en el acto realizado en 2 de octubre de 1987, en el Teatro Carlos Cariola. Convocado por las 7 asociaciones privadas de la salud no médicos," in: Colegio de Enfermeras de Chile A.G., 02.10.1987, quoted, in: Guzmán (2012), p. 64.
126. Contreras was mentioned for the first time in 1978. She worked in those days and during the 1980s as a lecturer in the nursing school of the University of Chile, in: Contreras Gúzman, Enfermera Docente del Departamento de Salud Pública, Salud Mental y Psiquitría, Facultad de Medicina Sur, Universidad de Chile, 1977: Las actividades y conductas del personal de Enfermería con pacientes mentales crónicos dentro de un contexto teórico de terapia basado en condicionamiento operante, in: *Enfermería*, No 57, 07-08-09-1978, p. 23–32.
127. Consejo Regional de Enfermeras de Santiago: Revista del Consejo Regional Santiago, No. 8, 08-09-1986, p. [3-4/6].
128. Colegio de Enfermeras de Chile: *Boletín Informativo*, 1987, No. 1, p. 12.
129. Marcha pacífica de los profesionales de la salud no médicos por el Centro de Santiago, in: Ibid; The only trace of nurses' actions was found in the bulletin of the *CECh*. Even the magazine *Coordinadora* (providing information about the activities of oppositional healthcare employees) did not mention the *CECh* activities, in: Colegio de Enfermeras de Chile: *Boletín Informativo*, 1987, No. 1, p. 12.
130. The protest led to a meeting of representatives of seven professional associations with the health minister. They could not reach an agreement, in: Ibid.

131. Ibid.
132. Enfermeras denuncian amenazas, in: *El Mercurio*, 13.02.1988, p. 7.
133. Guzmán (2012), p. 71-72.
134. Enfermeras denuncian amenazas, in: *El Mercurio*, 13.02.1988, p. 7
135. Ibid., p. 7.
136. Quote: "Llamadas telefónicas anónimas que manifiestan el ofrecimiento de muerte a funcionarias del gremio de enfermeras y la destrucción de éste. Además [...] últimamente han estado rondando el lugar individuos no identificados que hacen una ostentosa y manifiesta presencia en los alrededores de nuestro colegio, dice la dirigente Patricia Grau," in: "amedrentamiento volvió al Colegio de Enfermeras," in: *Fortín Mapocho*, 13.02.1988 [Museo de la Memoria, Fondo 00000617, Talloni Valdés Patricia].
137. Quote: "En las llamadas telefónicas se escuchaban además cintas grabadas de tableteos de ametralladoras," in: Acogen Recurso: Protección policial para Presidenta de Enfermeras. Medida favorecerá a Patricia Talloni, Hortensia Arizaballo y Jenny Vergara, in: *El Mercurio*, 19.02.1988, p. 7.
138. Enfermeras denuncian amenazas, in: *El Mercurio*, 13.02.1988, p. 7.
139. Ibid, p. 7.
140. Quote: "Rondas de periódicas para proteger la sede del Colegio de Enfermeras y recurrentes," in: Acogen Recurso: Protección policial para Presidenta de Enfermeras. Medida favorecerá a Patricia Talloni, Hortensia Arizaballo y Jenny Vergara, in: *El Mercurio*, February 19, 1988, p. 7; The security measures did not automatically guarantee feeling safe. Talloni commented on this: "I did not know who the guards were. I did not leave my house in the whole week," in: Guzmán (2012), p. 71-72.
141. According to Campos, there was no support from Santiago when he and his close collaborators opened the first *CECh* office in Talca, in: Interview with Luis Campos, Talca 2016.
142. Patricia Grau and the two former members of the regional council in Iquique commented that they had conflicts, but managed not to interrupt the communication between the national and the regional offices, in: Interviews with Sonia Cruz and Lidia Osorio Olivares, Santiago, March 2017.
143. Even the new directorate of the *CECh* could not stop the loss of members. In 1988, only 60 percent of the 2313 nurses were affiliated to *CECh*. Most of them worked in the following regions: Valparaíso (253), Maule (157), Araucanía (170), Los Lagos (205), and Santiago (960), in: Colegio de Enfermeras de Chile: Proyecto de Capcitación de Dirigentes Gremiales Del Colegio de Enfermeras de Chile A.G., Santiago 1988 [Museo de la Memoria, 51-81/81, Fondo Patricia Grau].

144. Talloni, Opgaard, and Grau commented that two lists ran for office, the list of the former directorate members, which they referred to as "the rightists," and their own list which was called the List for the Dignity of the Profession and the Defense of Health" (*Por la Dignidad de la Profesión y de la Defensa de la Salud*), in: Guzmán (2012), p. 65.
145. Huneeus (2014), p. 73.
146. Quote: "Bueno, para el plebiscito, nosotros salíamos a marchar por la salud, la vida y la democracia. Para nosotros esta cosa no era separada. [...] éramos parte de un todo, era colectivo," in: Ibid., p. 65.
147. Montivero Bruna, Sergio: Rechazo a exclusión de carreras de Salud, in: *El Mercurio*, 27.09.1987, p. 9.
148. *ICN* congresses in New Zealand, Panama, Ecuador, Mexico, and Madrid, in: Talloni: Día de la Enfermera, in: *Enfermería*, No. 93, 05-08-1989, p. 19–25, 22; In her speech in Madrid, Talloni criticized the military junta, in: Discursos [Museo de la Memoria, Fondo 00000617, Talloni Valdés Patricia].
149. Talloni: Día de la Enfermera, in: *Enfermería*, No. 93, 05-08-1989, p. 19–25, 24-25.
150. Since the beginning of Talloni's presidency, probably also because of Pincheira's retiring from all duties in the mid-1980s, the collaboration with the *FEPPEN* decreased. At least, we are left with that impression considering that this was mentioned only one more time for several years. After a congress in May 1988 in Argentina, Talloni described the event as a "revitalization" of the cooperation, in: Ibid., p. 24.
151. Cooperation with the Canadian Public Health Organization (CPHA) and with OXFAM, in: Noticolegio, in: *Enfermería*, No. 92, 01-04-1989, p. 42–43.
152. Asociaciones privadas crearon departamento de derechos humanos, in: *Fortín Mapocho*, 24.03.1986, p. 11.
153. The *CECh* criticized the "Anti-terrorist Law" (Ley 18.314 Antiterrorista) and made a plea to end pretrial detentions, in: Depto. Jurídico *CECh*: Indulto Presidencial a Patricia Herrero [Museo de la Memoria, Fondo 00000617, Talloni Valdés Patricia].
154. In 1987, Carmen Oye González passed away. *Enfermería* commemorated her "courage, commitment and honor," in: Colegio de Enfermeras de Chile: Palabras de Despidida a Carmen Oye, Enfermera jefe del Hospital Clínico José Joaquín Aguirre y ex Presidente del Colegio de Enfermeras de Chile (1979–1981), in: *Enfermería*, No. 90-91, 06-12-1987, p. 53–54; Oye's position as head nurse does not appear in the official organigram sent to the directorate of the university, in: Actas de la Junta Directiva, UCH 06-04, 1984, Sesión 65a, Exposición del Director del Hospital José Joaquín Aguirre, p. 2-47, 3; It seems that the denomination *enfermera jefe* (head nurse) was no longer common. Peake also used the name *enfermera coordinadora de hospital*, in: Resumen de la

Memoria Anual del Consejo General del Colegio de Enfermeras de Chile A.G. 1983-1984, in: *Enfermería*, Nos. 81-82, 07-12-1984, p. 42–47, 43.

155. According to the numbers given by Garrido in 1984, about 800 nurses worked in Chilean hospitals, in: Garrido Ballerino: Discurso de la Presidenta del Colegio de Enfermeras de Chile A.G. en la Ceremonia Solemne con que se conmemoró "El Día Mundial de la Enfermera," Mayo 1984, in: *Enfermería*, Nos. 81-82, 07-12-1984, p. 36–38, 36-37; According to the information given by the university directorate, 13.75 percent (110 nurses) worked in the *Hospital J.J. Aguirre*. Oye was also in charge of 683 nursing auxiliaries, in: Actas de la Junta Directiva, Sesiones 61-75, 1984, Sesión 65a, Exposición del Director del Hospital José Joaquín Aguirre, p. 2-47, 5.
156. The position of head nurse depended also on the political leaning of the candidate, as surfaced in a testimony by physician Gilda Gnecco, who worked in *Hospital J.J. Aguirre*. She reported about a nurse who, owing to her work for the military junta's secret service *DINA*, was entrusted all important decisions about staffing after September 11, 1973, in: Gnecco Tassara, Gilda: "Soy la 550," in: La dictadura de los sumarios (1974–1985). Universidad de Chile intervenida, Santiago [Editorial Universitaria] 2016, p. 195-198, 197; In 1984, Pincheira commented in *Enfermería* that an autonomous nursing management was common in the US and Canada but that was no longer the case in Chile. The *Directiva Permanente Interna No. 7* [Chap. 4] was only one step on the way to the reinstatement of an "internationally acknowledged nursing structure," in: Pincheira: Editorial, in: *Enfermería*, Nos. 81-82, 07-12-1984, p. 2.
157. All other institutions had two reporting lines, which would lead to a "doubled dependence," in: Resumen de la Memoria Anual del Consejo General del Colegio de Enfermeras de Chile A.G. 1983–1984, in: *Enfermería*, Nos. 81-82, 07-12-1984, p. 42–47, 47.
158. In public hospitals and private clinics it was physicians who sat in all positions of the highest management level but delegated some responsibilities on nurses. For instance, nurses administered the material and the auxiliary staff, in: Flores et al. (1999), p. 55-56.
159. In 1983, the *Sociedad Chilena de Enfermería en Pabellones Quirúrgicos* (operation theater), in 1984, the *Sociedad Chilena de Enfermería en Medicina Intensiva* (intensive care), and in 1987, the *Sociedad Chilena de Enfermería en Infectolo*gía (infection control).
160. Quote: "The actual technology has caused, among other things, an engrossment of a range of health professionals, badly called paramedical staff. They perform various tasks originally undertaken by nurses," in: Espinoza C., *CECh* Nacional. Depto. de Investigación et al.: Planteamientos Doctrinarios y Políticos de Acción Futura en Enfermería, in: *Enfermería*, No. 83, 01-02-03-1985, p. 3–12, 8.

161. La Enfermería en Crisis, in: Diario del sur, 1988 [Museo de la Memoria, Fondo 00000617, Talloni Valdés Patricia]; Another article, in: Patricia Talloni, presidenta la entidad: "El amedrentamiento volvió al Colegio de Enfermeras," in: *Fortín Mapocho*, 13.02.1988, in: Ibid.
162. Colegio Enfermeras de Chile: Boletín Informativo, No. 1, 1987, p. 6.
163. Between 1981 and 1987, the Chilean state accredited 23 vocational institutes, and between 1988 and 1989, the number rose to 34. Between January and March 1990, 23 new institutos profesionales started to operate, in: Bernasconi, Andrés; Rojas, Fernando: Informe sobre la educación superior en Chile: 1980-2003, in: Dirección de Bibliotecas y Recursos de Información, Temuco 2002 [Universidad de la Frontera] 2002, p. 1-204.
164. Figueroa (1991) [Museo de la Memoria, Fondo 1-10/81, Patricia Grau].
165. Until 1987, opinions of students only appeared when referring to technical aspects in hospitals or healthcare centers. The new national board tried to integrate them into its politics. In 1987, *CECh* organized the First National Meeting of Nursing Students, aiming at involving students in the last years of training, in: XI Congreso Nacional de Enfermeras/os. Coquimbo 1987 - Conclusiones y Recomendaciones, in: *Enfermería*, Nos. 90-91, 06-12-1987, p. 8–10, 10; In 1989, *Enfermería* reports about the nursing student María Raquel Villaroel, who "actively supported" the *CECh*, in: Talloni: Día de la *Enfermera*, No. 93, 05-08-1989, p. 19–25, 20-22;
166. Castellano Salas, Angela; Tagle Vargas, Cristina; Galdames Cabrera, Luz; Riquelme Pereira, Náyade; Landman Navarro, Cecilia; Peroni Parraguez, Sonia: Examen Nacional de Enfermería en Chile: Importancia y Desafíos, in: *Ciencia* y *Enfermería*, Vol. 17, No. 1, Concepción [Universidad de Concepción] 2011, p. 27-36, 28.
167. Castellano's were only estimates, in: Ibid, p. 28.
168. To compare, in the same timespan the number of midwives grew from 615 to 1535, in: Informe sobre brechas de personal de salud por Servicio de Salud, Santiago [Ministerio de Salud] 2016 p. 52, https://www.minsal.cl/wp-content/uploads/2015/08/Informe-Brechas-RHS-en-Sector-P%C3%BAblico_Marzo2016.pdf [22.05.2022].
169. The state increased budgets for the public health sector. Alongside the new wave of private universities, equipment for highly technical professions and the number of employees also increased; for example in audiology, from 205 in 2007 to 1185 in 2014, meaning a growth of 478 percent in a mere seven years, in: Ibid., p. 54.
170. Behn Theune et al. (2009), p. 89.
171. Castellano Salas et al. (2011), p. 28.
172. In the mid-1990s, María Figueroa became the first "emeritus professor in nursing," in: Behn Theune et al. (2009), p. 89.

173. Campos, Claudia; Vargas, Ximena; Milos, Paulina: Los servicios profesionales de la enfermera(o) en la legislación chilena, in: *Revista Médica Clínica Las Condes*, Vol. 29, No. 3, 2018, p. 270-277.
174. Behn Theune et al. (2009), p. 57.
175. Bachelet is a medical doctor by training. Her father was tortured during the dictatorship. For more information about her biography, please see Karnofsky, Eva; Potthast, Barbara: Michelle Bachelet, in: Mächtig, mutig und genial: Vierzig außergewöhnliche Frauen aus Lateinamerika, Berlin [Rotbuch] 2013; The name of the examination is *Examen Único Nacional de Conocimientos de Medicina, EUNACOM*, in: Castellano Salas et al. (2011), p. 31.
176. Ibid., p. 33.
177. *ACHIEEN* was supported by the Federation of the Nursing Students (*Federación de Estudiantes de Enfermería, FENEECH*). This can be seen as a sign of more involvement of nursing students in the development of the nursing profession.
178. Followed by *Universidad de Concepción* (semi-public) and *Universidad Mayor* (private). Universidad de Tarapacá (public) had the lowest results, in: La carrera de Enfermería en cifras: ¿Cuál es su proyección?, in: Emol.com, 25.10.2016, https://www.emol.com/noticias/Nacional/2016/10/25/828207/Enfermeria-en-cifras-Cual-es-su-proyeccion-futura.html [22.05.2022].
179. *Federación Nacional de Asociaciones de Enfermeras y Enfermeros de Chile, FENASEF.*
180. Conflicts arose out of this unclear situation. In 2004, the medical association contested the appointment of nurses as directors in Concepción, in: Behn Theune et al. (2009), p. 61.
181. Flores et al. (1999), p. 49.
182. The number of training hours rose from 1600 to 1800, in: Decreto 1.704, Aprueba reglamento para el ejercicio de las profesiones auxiliares de la medicina, odontología y química y farmacia que indica, 03.12.1994.
183. Decreto No. 90, Aprueba reglamento para el ejercicio de las profesiones auxiliares de medicina, odontología, química y farmacia y otras, y deroga Decretos No. 261 de 1978, y No. 1.704, de 1993, ambos del Ministerio de Salud, in: Ministerio de Salud, January17, 2017; 2500 hours to study in five semesters, in: González F., Tomás: Técnicos sin reconocimiento legal: Los TENS exigen su espacio, in: *Diario UChile*, 09.02.2019, https://radio.uchile.cl/2019/02/09/tecnicos-sin-reconocimiento-legal-los-tens-exigen-su-espacio/ [20.05.2022].
184. Since then they were able to reach level 12 instead of 16 in the Salary Scale. However, Flores et al. stated that in most of the cases nurses were not promoted higher up. Many of them would not even earn more than the auxiliary staff, in: Flores et al. (1999), p. 63.

185. Ayala, Ricardo A.; Fealy, Gerard M; Vanderstraeten, Raf; Bracke, Piet: Academisation of nursing: An ethnography of social transformation in Chile, in: *International Journal of Nursing Studies* 51, 2014, p. 603-611, 609.
186. Campos et al. (2018), p. 1.
187. According to Flores et al., because of their prestige university-trained nurses had a better standing in private clinics and would undertake fewer tasks considered to be auxiliary, like cleaning, or moving or washing patients, in: Flores et al. (1999), p. 63.
188. Clínicas de Chile A.G.: Dimensionamiento del Sector de Salud Privado en Chile, 2016, p. 70-71, http://www.clinicasdechile.cl/wp-content/uploads/2017/12/DimensionamientoSaludCifras2016.pdf [20.05.2022].
189. Informe sobre brechas de personal de salud por Servicio de Salud, Ministerio de Salud 2016, p. 57.
190. Flores et al. (1999), p. 61.
191. Behn Theune et al. (2009), p. 68.
192. Simonetti, Marta; Aiken, Linda H., Lake, Eileen T.: Nursing in Chilean Hospitals: A Research Agenda to Inform Health Policies and Improve Patient Outcomes, in: *Hispanic Health Care International*, Vol 17, No. 2, 2018, p. 79-88, https://journals.sagepub.com/doi/10.1177/1540415318819475 [20.05.2022]
193. In 2009, only 8000 out of 18,000 nurses were practicing, in: Behn Theune et al. (2009), p. 68.

Annex

Main Nursing Policy Shifts in Context

	MAIN LANDMARKS	ECONOMIC POLICY	NURSING POLICY
1880s	Spread of liberal ideas. War of the Pacific. Economy depended on exportation.		Charity relief
1890s	Civil war Rise of the working-class		Lobby by medical reformers
1900s	Birth of trade unions First steps towards work insurance	CLASSICAL ECONOMICS	Institutionalization of training in university Health work by Red Cross volunteers
1910s	Launch of the Panama Canal Economic turmoil. Centennial of independence.		Proliferation of university training
1920s	Consolidation of middle-class. Mandatory insurance for workers. New constitution.		Focus on public health
1930s	Reform by radical governments Great depression impacted the country		Requirements to enter nursing rose Est. First association of nurses (*AECh*)
1940s	Reform by radical governments Women's right to vote. Aid from the USA.		Health units started community care Training in North America through Rockefeller F.
1950s	Christian socialist ideas spread. Rise of associative movements, Est. NHS.	KEYNESIAN ECONOMICS	Est. Chilean Nurses Association (*CECh*). Fellowship was mandatory. Auxiliaries had a trade union.
1960s	Spread of Marxist ideas Aid from the USA		Special medical law excluded nurses. *Medicina curativa* Act.
1970s	Brief Socialist government. Coup d'état, Economic crises. Beginning of dictatorship		Front of Professionals Against Popular Unity. Adherence to military rule.
1980s	New constitution, major state reform. Economic crises.	NEO-LIBERAL	Associations become private associations. Rise of left-wing nurses. Proliferation of private universities.
1990s	Restoration of democracy Consolidation of state reform	ECONOMICS	Adoption of a managerial approach. Legal changes and curricular reform.

© The Author(s), under exclusive license to Springer Nature Switzerland AG 2023

M. Thulin, R. A. Ayala, *Nursing, Policy and Politics in Twentieth-century Chile*,
https://doi.org/10.1007/978-3-030-90835-5

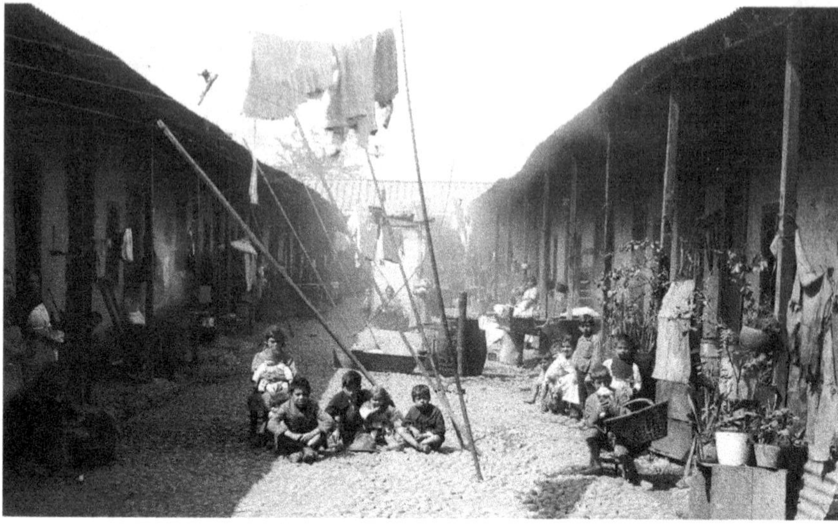

Picture 1 Life in Santiago's suburbs in the 1920s. Source: National Historical Museum

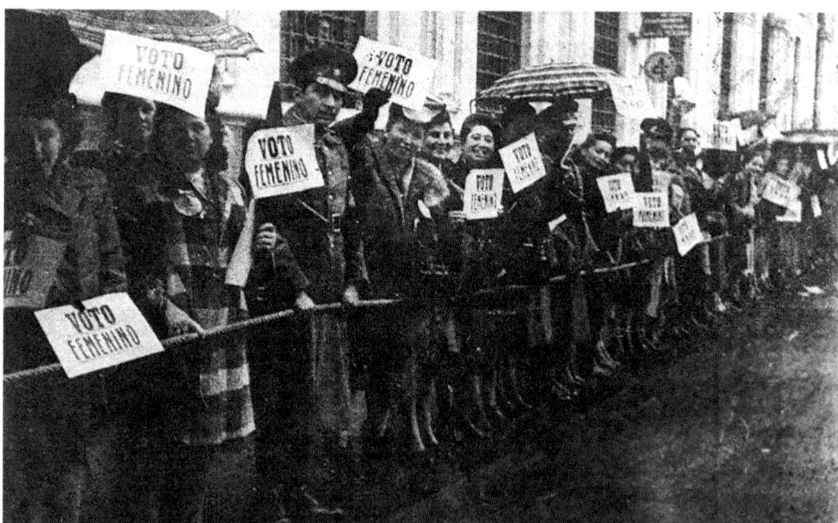

Picture 2 Nurses were close to the suffragette movement, especially through the Chilean Association of University-Trained Women. Chilean women voted for the first time in 1952

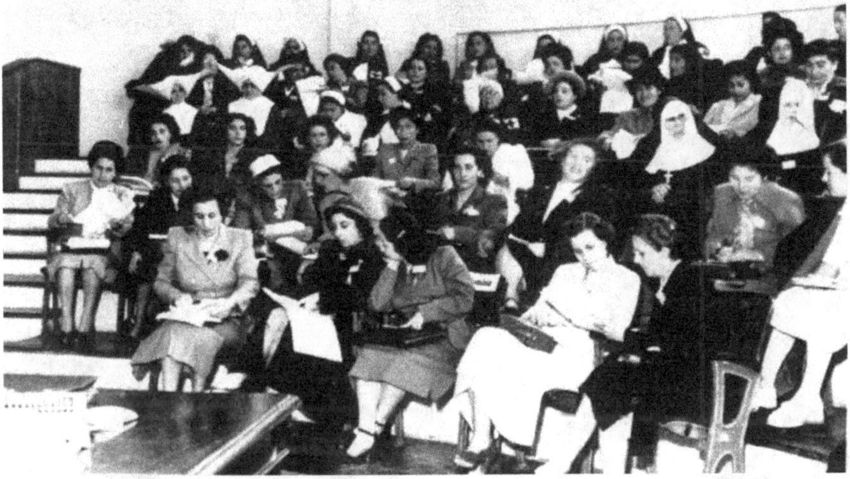

Picture 3 Nurses discussing the contents of the curriculum in a nursing conference in 1949. Chile's representative, Gladys Peake, the first from left to right, first row. Source: PAHO Final Report on the 2nd Nursing Congress held in 1949 in Peru, p. 96

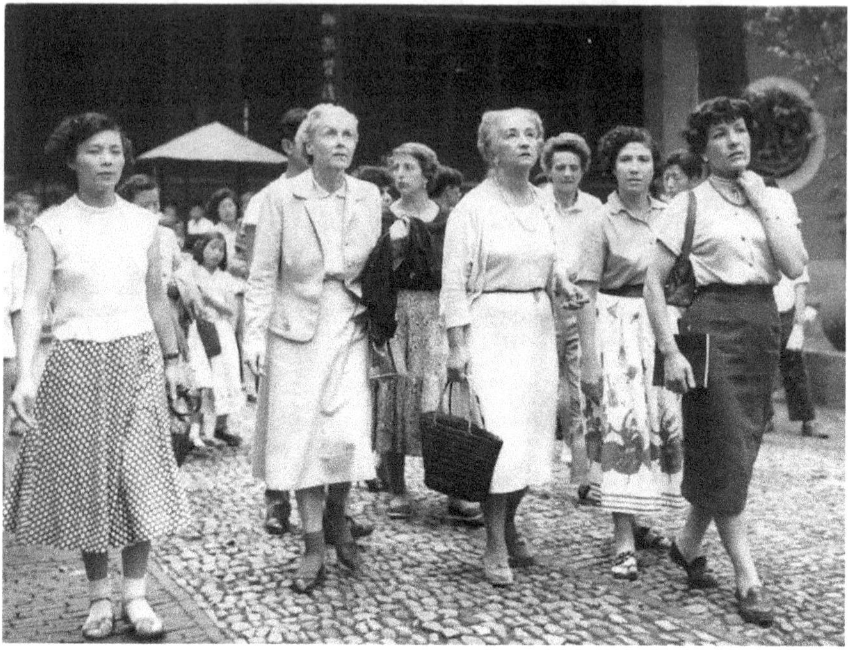

Picture 4 Irene Frei (center, second row, Ca. 1960), a trained social worker, Christian Democratic Representative and sister of President Frei Montalva, credited to have influenced the social welfare plan of his brother's presidency. Source: Casa Museo Eduardo Frei Montalva

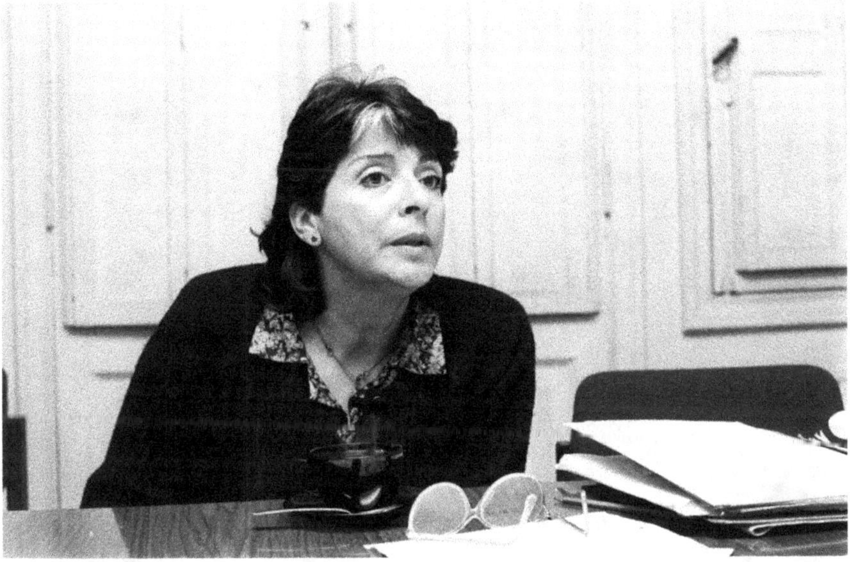

Picture 5 Nurse Patricia Talloni in a meeting at the Colegio de Enfermeras de Chile, 1989. Source: Archivo Fortín Mapocho

Index[1]

[1] Note: Page numbers followed by 'n' refer to notes.

© The Author(s), under exclusive license to Springer Nature Switzerland AG 2023

M. Thulin, R. A. Ayala, *Nursing, Policy and Politics in Twentieth-century Chile*,
https://doi.org/10.1007/978-3-030-90835-5

GPSR Compliance
The European Union's (EU) General Product Safety Regulation (GPSR) is a set of rules that requires consumer products to be safe and our obligations to ensure this.

If you have any concerns about our products, you can contact us on

ProductSafety@springernature.com

In case Publisher is established outside the EU, the EU authorized representative is:

Springer Nature Customer Service Center GmbH
Europaplatz 3
69115 Heidelberg, Germany

www.ingramcontent.com/pod-product-compliance
Lightning Source LLC
Chambersburg PA
CBHW071325270226
40259CB00058B/64
9783030908348